# Feminist Intersectional Therapy

# Feminist Intersectional Therapy

## Fourth-Wave Clinical Applications

*Edited by*

*Joanne Jodry, EdD, DMH*
*Monmouth University*

*Kathleen McCleskey, PhD*
*Longwood University*

ROWMAN & LITTLEFIELD
Lanham • Boulder • New York • London

Executive Acquisitions Editor: Jonathan Joyce
Assistant Acquisitions Editor: Sarah Rinehart
Sales and Marketing Inquiries: textbooks@rowman.com

Rowman & Littlefield
Bloomsbury Publishing Inc, 1385 Broadway, New York, NY 10018, USA
Bloomsbury Publishing Plc, 50 Bedford Square, London, WC1B 3DP, UK
Bloomsbury Publishing Ireland, 29 Earlsfort Terrace, Dublin 2, D02 AY28, Ireland
www.rowman.com

British Library Cataloguing in Publication Information Available

**Library of Congress Cataloging-in-Publication Data**
ISBN 978-1-5381-7977-2 (cloth : alk. Paper)
ISBN 978-1-5381-7978-9 (pbk. : alk. Paper)
ISBN 978-1-5381-7979-6 (electronic)

For product safety related questions contact productsafety@bloomsbury.com.

♾™ The paper used in this publication meets the minimum requirements of American National Standard for Information Sciences—Permanence of Paper for Printed Library Materials, ANSI/NISO Z39.48-1992.

*To my greatest feminist inspiration in life, my daughter, Mary Louisa Jodry, and my matriarchal lineage, Josephine Plunkett Jodry and Louisa Philomena Carey Plunkett, who have suffered and navigated patriarchal oppression throughout the last century and succeeded in raising feminists.*
*To my feminist mentor, Frances K. Trotman PhD, who first exposed me to feminist thinking in graduate school and mentored me into a feminist therapist. Lastly, to my dear friend, Courtney Deacon Lalotra, the founder of @OneLife2Love, who inspires me daily to live a brave meaningful life of service for those who are most oppressed.*

*—JJ*

*To my mother, Patricia Bergen Fry, who first introduced me to feminism and who always believed that I could do anything, despite the patriarchy. I would not be writing this book if not for her. To my husband, Pierce, who supports me in all my endeavors and who proudly stands with me as a feminist. Lastly, to my feminist mentor, Kathleen M. May, PhD, who helped me apply feminism to therapeutic work, and has been my teacher, my role model, and my friend.*

*—KM*

# BRIEF CONTENTS

# CONTENTS

## Part III  Specific Populations and Feminist Intersectional Therapy

## 14    Feminist Intersectional Therapy with BIPOC People 233

*David Julius Ford Jr., Sedaria LaNora Williams, Takeesha Hawkins, and Nicole Jackson Walker*

# PREFACE: ONE WAY, NOT *THE* WAY

*Feminist Intersectional Therapy: Fourth-Wave Clinical Applications* intends to aid practicing clinicians, supervisors, educators, and students in the mental health and related fields to have additional clinical tools to apply feminist intersectional therapy across disciplines. The editors of this book have been developing their feminist clinical constructs for decades. They have always hesitated to create theoretical frameworks or "techniques" in feminist therapy because adding structure could be contraindicated with the feminist theory itself. Creating models or techniques could be perceived as having patriarchal influences, the need for constructed hierarchies, and exact methods to be followed. It could also be viewed as attempts to be assimilated into the medical models of "evidence-based" exclusivity like other traditional theories. Lastly, feminist principles of honoring unique specific intersectional experiences could also be considered in conflict with creating sweeping general "frameworks." So, should this even be done? Anecdotally, one of the foremost reasons that the editors (who are higher education educators) decided to do this project is that clinicians and graduate students regularly claim that they do not know how to apply feminist theory. The editors wanted to create more options for fourth-wave clinical applications within feminist intersectional therapy, hoping that feminist clinical and critical thinking would become more mainstream for therapeutic usage. It is essential to note that this book provides ideas on applying feminist intersectional therapy from the collective thoughts of many contributors. Each chapter's model, application, and/or examples are *not* the only way or the right way; it is simply one way of conceptualizing and applying feminist intersectional theory. One of the beauties of the fourth wave of feminist intersectional therapy is that it is not rigid but collaborative, creative, and collective.

Feminist clinical therapy began by focusing on White women and heteronormative gender expressions in reaction to oppressive patriarchal psychological theories and practices being offered in mental health. Feminist therapy of the third and fourth wave has evolved in the last two decades to recognize that sex and gender conceptualizations were narrow definitions. This did not account for the intersectionality of each person's identities and the multiple oppressions that people suffer as a result of the associated cultural, social, and political expectations. This initial feminist focus on White-woman norming in reaction to White-man norming excluded and hurt people by using broad brushes of equality and inequality that were unrealistic for many women, particularly women of color.

With the third wave of feminist theory, feminists began to acknowledge that the complexities of intersectionality muddy the clinical waters when mental health systems attempt to label or categorize "normal" thoughts and behaviors. The evolution of the fourth wave of feminist theory and therapy has shifted to the understanding of unique identities, creating a complicated, privileged, and oppressive cultural, social, and political experience for everyone.

This book intends to build on those powerful feminist intersectional foundational roots and offer an additional clinical application layer with models and techniques to address these complexities, which often impact pain and suffering. The hope is that this fourth wave of inclusiveness strengthens feminist theory and feminist therapy, becomes more embraced by the masses for the betterment of society, and offers healing to the individuals suffering at the hands of the marginalizing and oppressive Eurocentric, heteronormative, Christian-dominant patriarchy. Now is the time.

But why now? With the rise of overt social oppression, divisiveness in politics, and personal social and cultural fears, the more clinicians who can conceptualize and apply feminist clinical theory, the better. Feminist intersectional therapy may help people think more critically and freely, breaking the chains of unhealthy, restricting cultural, social, and political norms. It could help illuminate the deeply embedded oppressive systems that impact people's lived experiences. Through becoming more critically conscious of these systems, norms, and expectations, feminist intersectional therapists invite people to reframe their personal experiences in light of this consciousness.

Feminist intersectional theory also seeks to disrupt and change oppressive systems. However, this does not mean that individuals will necessarily reject the oppressive systems and norms in which they have been immersed all their lives. Feminist clinicians do not recreate in therapy the same oppressive dynamics that individuals experience elsewhere; they do not require that clients think the same way they do. The goal of feminist intersectional therapy is to help people raise their consciousness, differentiate (not reject) from oppressive cultural, social, and political norms and systems, and make informed, higher conscious decisions free of Western patriarchal psychological and behavioral embedded conditioning.

The feminist intersectional clinical therapy is built on the shoulders of the feminist movement. This movement grew from the beginning of the activism of inequality in the West, predating Seneca Falls, 1848, to the suffragettes fighting for the right to vote. Next came the feminist movement of the 1960s fighting to gain equality in education, careers, and workplaces. Today, women and people with other oppressed identities are once again fighting for control over their bodies, reproductive rights, and other inequalities. Honoring the foremothers of these essential social justice movements is necessary to remember the sacrifice, bravery, and severe consequences these people suffered in the fight for equality, positively impacting the quality of modern life. At the same time, it is necessary to recognize that the earliest part of the movements did not acknowledge the intersectional multiple oppressions, especially the experiences of people of color, various affectional orientations, people of different abilities, non-Christians, people of lower socioeconomic status, and other identities that have social marginalization.

It is also essential to acknowledge the pioneers of feminist clinical therapy for standing up to a repressive patriarchal system that normed psychology from a Western patriarchal perspective. This non-exhaustive acknowledgment of feminist foremothers—such as Jean Baker Miller, Alice Walker, Laura Brown, Phyllis Chesler, Nancy Chodorow, Florence Denmark, Carolyn Enns, Olivia Espin, Carol Gilligan, Miriam Greenspan, bell hooks, Harriet Learner, Ellyn Kaschak, Lenore Walker, and Gloria Steinem—is what has allowed this book to exist as a collective addition to the clinical understanding of systemic inequality and oppressive cultural methodologies, and offers some possibilities for healing the psychic wounds caused by them.

As an important note, since this work has been a joint effort of collective feminist thought, not all authors agree with all ideas in this book or even within their authored chapters. Including all thoughts, even those with which some disagree, was essential to collective inclusion. The goal of this feminist intersectional book is to ignite additional critical thoughts of the reader, inspire creative clinical judgments to serve clients, and offer possible models and techniques for ease of use to move feminist therapy forward into a more saturated clinical usage.

This book is intended to be an essential handbook for clinical therapists, to be consumed in its entirety or in individual chapters as needed. The editors designed this book so clinicians could turn to the chapter they need and gain information with ease of clinical use, specifically within their practice areas. Therefore, each chapter stands alone in its comprehension of feminist therapy. Hence, there may be slight repetitiveness in fundamental understandings of feminist intersectional therapy (as interpreted by the authors and editors) between chapters.

Although this book's coeditors have had over two decades of study and experience immersed in feminist theory and therapy, there have been many discussions about the "Imposter Phenomenon" for each of us. No matter how much time, therapy, accomplishments, or validation we receive, the imposter phenomenon is still embedded in social messages and must be faced with the courage to produce, raise voices, and advocate. Who are we to have these opinions? Do we know enough to voice opinions that are incomplete or even wrong? What if Laura Brown or other foremothers read this book and think we are idiots? By the way, we hope they do read it! Nonetheless, we marched on.

—Joanne and Kat

# PART ONE

# Foundational Principles for Feminist Intersectional Therapy

# 1

# History of Feminist Theory: The Personal Is Political in Therapy

*Joanne Jodry, Emily R. Miller, Amy Nourie, and Barbara J. Shaya*

*Throughout the West, Eurocentric, Christian-dominant, heteronormative patriarchal views have dominated the narrative of history; narratives of oppressed intersectional identities were marginalized or never reported.*

## Historical Feminist Underpinnings to Feminist Clinical Theory

The history of feminist clinical therapy is grounded in a long, arduous feminist movement spattered with activism focused on equality for primarily Eurocentric women. Only in more recent history has the feminist movement recognized the multiple, intersectional oppression of all people. It is of note that, with minor exceptions, the historical feminist movement focused on and benefited White women. Brown (1991) wrote, "Feminist therapy, as a discipline, and many White feminist therapists as individuals have in the main excluded the realities and living presence of women of Color from our work, our theories and our writing" (p. 114). In just the past few decades, women of color, multiple oppressions, and intersectional identities were recognized and honored by the feminist movement. Ware (2015) points out, "Racism has proved to be an inescapable problem for White women; of all of the different factors that have divided feminists over the last twenty years, few have caused so much bitterness and resentment" (p. 18). As a note, the developmental evolution of the foremothers' fights for equality is honored by the authors in a historical context. The current critical thinking about it does not devalue the greatness of collective feminists who have contributed and sacrificed for the collective social changes for many women. Brown (2019) said, "Forgive yourself and your elders for the compromises that we have to make and will continue to make as we uncover, layer after layer after painful layer, heteropatriarchal white supremacist colonization of our psyches and our ideas" (p. 655).

There are volumes of documentation on feminist movements in the Western world. Some highlights of major contributions to frame the emergence of feminist clinical theory and its legacies in current practice will be the frame used. There is no intention nor claim that this history exploration is, in any manner, a comprehensive dive into the history of feminism, and there will undoubtedly be some contributors or events overlooked. In fact, like most historical accounts, the authors would like to acknowledge that it is incomplete and biased by the selective attention of the historian or historical manipulator.

In the 18th century, throughout European and American Western societies, notable works emerged postulating the equality of intelligence and social and cultural roles between sexes. Examples are books written by those like Mary Astell (1706), *Some Reflections Upon Marriage*, where she suggests that men and women are equally souls, and Mary Wollstonecraft (1792/2021), *A Vindication of the Rights of Woman*, calling for women to stop being dependent on men. Although there were early feminist movements in other parts of the world, a focus on the development of feminist movements in the United States, out of which feminist clinical theory was ultimately born, is offered.

The feminist movement gained momentum in the United States during the 1800s. Elizabeth Cady Stanton laid the groundwork for inventing "white feminism" (Schuller, 2021, p. 19). In 1860, during an address to the New York State Legislature, Susan B. Anthony and Elizabeth Cady Stanton stated, "The negro's skin and the woman's sex are both prima facie evidence that they are intended to be in subjection to the white Saxon man" (Schneir, 1994, p. 118). In early feminist history, it has been recorded that Stanton and Anthony often set up political comparisons between Black men and women. Stanton and Anthony stated, "The few social privileges which the man gives the woman, he makes up to the negro in civil rights" (Schneir, 1994, p. 118). Stanton also argued that women's right to vote was needed as an offset to the Black right to vote, "advancing the false choice voting rights for black men or voting rights for white women" (Schuller, 2021, p. 19). This comparison or competition between the voting rights of women and the voting rights of Black men recently freed from slavery may have played a role in setting the tone for the unfolding of the future of the feminist women's equal rights fight.

The feminist movements were often focused on and resulted in measured legislation, but that did not necessarily change the people's cultural norms, social behaviors, or internalized beliefs. As Ware (2015) suggests, although feminists have focused on social systems, political legislation, and so on, "[f]or many people, it confirmed the importance of changing consciousness from within, rather than concentrating on external structures of power" (p. 19). Some American legislation will be reviewed here with notations about the realities of social, cultural, and consciousness change.

In the 20th century, the feminist movement toward equality between the White sexes had some successes. Sadly, race, economics, gender and affectional orientations, and other oppressed identities were not swept up in the many early fights for equality. The legacy of the previous century prevailed, with continued social and cultural oppression remaining strong and dangerous to those oppressed. The early 20th century and the feminist movement began to reap legislative gains often described as "waves."

## Waves of Feminism

Feminism is often described through the metaphor of waves. The ocean and other large bodies of water ebb and flow, sometimes with large waves caused by a particularly devastating storm. At other times, the water is flat, barely rising and falling unless a boat passes, causing a small ripple of movement. Waves also erode the shore, sometimes completely changing the landscape, making some rocks very pointed and sharp while dulling others. This metaphor is valid for feminism as its movements act like waves. Historically, feminist movements have risen or fallen based on particularly impactful political, social, or cultural events and movements. The wave metaphor was popularized after Martha Weinman Lear wrote a 1968 *New York Times* article about the "new" feminism that she called "The Second Feminist Wave." Although describing feminism as occurring in waves has been criticized as privileging Western philosophies, excluding feminists of color (and promoting White feminism), and falsely creating a picture of unity among all feminists, the wave metaphor still prevails (Zeitz, 2008; Nicholson, 2010). Some also suggested discomfort because the rising and lowering of waves might indicate times when women were complacent about their oppressed status (Nicholson, 2010). Others might suggest that the ocean moves ceaselessly and is ever swelling with new tides and waves, which allows the movement to grow and create new and more inclusive strides with progress in the future. The metaphor of feminist waves will be used while acknowledging the issues associated with this language.

## First-Wave Feminism: Gender Equality

Describing the first wave of feminism as a quest for gender equality may be somewhat of a misnomer. Indeed, feminists of the first wave in the United States during the late 19th and early 20th centuries longed to gain gender equality. However, after taking cues from organizers in the temperance and abolitionist movements, first-wave feminists focused most of their efforts on one issue: voting rights (Crowhurst, 2022; Dicker & Piepmeier, 2016; Evans et al., 2005). Suffragists, including leaders such as Elizabeth Cady Stanton and Susan B. Anthony, believed accessing the right to vote would give women the best option to influence important legal and political issues, ultimately providing them a voice and a place at the table (Schneir, 1994). It is important to note here, however, that many women were not allowed to vote based on several factors, not just their gender. Women of color were excluded from the more typical and influential suffragist groups, often creating their own organizations while fighting to be heard and participate in marches and conventions (Dicker & Piepmeier, 2016).

Women were granted the right to vote in 1920 by the passage of the 19th Amendment. Of course, many women were still prevented from voting due to other marginalizing state laws, including literacy tests, complicated voter registration forms, and, most commonly, racial discrimination (Gidlow, 2018). While women were finally granted the right to vote, many feminists felt that that was not enough; there needed to be complete equal rights. In 1923, women's rights activists Alice Paul and Crystal Eastman proposed the Equal Rights Amendment (ERA), an amendment to the Constitution that would more explicitly prohibit discrimination on the basis of sex (Dicker & Piepmeier, 2016). For many years after this, the ERA was reintroduced to Congress but was not approved until 1971, during the second wave of feminism. Ultimately, despite various attempts at resurgence, the amendment has never been ratified (Zeitz, 2008).

## Second-Wave Feminism: Feminist Therapy Emerges

The second wave of feminism is usually defined by the social movements of the 1960s through the 1980s. During this time, Betty Friedan questioned gender equity and women's fulfillment in *The Feminine Mystique* (1963). Gloria Steinem emerged as a feminist leader with a renewed focus on women's economic, social, and civil rights. The second wave signaled to White, middle-class women that they should be "unwilling to be treated like second-class citizens in the boardroom, in education, or in bed" (Thompson, 2002, p. 338). Although these feminists took their cues from the coalition-building of the civil rights movement, the second wave has been criticized for excluding women of color and ignoring women's differences, oppression, and privilege based on the intersectionality within race, class, social standing, sexuality, and so on (Brown, 2018).

The second-wave feminist movement in the United States during the 1960s and 1970s would not have been the same without the contributions of many often-overlooked, but no less significant, women of color. Alice Walker (1983) introduced the term "womanist" in her work; the word womanist helped to define the Black woman's experience specifically. Cultural critic bell hooks (2015) encouraged love, justice, and humanity in many of her works, including her 1984 feminist primer *Feminist Theory: From Margin to Center*.

The second wave of feminism in the United States focused on women's health, including issues related to reproduction, abortion, sexuality, and violence against women. In 1973, the Boston Women's Health Collective published the first commercial edition of the book *Our Bodies, Ourselves*, which included first-person accounts of women freely discussing health issues and experiences. It was around this time, in the late 1960s, that feminist therapy emerged, challenging the accepted norms and stereotypes that created the dominant narrative of women.

## Feminist Clinical Theory Emerges: The Personal Is Political

Some consider Adler (1927/2009) to be a forerunner to feminist therapy due to his early therapeutic concept around egalitarian relationships and more notably, around "masculine protest." Adler defined "masculine protest" as "a reaction, by either sex, to the prejudices of our society about masculinity and femininity" (Adler, 2009, p. 231). Likewise, some might consider neo-Freudian psychologist Karen Horney's groundbreaking writings (1967/1993) *Feminine Psychology* (a collection of works from 1922 to 1937) as early feminist theory underpinning. Her early advocacy for understanding the feminine experience was notable with such concepts as "womb envy" in reaction to some of Freud's patriarchal-centered theory. However, Horney's work was also based on psychoanalytic theory, and since many feminists rejected the psychoanalyst approach as a patriarchal theoretical construct, Horney's work might inspire conflicted views.

### *Feminist Clinical Theory Takes Root*

As the women's rights and civil rights movements were taking hold to effectuate change toward equality in America, many psychologists (e.g., Weisstein, 1968) were noting that psychology was formed and normed by the males' experience of women and had very little to do with understanding the narrative or lived experiences of actual women. Additionally, the American Psychological Association (APA) was not addressing the concerns brought up by members to address the needs of women; a group broke off from the APA to form a new organization, the Association of Women in Psychology (AWP), in 1969 (Tiefer, 1991). Tiefer (1991) reported that the initial group consisted of "26 women and one man when they met in Chicago to create a formal organizational structure" (p. 6). Although other organizations emerged (e.g., the Committee of Women in Psychology, 1973), the AWP has been a consistent foundation and birthplace of collective feminist thought that has emerged as feminist theory (Tiefer,1991). Through collective feminist clinical thoughts, groundbreaking publications that focused on counseling women differently from men, and the growth of feminist clinical organizations to discuss these thoughts, clinical feminist theory emerged as a psychology theory. This new feminist clinical theory focused on healing psychic wounds created by the social, cultural, and political patriarchal norms.

### Second-Wave Feminist Developmental Model

Downing and Roush (1985) created a developmental model for positive feminist identity development foundational to a basic understanding of how the feminist consciousness evolves. This *Feminist Identity Development Model* has been reviewed and used by many feminists across disciplines over the decades (Dicker & Piepmeier, 2016; Marine & Lewis, 2014; Enns, 2012; Moradi et al., 2002). This model provided a construct for developing awareness and a deeper understanding of gendered social oppression and hierarchies, leading to an awakening as women embrace their feminist identity. This feminist identity model seems relevant today as an explanation of how one develops a higher consciousness that evolves into feminist thinking. Like many second-wave feminist clinical underpinnings, this model also does not account for the intersectionality and specific challenges faced by those with multiple oppressions.

## Third-Wave Feminism Evolves: Multiple Oppressions

Rebecca Walker (1992), the daughter of Alice Walker, is often credited for beginning the conversation about the third wave of feminism through an article she wrote in *Ms. Magazine*. As discussed previously, the waves of the feminist movement and, hence, feminist clinical therapy are very fluid and difficult to define. For clarity, we will refer to the third wave of the feminist movement beginning in the early 1990s, recognizing this as a source of reference and not a hard date of birth. Walker's article addressed a defining moment in American history, specifically for women of Generation X: the 1991 Clarence Thomas Supreme Court nomination hearings in the U.S. Senate. For many, this was the first time people heard a national conversation about sexual harassment and, almost definitely, the first time people saw U.S. senators ask a Black Supreme Court nominee about his sexual proclivities. Anita Hill, a professor, writer, and Yale law school graduate, became infamous and mocked for her brave allegations in these hearings. At the same time, Clarence Thomas currently sits on the highest court in the country. Walker (1992) stated, "He was promoted. She was repudiated," finally realizing that "I will not be silenced. I intend to fight back" (p. 86).

This new wave of feminism brought multiple oppressions into the mainstream discussion, later termed *intersectionality* by legal scholar Kimberlé Crenshaw (1991). The third wave was, once again, overtly political and now moved toward shared identities and identity politics. Black feminism, specifically, argued the relationship between race, gender, and class and the resulting oppression and "matrix of domination" (Collins, 2000). Feminists in the third wave embraced new technologies to express their views, using blogs and zines as a tool for their resistance (National Women's History Museum, 2020). Musical subcultures also abounded with the popularity of feminist punk bands in the Riot Grrrl movement and lesbian artists, bringing in a new discussion of LGBTQ+ identities. Sometimes criticized as an attempt to construct universal womanhood, the third wave also brought hip-hop feminism and Black female rappers into popularity with groundbreaking artists such as Missy Elliott, Queen Latifah, and Lauryn Hill, as well as female-led musical groups like Salt-N-Pepa and TLC (Gillis & Munford, 2004).

### Third-Wave Feminist Clinical Theory Evolves

Although feminist clinical therapy was initially developed as a therapy for women, by women, in the third wave, feminist clinicians had begun to evolve feminist therapy by addressing the effects of power and oppression on the mental health of any individual, recognizing the complexity of multiple oppressions, not simply sex, and gender. Feminist clinical theory began to expand beyond the White, educated, middle-class consciousness of the collective founding foremothers. Tiefer (2008) states, "AWP was undeniably a white woman organization" (p. 9). She also reported that in 1989, the Women of Color caucus for AWP insisted that AWP more actively include women of color instead of just being "open" to all women.

The third wave is also notable for clinically evolving toward the concepts of the psychological impacts of multiple oppressions of people of nondominant race, sexuality, and so on. Feminist clinical theory had begun to understand the importance of considering the individual's unique experience through multiple oppressions and privileges and the consequent impact on the individual's mental health, capabilities, opportunities, and motivations as opposed to just sex and gender. Brown (2018) suggested,

> It was around this time that more feminist therapists began to conceptualize women in the context not simply of generic patriarchy but of specific cultures and milieus and to ask how feminist models of responding to distress could be informed by the experiences of women from the margins of dominate society. (p. 28)

This later came to be known as *intersectionality* (Crenshaw, 1991).

# Feminist Clinicians' Rejection of Patriarchal Therapeutic Systems of Oppression

The oft-stated phrase "the personal is political" (Hanisch, 1969) refers to the feminist belief that oppression is rooted in systemic, societal, and historical contexts that must be addressed at the sociopolitical level. The colonization legacy of all current social and political systems is rooted in Eurocentric, heteronormative, Christian-dominant patriarchal norms, including the mental health systems (Mullan, 2023). This also makes "the political very personal" in the human psyche due to the social and cultural oppression that causes lived pain. The systems, including the mental health system, have implicit and explicit inequities. Brown (1992) suggested that the psychological impacts of people living in oppressive conditions could be called "oppression artifact disorders," and they were "embedded in the framework of the culture in which an individual develops" (p. 223).

Traditional psychological theories that are the underpinnings of the mental health professions were historically normed from constricted views and have been developed and interpreted by the White, Eurocentric, heteronormative patriarchal views of normal. Cultural, social, and political behaviors normed on patriarchal views have also historically infiltrated psychological research, clinical diagnosis, treatment, and overall perceptions of "normal" (Brown, 1992; Brown, 2018; Enns, 2018).

# Patriarchal Clinical Theories Conceived in Eurocentric Norms

## Medical Model: Statistics Norming of Narratives Experiences

Historically, concepts of the etiologies and treatments of mental illness have evolved from beliefs of evil possession and sin to an understanding of science and biology as explanations for mental abnormality (Hayes, 2024; Coleman, 1956; Szasz, 2010). As science has taken the lead for explanation in the mental health discipline, a medical model has emerged as the system that often lays standards, infiltrates education, and controls treatments. The current medical and mental health system in the United States is couched in capitalism, profits, and the categorization of people. Insurance companies, or insurance systems, are not designed to lose money, and they have been influential through the past decades in creating statistically driven "evidence-based" mandates, often as the only acceptable treatment modality. Educational and licensure standards within the various clinical therapy professions direct the teaching and use of the Diagnostic and Statistical Manual of Mental Disorders (DSM) diagnosis model and the use of evidence-based, often manualized, treatment protocols. This essentially means research-based statistical probabilities are more acceptable within the medical model systems when working with people over their perceptions, oppressive existence, and lived experiences. The only true objective, measurable human condition is behavior. Therefore, the medical model encourages measurable behavioral changes based on statistical probabilities. Feminist therapists argue that statistics based on norms of the dominant majority contribute to the psychopathology that is often diagnosed (Brown, 2018; Evans et al., 2011). Evans et al. (2011) recapped a feminist therapy posture: "The definition of psychological wellness or mental health embraces the beliefs and values of the group of people who control the social, political, and economic arenas—White, middle and upper class, heterosexual, able-bodied, Protestant males" (p. 67).

Little room is left for people outside the normal curve . . . in the margins (hooks, 2015). Feminist clinicians believe individual narratives and lived experiences are therapeutically honored and curative over statistical probabilities (Brown, 2018; Mullan, 2023; Evans et al., 2011). The feminist therapeutic relationship is based on understanding the client's intersectional existence in an oppressive world of colonized systems with White supremacy underpinnings (Mullan, 2023). In other words, the feminist therapist believes the client's experience without judging what is "normal."

The Eurocentric, heteronormative, Christian-dominant patriarchal majority's judgment of mental health "norms" has made many egregious errors in the past around diagnosis and what was considered normal behavior and what was psychopathology. The current majority view of society lingers in remnants from the history of mental illness treatment and continues to decide psychopathology based on majority views. Mullan (2023) suggests that the current system of mental health is "the systemic suppression of emotional discharge and the invalidation of oppressed people's minds" (p. 9). Szasz (2010) has long proposed that the concepts around mental illness are social constructs that were created to promote and expand psychiatry in the medical field.

## The Oppressive Nature of 20th-Century Patriarchal Diagnosis

Historically, the dominant majority view of psychopathology has subjected people to what is now considered torture by using cures, such as bloodletting, drilling holes in heads, immersing in cold water, and primitive shock treatments for what might have been considered simply bad or odd behaviors (Hayes, 2024; Coleman, 1956). Once diagnosed, people were often placed in asylums. Women, people of color, and people in lower socioeconomic positions have often been the specific targets of these patriarchal declarations of mental disobedience or abnormality and poor access to quality help (Maass, 2022; Brown, 2018). Although some mental health disciplines (e.g., social work, counseling, etc.) have shifted the conversation in literature from the medical model construct to clinical conceptualizations of personal strength and wellness, the healthcare system remains in place with continued restrictive barriers. This is often an obstacle for feminist clinicians.

Perhaps the one of most egregious tools of systemic patriarchal subjugation is the pathologizing of oppressed populations using the DSM (American Psychiatric Association, 1952; American Psychiatric Association, 1980; American Psychiatric Association, 1987; American Psychiatric Association, 1994; American Psychiatric Association, 2013) to guide the process of diagnosis. Western society began mental diagnosis to classify human suffering that is common to all human experience. From the inception of the first DSM to its current edition, the number of diagnoses categorizing people as abnormal has grown by 192%. The first DSM (1952) had 102 mental disorder diagnoses, while the 5th edition DSM (2013) had 298 diagnoses (Surís et al., 2016). Historically, there have been diagnoses such as those related to enslaved people's desire for freedom, women's emotional reactions to traumatic environmental events, people who did not identify as heterosexual, and so on. Although these diagnoses may seem outrageous to clinicians today, are we sure that current diagnoses will not seem outrageous 100 years from now?

# Final Thoughts

While all theories are situated in history, not all theories are developed as a reaction to history. Feminist theory was. Consequently, feminist theory and therapy continue to evolve as social, cultural and political constructs and systems change. Therefore, not only understanding history but remaining current regarding intersectional privileges and oppression must remain in the forefront of the fourth-wave feminist clinician.

# What If?

What if the U.S. Constitution did not mention gender and used the word "persons"?

What would the United States be like today if there had been no slavery?

What if the education system allowed for more free thought instead of the current rote learning process that evolved from the patriarchal educational legacy? What if there were no grades, only thoughts in school?

What if women and people of color had been more valued in history and had been the authors of history? How would equality be different today?

What if a diagnosis had never been developed as part of the mental health system? How would therapy be different?

# References

Adler, A. (2009). *Understanding human nature*. OneWorld. (Original work published 1927)

American Psychiatric Association. (1952). *Diagnostic and statistical manual of mental disorders* (1st ed.). American Psychiatric Publishing.

American Psychiatric Association. (1980). *Diagnostic and statistical manual of mental disorders (DSM-III)*. American Psychiatric Association.

American Psychiatric Association. (1987). *Diagnostic and statistical manual of mental disorders (III-R)*. American Psychiatric Publishing.

American Psychiatric Association. (1994). *Diagnostic and statistical manual of mental disorders: DSM-IV* (4th ed.). American Psychiatric Association.

American Psychiatric Association. (2013). *Diagnostic and statistical manual of mental disorders* (5th ed.). American Psychiatric Association.

American Psychiatric Association. (2022). *Diagnostic and statistical manual of mental disorders* (5th ed.). American Psychiatric Association.

Astell, M. (1706). *Some reflections upon marriage* (4th ed.). Printer for William Parker.

Boston Women's Health Book Collective. (1973). *Our bodies, ourselves*. Simon & Schuster.

Brown, L. S. (1991). Antiracism as an ethical imperative: An example from feminist therapy. *Ethics and Behavior, 1*(2), 113–127.

Brown, L. S. (1992). A feminist critique of personality disorders. In L. S. Brown & M. Ballou (Eds.), *Personality and pathology: Feminist reappraisals* (pp. 206–228). Guilford.

Brown, L. S. (2004). *Subversive dialogues: Theory in feminist therapy*. Basic Books.

Brown, L. S. (2006). Still subversive after all these years: The relevance of feminist therapy in the age of evidence-based practice. *Psychology of Women Quarterly, 30*(1), 15–24. https://doi.org/10.1111/j.1471-6402.2006.00258.x

Brown, L. S. (2016). *Supervision essentials for the feminist psychotherapy model of supervision*. American Psychological Association.

Brown, L. S. (2018). *Feminist therapy* (2nd ed.). American Psychological Association.

Brown, L. S. (2019). Celebrating the fiftieth anniversary of the Association for Women in Psychology: A life in feminist psychology: A long and interesting journey from Ft. Wayne to Newport (Herstory). *Sex Roles, 80*, 647–655. https://doi.org/10.1007/s11199-019-01044-w

Coleman, J. C. (1956). *Abnormal psychology and modern life*. Scott, Foresman and Company

Collins, P. H. (2000). *Black feminist thought*. Routledge.

Crenshaw, K. W. (1991). *Stanford Law Review, 43*(6), 1241–1299.

Crowhurst, A. (2022). *Badly behaved women*. Welbeck.

Dicker, R., & Piepmeier, A. (Eds.). (2016). *Catching a wave: Reclaiming feminism for the 21st century*. Northeastern University Press.

Downing, N. E., & Roush, K. L. (1985). From passive acceptance to active commitment: A model of feminist identity development for women. *The Counseling Psychologist, 13*, 695–709.

Enns, C. Z. (2018). Feminist therapy and empowerment. In C. B. Travis, J. W. White, A. Rutherford, W. S. Williams, S. L. Cook, & K. F. Wyche (Eds.), *APA handbook of the psychology of women: Perspectives on women's private and public lives* (pp. 3–19). American Psychological Association. https://doi.org/10.1037/0000060-001

Evans, K. M., Kincade, E. A., Marbley, A. F., & Seem, S. R. (2005). Feminism and feminist therapy: Lessons from the past and hopes for the future. *Journal of Counseling & Development, 83*(3), 269–277. https://onlinelibrary.wiley.com/doi/pdf/10.1002/j.1556-6678.2005.tb00342.x?casa_token=hHSt_MEeUccAAAAA%3AL410QLgqU9o8cmM1gF9f0x4_OR5BePy0jUUw-kwv6Gvo_8xaNMQiFMorV0_PM-hZ0bQqIt530HwOPw

Evans, K. M., Kincade, E. A., & Seem, S. R. (2011). *Introduction to feminist theory*. SAGE.

Friedan, B. (1963). *The feminine mystique*. W. W. Norton.

Gidlow, L. (2018). The sequel: The Fifteenth Amendment, the Nineteenth Amendment, and southern Black women's struggle to vote. *The Journal of the Gilded Age and Progressive Era, 17*(3), 433–449. https://www.cambridge.org/core/services/aop-cambridge-core/content/view/9EDB82609 6C0353E6FE12E3E345FC5CF/S1537781418000051a.pdf/sequel_the_fifteenth_amendment_the_ nineteenth_amendment_and_southern_black_womens_struggle_to_vote.pdf

Gillis, S., & Munford, R. (2004). Genealogies and generations: The politics and praxis of third wave feminism. *Women's History Review, 13*(2), 165–182.

Hanisch, C. (1969, February). *The personal is political*. www.carolhanisch.org. https://www. carolhanisch.org/CHwritings/PIP.html

Harper, I. H. (2020). *The life and work of Susan B. Anthony* (Vol. 3). CosimoClassics. (Original work published 1899)

Hayes. N. (2024). *A little history of psychology*. Yale University Press.

hooks, b. (2015). *Feminist theory: From margin to center*. Routledge.

Horney, K. (1993). *Feminine psychology*. W. W. Norton. (Original work published 1967)

Lear, M. W. (1968, March 10). The second feminist wave. *New York Times*. https://www.nytimes. com/1968/03/10/archives/the-second-feminist-wave.html

Maass, V. S. (2022). *Feminist psychology*. Praeger.

Marine, S., & Lewis, R. (2014). I'm in this for real: Revisiting young women's feminist becoming. *Women's Studies International Forum, 47*(A), 11–22.

Moradi, B., Subich, L. M., & Phillips, J. C. (2002). Revisiting feminist identity development theory, research and practice. *The Counseling Psychologist, 30*(1), 6–43.

Mullan, J. (2023). *Decolonizing therapy: Oppression, historical trauma, and politicizing your practice*. W. W. Norton.

National Women's History Museum. (2020, June 23). Feminism: The third wave. https://www. womenshistory.org/exhibits/feminism-third-wave

Nicholson, L. (2010). Feminism in "waves": Useful metaphor or not? *New Politics, 12*(4), 34–39.

Schneir, M. (1994). *Feminism: The essential historical writings*. Vintage.

Schuller, K. (2021). *The trouble with White women: A counterhistory of feminism*. Bold Type Books.

Surís, A., Holliday, R., & North, C. S. (2016). The evolution of the classification of psychiatric disorders. *Behavioral Sciences, 6*(1), 1–10. https://www.mdpi.com/2076-328X/6/1/5

Szasz, T. S. (2010). *The myth of mental illness*. Harper Perennial.

Thompson, B. (2002). Multiracial feminism: Recasting the chronology of second-wave feminism. *Feminist Studies, 28*(2), 337–360.

Tiefer, L. (2008). A brief history of the Association of Women in Psychology:1991–2008. *Association of Women in Psychology. AWP Herstory*. https://www.awpsych.org/awp_herstory.php

Tiefer, L. (1991). A brief history of the Association of Women in Psychology: 1969–1991. *Psychology of Women Quarterly, 15*, 635–649. doi:10.1111/j.1471–6402.1991.tb00436.x

Walker, A. (1983). *In search of our mothers' gardens: Womanist prose*. Mariner Books.

Walker, R. (1992). Becoming the 3rd wave. *MS: Spring 2002, 12*(2), 86–87.

Ware, V. (2015). *Beyond the pale: White women, racism, and history*. Verso Books.

Weisstein, N. (1968). *Kinder, Kuche, Kirche as scientific law: Psychology constructs the female*. https:// www.bibliotechecivichepadova.it/sites/default/files/opera/documenti/sezione-6-serie-8-175.pdf

Wollstonecraft, M. (2021). *A vindication of the rights of woman*. Affordable Classics. (Original work published 1792)

Zeitz, J. (2008). Rejecting the center: Radical grassroots politics in the 1970s—Second-wave feminism as a case study. *Journal of Contemporary History, 43*(4), 673–688.

# 2

# Fourth-Wave Feminist Intersectional Theory Foundations

## *Joanne Jodry and Kathleen McCleskey*

*Feminist theory has evolved to understand that all people's experiences, rights, power, and oppression are not the same, and without honoring intersectional identities, there is no true feminist therapy.*

The feminist intersectional clinical theory has risen from the recognition that social, political, and cultural systems born in Eurocentric, heteronormative, Christian-dominant, patriarchal roots have psychological effects and effects on the development and well-being of individuals oppressed by the systems created and reinforced by these norms (Garcia, 2021; Bagshaw, 2019; Brown, 2018; Disch & Hawkesworth, 2016; Evans et al., 2011; Chaplin, 1999). Brown (2018) stated, "Feminist therapy asserts that patriarchal systems surrounding most human life intentionally or unintentionally systematically and structurally disempower almost all people on one or more of these variables, such that this paradigm of a powerful person is entirely aspirational" (p. 44). Oppressed individuals or groups with marginalized intersectional identities are often kept from reaching their full potential due to the psychological impact of oppression and the normalization of subjugation that is created within society. Privileged individuals or groups with privileged intersectional identities might not consciously recognize their privilege. The privileged intersectional parts of people may be internalized, similar to internalized oppression (Hardy, 2023) or learned helplessness (Maier & Seligman, 2016). This internalized privilege may present as justification for why the macrosystems are equal in attempts to deny their own advantage or to bolster their accomplishments. These concepts of privilege and oppression may be conscious and unconscious, implicit and explicit, embedded and learned, and embraced or defended. In the Western world, there is a developmentally passive social and cultural assimilation to the Eurocentric, heteronormative, Christian-dominant, patriarchal norms that begin at birth (Brown, 2018; Downing and Roush, 1985). Many people have not had the opportunity or exposure to be able to examine these issues consciously with a full understanding of the possible influence and impact the social and cultural norms may have had on their personal limitations and disempowerment. Feminist fourth-wave intersectional theory attempts to help clients(s) understand and become fully conscious of their privilege, oppressions, and power within the ecosystem. *Fourth-wave feminist intersectional theory attempts to raise consciousness and bring awareness to help the client(s) identify and strengthen areas of empowerment and navigate the best possible well-being for the most conscious, fully functioning life.*

## How Does Acceptance of Oppression Happen?

Through a natural process of human generational existence and personal development, people organically acculturate and enculturate to their environment. Many people never become conscious to or feel the need to examine that natural process that evolves as "normal and right." This assimilation process happens on all levels through an individual's ecosystem. A person can go a lifetime and never question that process. In contrast, if a person does begin to question and seek a more conscious awareness that informs their future selves, a fuller intentional identity development may follow. This is in alignment with the goals of feminist intersectional clinical theory.

Downing and Roush (1985) created a model for feminist identity development that has been an underpinning of basic understanding in feminist counseling and shows how a feminist awareness evolves. This model has been reviewed and used by many over the decades (Dicker & Piepmeier, 2016; Enns, 2012; Kelly, 2015; Marine & Lewis, 2014; Moradi et al., 2002).

Downing and Roush (1985) suggested a 5-stage feminist identity model inspired by the works of Cross's (1971) Positive Black Identity Development. Downing and Roush (1985). began with *Stage 1: Passive acceptance.* In this stage, "a woman is either unaware of or denies the individual, institutional and cultural prejudice and discrimination against her" (p. 698). A woman either openly accepts the position of White male superiority or enjoys her personal comfort in her feminine role as a minority voice. In *Stage 2: Revelation,* Downing and Roush (1985) suggested that something or a series of somethings happen that a woman can no longer "ignore or deny," which causes a woman to have a revelation toward awareness of oppression, unfairness, and feminist thoughts. (p. 698). In *Stage 3: Embeddedness-Emanation,* the developers suggested that noticing the embeddedness and moving from it to emanation is very difficult due to the interconnectedness to the dominant culture through marriage, roles of mother, sisters, lovers, and so on. They also suggested this was "more difficult for Caucasian women" (p. 701). Perhaps this is because they experience less oppression than women of color. In *Stage 4: Synthesis,* Downing and Roush (1985) suggested that in the stage, "[Women] are able to transcend traditional sex roles, make choices for themselves based on well-defined personal values, and evaluate men on an individual, rather than stereotypical basis" (p. 702). In this final *Stage 5: Active Commitment*, people "select issues carefully based on their unique talents and the possibility of both personal gratification and effecting social change" (p. 702).

## Intersectional Feminist Identity Development Model: Oppression Realized

This new Intersectional Feminist Identity Development Model complements Downing and Roush's (1985) work and builds on it to consider fourth-wave advances. This model will focus not on women and gender but on intersectional development toward fourth-wave feminist thinking, explaining how social, cultural, and political oppressive norms and hierarchies of power maintain themselves if not examined clinically or socially.

## Birth: Immersion and Assimilation

In this stage, a child often enters the world with an advanced declaration of the child's sex and gender. Social norms in the West have even normalized having a "gender reveal party" while the child is still in the womb. Assumptions about clothing, characteristics, parental dreams/fears, and future expectations often begin before birth. At birth, the child is announced with sex/gender, and the world begins to immerse them in a manner with gender-reinforcing words and behaviors. Likewise, a child born with existing intersectional multiple privileges and oppressions has those identities reinforced as well. Socioeconomic status, race, family constellations and support, parental affectional orientation status, parental emotional availability, and so on all begin to influence the child from the moment of birth intersectionally. Through parental messaging and the ability, or not, to create safety for the child, additional messaging is received by the infant.

## Toddler: Safety in Learning and Knowing

The toddler receives messages that become embedded in their psyche about normal and correct behavior. Parenting styles differ; many parents attempt to have their toddler fit into normal decorum and acceptable social conforming manners. For example, share your toys, behave in public, listen to adults, and so forth. Conforming behaviors often receive reward and approval through a child's developing lens, while nonconforming behaviors receive punishment and disapproval from the family and ecosystem. Therefore, in functional households, a child might naturally assimilate to conforming. This is a stage of "knowing." Many children with predictable households may begin to embed the following into the consciousness: "I know I am right and will be safe if I do this." Is it possible that this "knowing" grows into adulthood with the "need to know," creating the judgment of defensive adults? Although a toddler's brain function is limited and concrete, the child might also notice how different people are treated differently in this stage (Piaget, 1968). Perhaps siblings' cousins or playmates of different genders, family constellations, races, and so on could make a child recognize a rudimentary sense of the unfairness of intersectional privileges and oppressions. The child might recognize concrete differences without knowing "why," but the messages are still embedded.

## Childhood: Ecosystem: Us and Them

Once a child interacts independently with some ecosystems (schools, churches, social groups, etc.), labels, categorization, comparison, and judgment begin externally and internally. There begins a process of us and them. Although the education system makes strides toward equality, it sets the tone for comparison between and among children. Grades, groups, teams, and all other activities define children according to their developing intersectional identity formation of intelligence, likability, and talents. Children may try to fit in with peers, gain adult favor, or reject it all. Children in this stage learn what society likes and whether they are favored or unfavored in their micro and macro systems. For example, depending on the child's intersectional identities and environment, the assimilation process can yield favor in a micro but not a macro system. Either way, the child begins to sort through society's intersectional privileges and oppressions; even if this is not conscious or they do not have the language to describe it, they begin to understand where they fit in the hierarchies of the social systems.

## Teens: Privileged or Oppression. Identity Forms Groups In and Out

By the time a Western child becomes a teenager, they have learned social expectations: *raise your hand in class* (to keep order); *respect adults* (even if some are not respectable); *school is everything* (even if you have no food at home). They have learned how society judges them as popular or not, loud/quiet, intelligent or not, attractive or not, privileged/favored or not, and so forth. Since teenagers have more brain development than younger children and can think abstractly at a higher level than a child (Piaget, 1968), they begin to question their environments. They either embrace or reject the labels and categories they have been put into by the social environment. Arguably, the teenager who embraces the favor of society may have the most challenging existence, needing to maintain that favor. Conversely, the student who rejects their position can get caught in a lifetime of rejecting many aspects of life. In this stage, if a child is exposed to feminist intersectional thinking, it may begin to impact them in exploring their identity (Erikson,1980). Disappointingly, most Eurocentric, heteronormative Christian-dominant patriarchal systems are set up to maintain the status quo, and often teens are exposed to the social norms of conformity.

## Young Adults: Limits Known and Accepted: Trying Your Place in the System

"Adulting" begins at different ages for different people, depending on privilege and oppression of the environment. For our purposes, we will refer to this stage as when the person begins to take responsibility for themselves, make decisions, and suffer the consequences of their choices. When raised in Western society and reaching adulthood, many people have embedded beliefs that life's primary goal is to succeed in capitalism. All of the oppressive constructs and systems in place have messaged the developing person to conform to the patriarchal norms. Depending on their intersectional identities, young adults may have received messages from their ecosystems to dress a certain way, wear their hair a certain way, speak a certain way, go to college, and work without consideration for their health or personal life, show that they are better than their coworkers, and make as much money as possible to look and feel successful. Depending on how committed the person is to their assimilated beliefs, they may go their whole life with these goals of financial, social, and cultural achievement without examining the macro system. Arguably, many cultural and social systems may not contribute to empathy for others, continuing the focus of competition born in early developmental stages.

## Adults: Living in Action

Many people follow the environmentally learned path of success: assimilating to social and cultural norms to define success and happiness. Often, that might include purchasing things, climbing into job opportunities, building romantic relationships, and finding the right image to project success. People will live according to their constructs. If a person has embraced a consciousness-raising experience, that added experience may offer an opportunity to redefine meaning and happiness in life.

## Consciousness Raising: Seeing It Everywhere

Sometimes, consciousness awakening happens to people. It can be any encounter anywhere with a high school teacher, a church leader, or a friend with a deep awareness that brings an awareness of the privileges and oppressions of the Eurocentric, heteronormative, Christian-dominant patriarchal norms. An event can happen that triggers a conscious raising as well. It can be a personal event that triggers a person's awareness or a social or cultural macro event. It is possible to be exposed to feminist thinking without even recognizing it. A political, social, or cultural injustice can be so evident that it breaks through the assimilation of people "knowing." An example may have been the death of George Floyd in May of 2020, which may have been a conscious-raising event for many people of different privileges and oppressions.

## Choices: Deciding What to Do with Awareness

Once consciousness is raised around injustices, intersectional identities, inequality, bias, and so on, it can go back down in the consciousness as quickly as it rises. Although we cannot "unring" some bells, perhaps the mind can decide to go back to the place of "knowing," which brings the person a sense of safety and peace. Once consciousness has risen, the person must decide what to do with this new awareness. If the person embraces their raised consciousness and begins to look at how Eurocentric, heteronormative, Christian-dominant patriarchal norms have permeated the social, cultural, and political systems that rule society, they may begin to see it everywhere throughout their ecosystem. Once it becomes blatantly evident to the person, returning to the assimilated naivete is hard. Now, a person needs to decide how they may want to adjust or not to their new awareness. This might include further education, finding and becoming a mentor, therapy with a feminist therapist, and so on. As a feminist with differentiated choices, a person may quietly choose to expose their family and friends to these ideas, they may march and protest more radically, or choose to do nothing—all equal choices.

## Finding Power and Freedom: Tribe

In the intersectional feminist development model, as with any consciousness-raising model, the goal is freedom from the constraints of living/thinking in the established Eurocentric, heteronormative, Christian-dominant, patriarchal norms that oppress people. Freedom can come from breaking social expectations and judgments and moving toward a more meaningful existence not couched in assimilations to ecosystems. Recognition of intersectional identities and strengths can lead a person to choices with the awareness of social interactions filled with privileges and oppressions. For many people, it seems impossible to reject social and cultural norms and still become successful; that is not the only choice. Sometimes, there are ways to navigate oppressive systems for one's benefit. In the feminist development, it might be helpful to find a tribe to help steer these very tedious positions.

The *Intersectional Feminist Identity Development Model* can be used to conceptualize and examine people's privileges and oppressions within the systems. It is important to honor where the person is in their development and not attempt to move them linearly through their consciousness-raising processes. Resistances should be met with honor. Examining society's impact on people's intersectional identities may be an overwhelming experience. The individual sets their pace and makes all decisions with awareness.

# Living Legacy of Oppressive Systems Today: Understanding Social Positioning

As discussed, the historical Western patriarchal culture has informed all of the cultural and social systems that create the macro environment in which people develop and live. Although much cultural and social consciousness has created more equality throughout Western history, there is still much work to do to remove the power differentials and lack of equality that continue to oppress people today and impact their future potential for meaning and growth.

## Wage Gaps

Pew Research (2023) reported, "The gender wage gap has remained relatively stable in the United States over the past 20 years or so" (Pew, 2023). They reported that in 2022, women earned an average of 82% of what men earned, which is slightly up from 2002, when women earned 80% of what men earned. Additionally, 28% of men are likely to be the top boss, compared to 21% of women. Of course, this does not account for the intersectional wage gap differences. Chapman and Benis (2017) studied intersectional wage gaps and found the following: "The gender wage gap is not uniform across racial groupings, with African Americans and Latinx groupings having significantly higher wage gaps than their white, non-Hispanic peers" (p. 85).

## Educational Systems

Many public and private educational systems train children and teens with the information that maintains the status quo of the systems. Depending on the schools' geographic area, most educational systems follow the Christian holiday schedules with vacation days off to celebrate (Christmas and Easter week). Children who do not follow that Christian schedule might encounter internal and external marginalization, discrimination, and even anxiety. Additionally, sex and gender are often clearly divided in the school systems around abilities, subject matters, or even social expectations. The intersectionality of students from oppressed groups, consciously and unconsciously, does not allow marginalized students the same opportunities as their privileged peers. Potter and Morris (2017) studied the overall accumulated experiences in the education systems between White and historically disadvantaged racial/ethnic minority children and its impact on achievement. They found that these differences in accumulated experiences and their perceptions of them accounted for a "moderate portion of the gap in reading and math gains between White and historically disadvantaged minority children" (p. 132).

## STEM and Girls

It is difficult to forget Harvard president Summers's (2005) speech suggesting that "in the special case of science and engineering, there are issues of intrinsic aptitude, and particularly of variability of aptitude, and that those considerations are reinforced by what are lesser factors involving socialization and continuing discrimination" (par. 30). Jungert et al. (2019) challenged the lack of aptitude as an explanation why so few women were in STEM (science, technology, engineering, and mathematics). The study suggested that the major difference between genders' learning STEM was a higher correlation for girls between anxiety and self-efficacy. This may have implications for teaching styles and social and cultural expectations. According to the U.S. Census (2021), by 2019, 27% of STEM workers were women, while women comprised 48% of the workforce. Men made up 73% of the STEM workers and only represented 52% of the workforce.

## Teacher Studies around Living up to Expectation

Historically, there have been consistent studies showing the relationship between teachers' expectations and students' performance (Benner et al., 2021; Johnston et al., 2021; Timmermans et al., 2016). How do teachers form these expectations? Experience in the patriarchal systems (cultural norms for concepts of "respect"; the educational systems based on grades and comparisons; labeling and ranking of students, etc.) that they have experienced, assimilated, and embraced. Not surprisingly, Sorhagen (2013) also found significant teacher misperception in math and language skills based on the families' income. Like all other people, teachers are a product of the environment and form judgments based on these systemic "norms of right and wrong." This may set even the youngest students on a trajectory of success or failure, self-efficacy, or low self-esteem based on the teacher's patriarchal acculturation.

## Meritocracy

Historically, American children are taught that Americans live up to the ideals of America. The United States has deep values as a meritocracy—described as a place where any person can achieve their goals if they try hard enough (McNamee & Miller, 2009). This view assumes that all people have equal access to the same resources—that, in effect, there is a level playing field and that each person has the same starting position in achieving goals. In other words, equality is already in place. From this perspective, examples are frequently given of people from minoritized populations who have achieved visible success, such as Barack Obama, who personifies the ability of anyone, regardless of race, to achieve the American dream (Kwate & Meyer, 2010). Holding up these examples serves two important purposes. First, it reinforces the message that opportunity is available to all. Insidiously, it also reinforced the idea that all other marginalized individuals from the same groups are just not working hard enough or are not motivated enough (Hardy, 2023). Taken together, these social messages reinforce achievement (or lack of achievement) as residing solely within the individual and without assessing any systemic impacts on achievement, such as lack of resources or opportunities (Hardy, 2023). For some individuals who endorse meritocracy, this can also encourage them to turn inward toward believing it is their own inadequacy since the larger majority agrees with the truth of equality for all (Hardy, 2023; Kwate & Meyer, 2010). Believing that equality exists in all situations must make the individual at fault. Internalizing these social messages can cause an "oppressor within" (Hardy, 2023, p. 42). Hardy (2023) states, "The unconscious internalization of messages about the inherent inferiority of the oppressed and the corresponding superiority of the oppressor is inevitable and predictable" (p. 44).

## Legal System

Currently, African Americans and other non-white groups dominate the incarcerated populations in the prison systems. According to Pew Research (2023), "As of 2022, Black people were admitted to jail at more than four times the rate of White people and stayed in jail for 12 more days on average across the 595-jail sample" (para 4). Additionally, Black people made up 12% of the local population but 26% of the jail population (Pew, 2023). However, there are many contributing factors to who is being incarcerated. Gase et al. (2016) conducted an extensive study (n=12752) attempting to investigate the racial and ethnic disparities in arrest. Their study found a "[s]ignificantly higher likelihood of having ever been arrested among blacks, when compared to whites, even after controlling for a range of delinquent behaviors" (p. 296). They also suggested that neighborhood racial composition due to the historically differing conditions of economic, social, and political resources may be one of the reasons for the disparities (Gase et al., 2016, p. 309). Additionally, feminist therapists might suggest that the historical Eurocentric, heteronormative, Christian-dominant White patriarchal cultural and systemic influence contributes to the police officers' decisions at the point of arrest.

## Oppressive Politics: The Political Is Personal

The history of the political system, laws created, and privileges given have been historically designed by the Eurocentric, heteronormative, Christian-dominant, White man's lived experience and perceptions. This is the political system that exists currently, and although there have been inroads with some non-Christians and people of color in recent history, the more significant majority that is still electable falls within the existing White-privileged group. For example, according to the Center for American Women and Politics (CAWP), in 2024, women make up 25% of the Senate and 28.7% of the House of Representatives. Additionally, Pew Research (2023) reports that people reporting as "nonwhite" make up 12% of the Senate and 28% of the House of Representatives. Often when people from oppressed groups gain some political power, oppressive reactions might be the response (e.g., gerrymandering geography, decreasing voting sites, creating lines for people who cannot afford to take off from work or stand in lines for hours to vote, and attempts to confuse and conflate issues with untrue talking points). Politics is power, and the *personal is political*.

## Multicultural Systems

There is traditionally an American narrative that America is the best country, often noting its "melting pot" of multicultural historical immigration. As a result of the Civil Rights Movement of the 1960s, concepts of multiculturalism, inclusion, equality, and equity are often integrated into the educational systems (Kirylo, 2017). Nevertheless, politically, legislatively, and culturally, there remain clear hierarchies and labels of people to categorize their worth. For many people, there is a desire for power over other groups to gain favor and capitalistic gains, the desire to keep massive asylum seekers out of the United States, and an overall lack of empathy for another's oppressive experience. This may or may not be the dominant sentiment, but it exists and permeates many constructs and systems of the West's macro and micro ecosystems. The intersectional oppressive identities are often most impacted by the hypocrisy and incongruence between ideal selves (of full equality) and realities (desire for superiority). When investigating intersectional oppression, the influence of the Eurocentric, heteronormative, dominant-Christian patriarchy is still evident as the primary influencer of "normal" on the personal development, social standards, and cultural expectations that one might hold for oneself.

## Parental Norms

Parents often raise children to acculturate and accelerate societal achievement. There is a collective Western thought that children should/must be educated most often in a school system. Depending on the parents' socioeconomic status, there may be choices of prestige, hierarchies, and different arenas for their children to compete within. Parents and the social systems teach children to compete with each other at an early age. This can be seen in parental behaviors like buying the latest stylish clothing for children and ensuring they have the same things the other kids are purchasing to fit into the system they live within. In addition to the love and support parents give their children, one of the main goals of parenting is to raise them to be "happy." A patriarchal historical view of the path to happiness in Western culture is often through financial success, esteem, and power. Where does this leave the children and families without financial means to compete? What happens to children who have to tell their classmates that they got nothing from Santa (especially because Santa comes only for good children)? Is this equitable and giving each person equal opportunity as they grow into adulthood? Nevertheless, asking a parent to abandon this idea of Santa or not let their child have anything that everyone in the class does would likely be met with much resistance. Arguably, many Western parents tend to raise their children with entitlements to their birthright of privileges or acceptances of their oppression.

## Capitalism as a Meaning of Life

The driving force in many of the Western systems is capitalism. Capitalism might even be considered the religion of Western society since it often dominates Western patriarchal ideas around success and happiness. Although in the United States, about 90% of the population identified as Christian, by 2022, that number had fallen to 63% (Pew, 2022). It might seem that even in some spiritual circles, capitalism plays a primary role related to self-protection, "America first," hierarchies of wealth, paying taxes, and so on. When making many life decisions around career, marriage, having children, where to live, and the like, often the primary consideration is money due to the embedded values of patriarchal financial systems. Social, cultural, and political systems have created and promoted hierarchies around money and power.

About 4 in 10 people report their jobs as essential to their identities (Pew, 2023). Yet, according to Pew (2023), only about 51% of people are satisfied with their jobs. Many people are in jobs that they do not find fulfilling, yet those who are unsatisfied continue to do their jobs and assimilate into patriarchal capitalist-driven norms where capitalism is viewed as a superior way of living as opposed to other ideologies like socialism. Pew (2019) reported that 55% of Americans have a negative view of socialism, and 65% have a favorable view of capitalism. Ideals of capitalism as a patriarchal construct often serve to oppress the marginalized intersectional identities of the masses while rewarding the privileged by promoting the propaganda that anyone can get ahead with hard work (Hardy, 2023). In fact, this notion can potentially lead to suffering of learned helplessness (Maier & Seligman, 2016; Seligman & Maier, 1967) and/or internalized devaluation (Hardy, 2023).

# Intersectional Human Experience: Oppressive Systemic Impact on the Psyche

## Multiple Oppressions and Intersectionality

Justifiably, feminist intersectional theory has been historically criticized for lumping women together as an equal group normed on White, middle-class women. As we know, there are so many identity variables to woman's lived experience, like race, economic status, abilities, and so on that impact the privilege and oppression of a woman. During the third wave of the feminist movement, the introduction of the conceptualizations of multiple oppression and intersectionality to feminist theory had a significant impact on clinical feminist therapy (Collins, 1990; Crenshaw, 1991). The concept of intersectionality comes from Black feminist thought. Crenshaw (1989) originally presented it as the nuanced and exponentially oppressive effect of being both Black and female in terms of legal decisions. Intersectionality suggests that examining a person's oppressed social locations singly does not adequately capture the lived experience of having multiple oppressed social identities and how those intersections impact experiences. So, the gendered experiences of White women, Black women, and trans women cannot be viewed as being identical. Without adding other intersecting identities, gender (or other social identities) become reductionist frames.

Over time, intersectionality has been applied to many areas outside of legal studies. An intersectional perspective invites clinicians to consider how a person's identities (including those of the therapist) intertwine in different spheres of life, how multiple identities are valued or oppressed in varying relational situations, and how systems are likely to take reductionist views of identities, viewing them as single pieces of a person (race, gender, ability, etc.) rather than as interrelated aspects of the self. For example, an Asian transgender male who uses a wheelchair may, in the same moment, experience the intersection of racism, sexism, and ableism.

Intersectional thought has been deeply related to social justice and critiques of existing social systems. For example, Collins et al. (2021) identify four premises to frame projects on intersectionality. These include understanding social identities as being "markers of power" (p. 694) that are co-constructive and interdependent; recognizing that relationally, intersecting identities reflect nuances of power differences; that people, singly and as groups, experience and assess their lived experiences through these experiences of intersectional power; and that social problems at any level of people or society cannot be solved unless these intersectional foundations are used to understand problems and to create solutions. Using an intersectional lens allows clinicians and clients to explore the complexity of social identities and how multiplicative oppressions can manifest.

## Critical Race Theory

Critical race theory (CRT) is a theory that also originated in legal thought (Crenshaw, 1989, 1991). CRT examines how race, in particular, has been used over time in complex ways to reinforce White supremacy at the expense of people of color, particularly African Americans. CRT has illustrated the myriad ways that the system of White supremacy is deeply embedded into dominant systems in the United States and demonstrates how laws, policies, and processes continue to buttress White supremacy despite laws and policies that, on their face, are colorblind. CRT is a theory that has illuminated for many people how systems work to keep the status quo of White dominance. CRT has also become a lightning-rod concept in the political arena with concerns about how it rewrites history and inculcates students, even in elementary schools, into liberal thought (see, e.g., Burns, 2022).

In the therapeutic world, CRT has been included in higher education curricula as multicultural and social justice foundations have evolved. There may already be a clear understanding that individuals and groups must be viewed in terms of their societal power during all phases of helping. However, CRT asserts that racialization still occurs on a deep level even if, on the surface, programs or individual clinicians espouse multicultural values (Trahan & Lemberger, 2014). Therefore, like intersectionality, CRT provides a context for contextualizing a client's experiences and informs how clinicians, particularly clinicians from the dominant culture, address race within clients' lives and the therapeutic relationship.

## White Fragility

"White fragility" is a term created by DiAngelo (2011) to describe the reactions and responses of White people to evidence of White supremacy and of their continued participation in systems or practices that reinforce it. Because White people have been the dominant social group in the United States, White people have been unaccustomed to considering themselves through the lens of race or viewing systems as being racially privileged to them. In addition, White people may view racism as being on a *good–bad* or *racist–not racist* binary such that any uncovering of bias or racist thoughts or behaviors would make them immoral and racist people (DiAngelo, 2018).

DiAngelo (2011, 2018) describes the impacts of White fragility as harmful to both people of color and White people. When a White person reacts emotionally to being asked to consider implicit bias, for example, the reaction can derail further discussion of implicit bias (DiAngelo, 2018; Hamad, 2020). Hamad (2020) has called this often-unconscious reaction "White tears." These reactions can also center the experience of Whiteness rather than centering the lived experiences of people of color. The result, in this example, can be a reinforcement of the status quo—shutting down honest and painful explorations of continued White privilege. White fragility and White tears can serve as an often-unconscious protection for individual White persons and also for the system of White supremacy (DiAngelo, 2018; Hamad, 2020). It may also reinforce the good–bad binary of racism for White people rather than opening contemplation of how living in a racialized society can profoundly impact people.

In the therapeutic environment, White fragility may be seen as a defense mechanism that is used to shield Whites from the discomfort of being racially challenged (Keramidas, 2021). It can also be viewed through the lens of emotional regulation theory (Ford et al., 2022). From a feminist perspective, White fragility is a manifestation of how deeply embedded the patriarchal system of oppression is and how upsetting it is to challenge those who hold more privilege and power.

## Ecosystem Disorder?

The psychological construct of the "ego" is one way to think of the complicated creation of reality versus personal truth that each person develops (and might be called personality). The ego attempts to make sense of the world, to mitigate between the instincts of the id and the ideals of the superego, to create a safe feeling of knowing and will defend that knowledge with defense mechanisms. Therefore, if it is a normal adaptation to assimilate into society, how can someone have a personality disorder? Would it not seem true that the person not functioning to the best of their ability was exposed to an *ecosystem disorder*? This person is "disordered" in how they fit into society and labeled as borderline, narcissistic, and so on in the medical model system. However, this disordered person may simply be adapting to the disordered ecosystem that surrounds them. A feminist therapist sees the oppressive, abusive, rejecting systems as the disorder as opposed to the individual pathology assigned to the normal adaptation to the unjust systems. Hence, *ecosystem disorder might be the most appropriate diagnosis that exists.*

# Guiding Feminist Principles of Fourth-Wave Feminist Intersectional Therapy

## Individual Strength-Based Theory

Feminist theory places the highest value on the individual's experiences and the perception of those experiences over statistical probabilities of what is normal (Brown, 2018; Evans et al., 2011). Feminist intersectional theory accepts all consciousness and experiences as believable, equal, and valuable. Feminist intersectional therapy views the client from a lens of survival with resilience from growing up in oppressive and often dysfunctional, accepted cultural and social norms. Building on that strength of adaptive existence underpins feminist theory (Brown, 2018; Evans et al., 2011). For example, a client diagnosed with a "personality disorder" might be seen as adaptive, having developed coping mechanisms for their personality to organize itself in a manner to survive their early experiences.

## Transparency

Many clients seek therapy to look for answers from wise people. The media has promoted that concept with no shortage of advice, often from mental health professionals. The mental health profession does not discourage this thinking with advertisements encouraging people to "seek help." Patriarchal systems, licenses, medical models, and so on might give people the confidence to seek answers about how to run their lives from people trained in psychological principles. When clients come seeking help, they often think there is a right way to be or to do things (often guided by patriarchal normed thoughts), and perhaps the clinician can give them the answer. They often think there are some magical words or analyses that clinicians have as a secret from the rest of the world. It is up to the feminist clinician to demystify the therapeutic process and empower the client to understand that this is an equally shared process, but they are the magic that makes the changes they seek. The magic is in the empowerment; only the client can decide what to do with the power.

## Oppression Affects Pathology and Potential

Szasz (1974/2010) suggested that the constructs of psychopathy are a myth that has been born in the confines of a restrictive mental health system. Feminist theorists would agree that labeling people, either with diagnosis or other limiting distinctions, can hold them back from their potential. Brown (2018) suggested that "formal diagnostic systems are all simply socially constructed taxonomies for organizing and grouping people's manifest expressions of distress, diagnosis as practiced is commonly a strategy for reification and objectification of the client and pathologizes their pretherapy strategies for increasing power by whatever means available" (p. 67).

The pathological label often carries a social stigma that puts a person in a position to be judged by larger social and cultural communities; this can impair a person's future opportunities. For example, mental health name-calling (e.g., you are psychotic, narcissistic, etc.) is often used in societies as insults and criticisms. The stigmatized word "crazy" is one way people marginalize an individual or concept to dismiss the complexity of human existence or of an argument. The Western clinical mental health system and higher clinical education systems are often based on the medical model, scientific outcomes (statistics and probabilities), and specific "evidence-based" techniques. Feminist theory rejects the patriarchal medical model and the patriarchal clinical, educational system since it categorizes, labels, and marginalizes the human experience.

## Egalitarian Therapeutic Fellow Travelers

Yalom (1980) said,

> There are technical manuals that teach student therapists methods of conveying empathy, genuineness, and positive regard. To an existential therapist, when "technique" is made paramount, everything is lost because the very essence of the authentic relationship is that one does not manipulate but turns toward another with one's whole being. (p. 410)

In alignment with Yalom (1980), the feminist intersectional therapeutic relationship rejects hierarchies and views the client as capable, whole, strong, and truly equal, and highly esteemed (Brown, 2018). The client knows themselves better than the therapist knows them (Rogers, 1961/1995). Society often places people in hierarchical positions of power when they have a higher (or specific) education, higher income, prestigious family history or have attained a level of fame. The natural inference for a client is that the feminist therapist has the power and knowledge to help them due to their higher education. There must be complete transparency of the therapeutic process and the shift of expertise back to the client throughout the relationship. The feminist therapeutic power dynamics must be a continual conversation throughout therapy. Self-disclosure can be used intentionally and strategically as a therapeutic tool, being mindful not to fall into self-deprecation or nontherapeutic disclosure as a means to equalize power. Feminist theory attempts to level the therapeutic power by acknowledging, monitoring, and sharing the power throughout the process. As stated, there must be constant check-in with the client so that the feminist clinician's thoughts and words do not hold more power than their own. The goal is to empower the client by raising and discussing higher consciousness matters by examining their intersectional identities related to social, cultural, and political privileges and oppressions to navigate a better future outcome. An important vehicle for this empowerment is a genuinely collaborative relationship where honesty and power sharing are consciously sought and affirmed.

## Raising Consciousness

If there had to be one goal of feminist intersectional theory, it might be to join the clients in raising their consciousness to a deeper understanding of how Eurocentric, heteronormative,

Christian-dominant, patriarchal systems and norms have influenced their conscious and unconscious beliefs and experiences. Western society, like most societies, has conditioned people into their explicit and implicit beliefs about normal and abnormal, right and wrong, and so on, which automatically establishes a cognitive frame to interpret life events. Many life choices are built on that foundation filled with socially driven self-beliefs, limitations, and internalized functional or dysfunctional messages. Questioning that foundation can be a very frightening experience for people. The goal of feminist intersectional therapy is to respect the foundation while allowing the client to understand its origins, the systems that maintain it, and whether they would like to choose to keep the beliefs, assumptions, and norms associated with it. As with any beliefs, the clinician must proceed at the client's pace, honoring and exploring any resistance to new thoughts. Once the client understands how beliefs may have been infused and never examined, the therapist has facilitated raising consciousness. The client then has a freer sense of what to do with decisions. Raising consciousness may allow clients more freedom of thought and choices to make unconventional decisions or stay with the ones already in place. The difference is that the client is now fully conscious of the choice; it was not simply unconsciously embedded in their development.

## Recognition and Exploration of Existing Power

What is power, and how does one recognize it? Oppression is a limitation of freedom behaviorally, psychologically, and existentially. Often, we are oppressed behaviorally, and opportunity is not available (e.g., poverty, support, bias, expectations, etc.). Learned helplessness (Maier & Seligman, 2016), embedded perceptions, and assimilation to the oppressor are examples of how we can psychologically become oppressed. We can also be oppressed existentially through our assimilation to oppressive experiences. Examples might include being raised with capitalism as a focus of success instead of creativity. Power is a perception of, and may be the ability to move past, oppression. Power can be thought about, felt, and behaved upon; any of these may be impacted by one's intersectional identity. Having more power typically provides more life choices. Power can occur in multiple spaces and parts of life, and clients may hold great power in all spheres, little power in all spheres, or a combination of power and powerlessness, depending on the sphere and their intersectional privileges and oppressions. Therefore, it is essential to note that not everyone's circumstances will allow them to behave with power safely in their environment, and that needs to be considered when working with clients. For example, it may be unsafe for a person of color to speak out at a White supremacy gathering.

## Empowerment

Em"power"ment is another goal of feminist intersectional theory. Brown (2018) defined empowerment as "[a]ny process by which an individual either (a) becomes aware of, and able to use, power already available or (b) gains access to new ways of being powerful" (p. 151). A bedrock goal of feminist therapy is helping the client to examine their consciousness and find or help create their power and associated perceptions that align with it. In all relationships, there are levels of power and control. Examining relationships in the client's life is essential so that the client can see where they hold power and where they may want to exert more power. This can be done through discovering (consciously and unconsciously) why a differential of power exists in any relationship. Often, disempowering feelings are couched in social and cultural norms (e.g., respect for elders, respect for positions, respect for authority, etc.). They may also be couched in fear (e.g., they pay my salary; they will not love me; I may be abandoned). With this bedrock feminist recognition, the client can decide if they would like to pursue more power in a relationship or not. If so, the clinician can collaborate on empowerment strategies in specific situations.

## Intersectionality and Multiple Oppressions

With the third-wave evolution of feminist collective thoughts of multiple oppression and intersectionality, feminist theory has become more inclusive, honoring even more the distinction between people's existence and experiences in society. This allows for more understanding of the individual challenges and impacts that cultural and social systems have on clients. Having a focus on intersectional examinations ensures a spectrum of perspectives and lived experiences are honored and navigated.

## Advocacy

The roots of feminist theory grew from social justice and advocacy (Brown, 2018; Tiefer, 1991). Feminist theory advocacy is often associated with large movements like the women's rights movement, civil rights movement, Black Lives Matter, and so forth. Clinical advocacy is different from that of a macro construct. Part of feminist intersectional clinical theory certainly encourages advocacy, but the definition therapeutically may be different. Advocacy can vary between self-care and running for political office to make changes. A client can advocate by finding their voice occasionally in certain situations. That could mean parenting with power, asking for a raise at work, or asserting themselves in any relationship. Of course, if a client initiates a more extensive external advocacy, that can also be empowering. The client's advocacy is solely up to them without the feminist therapist's influence. The goal has been met if they choose to behave with full consciousness and empowerment. If the mental health professional pushes for a specific type of advocacy, that may be disempowering and defeat the therapeutic ambitions of feminist therapy of empowerment and autonomy.

# Stand-Alone Theory or Addendum to Other Theories

Feminist therapy, as related to traditional clinical theories, often meets with marginalization in the academy built on hierarchies, competition, and power. This may have contributed to the lack of widespread adoption of feminist theory as opposed to "evidence-based" theories, such as cognitive behavioral theory, have received. If clinical mental health students are even exposed to the feminist theory, they may see it as a philosophical construct or an addendum to other existing traditional patriarchal-founded theories. Many clinicians have a weak understanding of feminist theory, or in some cases none, due to a lack of exposure (Jodry, 2011). Jodry (2011) suggests that several factors may have contributed to this lack of embracing feminist theory as a stand-alone theory: (1) The word "feminist" might feel exclusive to women and perhaps even to White women; (2) feminine constructs are devalued in a patriarchal society; (3) there is no "founder" who can be followed for specific instructions on the clinical application; (4) there is a lack of "techniques" associated with the theory unlike other more traditional theories; (5) equalizing therapeutic power may be uncomfortable; (6) feminist theory is intersectionally complex (and often counterintuitive) to research in traditional quantitative manners since categories and labels are rejected as reductive and individual narratives are honored; and (7) marginalized groups who might most benefit from feminist theory are often not as powerful or accepted by the mainstream.

Traditionally and historically, feminist theory has been loosely woven with collective thoughts, which might have lent itself to being more of an addendum theory than a more fully constructed theory with a definitive founder, techniques, and disciples. Chaplin (1999) wrote, "Feminist counselling is a process, not a technique or theory. I can allow myself to make connections between different approaches, finding similarities as well as differences, taking what is useful and leaving what feels oppressive" (p. 17). Many clinicians have pieced together their clinical theories, and feminist theory may have been a backdrop or philosophical underpinning, but not a stand-alone theory for most.

Fourth-wave feminist intersectional therapy will offer models and conceptualizations to allow the feminist clinical practitioner ideas of application, if desired. Unlike most other theories, no "founder" can be followed for specific instructions on clinical practice application. Feminist therapy was born in collectivist thought, and it tends to make this theory and therapy more challenging to teach clinically. There is no "here is how to apply" feminist theory to budding mental health graduate students. This book intends to become another voice in the collective by adding feminist intersectional theory and therapy and offering some application ideas for the practitioners to conceptualize and the feminist intersectional educators to convey in clinical classes.

It is important to note that these models, "techniques," and other applications are just one way to apply feminist intersectional therapy as imagined by these feminist therapists. It is not the only way. The authors hope that this book sparks additional feminist creative thinking and that clinicians use it to allow for collective expansion of the stand-alone theory while not losing the most essential factor of the individual relationship and experience of the client.

# Current Literature on Efficacy of Traditional Feminist Therapy

While there have not been large-scale outcome studies with feminist therapy, this does not mean that feminist therapy is not helpful or effective. There are some challenges with researching feminist therapy, including that this is not a well-defined, manualized approach. As with other "harder to research" approaches, a smaller evidence base is not evidence that this approach does not work. Feminist clinicians and researchers value quantitative research, but they also value qualitative research, case studies, and the knowledge that comes from their clients (Brown, 2006). These different sources of knowledge are all valid. Honoring individual knowledge is embedded in feminist thought so it is no surprise that research approaches that include that are prized.

While there are individual studies showing feminist therapy as being effective with clients (see, e.g., Stevens et al., 2018; Tone et al., 2022), a different approach has been to examine the hallmark aspects of feminist therapy and research the effectiveness. Specific aspects of feminist therapy examined have included its focus on power and oppression, both in terms of how these practices impact mental health and on how they are addressed in therapy. The egalitarian relationship, consciousness raising, and client empowerment—all of these have been shown in studies to decrease symptoms and/or to increase positive outcomes of treatment (Conlin, 2017). Similarly, feminist therapy approaches can be examined through a common factors lens that identifies therapeutic practices that, regardless of theoretical orientation, have been shown to be effective. From this perspective, feminist therapy practices that align with common factors include the cultural responsiveness of feminist therapy and its attention to oppression, power, and social identities, as well as the deeply collaborative egalitarian therapeutic relationship that emphasizes client empowerment and privileging clients' voices (Brown, 2018).

## Criticisms of Feminist (Intersectional) Theory

The word "feminist" might feel exclusive to women and perhaps even to White, middle-class women. Historically, the rejection of patriarchal norms was in reaction solely to constructs and practices related to sex and gender. Early feminists normed their new clinical collective perspective from a lens that did not include multiple oppressions and intersectionality. Gendered perspectives are still a part of feminist theory—for example, the "feminine" is still devalued and often seen as less than the "masculine" in dominant U.S. culture. Examples of this can often be seen in the following: female-dominated jobs are often less prestigious and lower paid; crying is associated with femininity and is often seen as weak, particularly in males; and feminine sexuality is often used as a way to shame and degrade women while masculine sexuality bolsters men's images and status.

The word "feminist" can also seem divisive and may garner negative reactions from some as radical, hateful, man-hating, or other propaganda that has been associated with feminism to discredit the fight for equality across history. Many clients and clinicians have been exposed to this propaganda and have ingrained conscious and unconscious negative reactions to these ideas. Images of unrest and anxiety may be associated with thoughts of feminism. Therefore, some people may naturally reject any concepts related to this theory.

Feminist theory has been viewed as a philosophy more than a clinical practice due to its lack of application. As stated earlier, this theory has traditionally been perceived as difficult to apply because it has loose constructs with no hierarchies or founders who give specific techniques for using this theory. What it means to be a feminist clinician can vary person-by-person as practitioners can subscribe to the basic tenets of feminist theory and identify as feminist while making this approach their own. There has been no credentialing of feminist therapists through an educational body to date. Much like existential theory, born from philosophy, there is great merit to the basic constructs therapeutically, but the lack of application makes it challenging to research and use clinically. Yalom's (1980) *Existential Psychotherapy* attempts to add more teachable constructs but still remains difficult to use as a free-standing approach. Feminist therapy has similar challenges.

Feminist therapy does not fit with the Western medical model that dominates mental health with its emphasis on diagnosing through the patriarchal-driven *Diagnostic and Statistical Manual of Mental Disorders* (DSM), which states what is normal or not in human behavior. The Western medical model also emphasizes the capitalistically driven "evidence-based" approach, known as behavior outcomes. How does a feminist theorist who honors the individual experience and rejects many parts of the patriarchal categorization and cookie-cutter treatments navigate within this world?

Equalizing therapeutic power may be uncomfortable. When one person comes to another seeking help, there is an implied power differential. The person most in need usually does not have the most power. Helping the client feel empowered often includes the clinician's need to equalize the power. This can be uncomfortable for clinicians. Often, feminist practitioners try to demystify the experience and lower their power in the room, moving it more toward the client. This is sometimes created by self-disclosure. If the feminist clinician is not careful with this self-disclosure, this can be seen as self-deprecation, low self-esteem, or perhaps worse, incompetency as a therapist. Patriarchal social structures place people in hierarchical positions of power, and breaking hierarchies can be uncomfortable and misunderstood by both the clinician and the clients.

Since feminist therapy honors the individual story and scientific journals place more value on normal curves, feminist theory is difficult to research in a traditional quantitative manner. This often makes it difficult for feminist scholars to become published in journals that place high value on grouping people to compare and contrast them. Therefore, feminist theory is often criticized for not having high levels of "evidence-based" research. Likewise, some academic institutions might place more value on certain quantitative analyses for ideas around tenure and promotion. This can lead to a marginalization of the feminist academic and clinical theorist and a relegation of their way of knowing.

# Summary

Feminist intersectional therapy, born from the historical feminist movements, has evolved into a much-needed therapeutic construct for modern society. This theory has evolved from being focused on sex and gender to recognizing the fullness of multiple oppressions and intersectionality for a deeper understanding of the client's experiences. The underpinning principles outlined in this chapter of feminist therapy include the evolution to the fourth-wave feminist concepts of multiple oppressions and intersectionality. This book intends to become another voice in the collective by adding feminist intersectional theory and therapy and offering some application ideas for the practitioners to conceptualize and the feminist intersectional educators to convey in clinical classes. The authors believe that these underpinning principles of feminist theory are essential to be embraced right now, given the trends in Western society toward tribalism, inequality, hierarchies, and unkindness.

# What If?

What if equity and equality actually existed in the systems? If people had equal esteem in society? How would that change mental health and the human experience?

What if hierarchies of capitalism were dismantled and systems were focused on existential and/or spiritual growth over ego-driven desires and competition? How would the world be different?

What if feminist theory became more of a mainstream theory and was taught and used as often as cognitive behavior therapy? Would that change anything in mental health? Society? Education?

What if telehealth becomes the only modality for therapy (because it is more cost effective and convenient for everyone)? What impact might that have on feminist theory?

What if society continues to develop technology and therapy and AI begins to take over the therapy? What might happen to concepts of feminist intersectional theory?

# References

Bagshaw, J. L. (2019). *The feminist handbook*. New Harbinger Publications.

Benner, A. D., Fernandez, C. C., Hou, Y., & Gonzalez, C. S. (2021). Parent and teacher educational expectations and adolescent academic performance: Mechanisms of influence. *Journal of Community Psychology, 49*, 2679–2703. http://doi.org/10.1002/jcop.22644

Brown, L. S. (2006). Still subversive after all these years: The relevance of feminist therapy in the age of evidence-based practice. *Psychology of Women Quarterly, 30*(1), 15–24. https://doi.org/10.1111/j.1471-6402.2006.00258.x

Brown, L. (2018). *Feminist therapy* (2nd ed.). American Psychological Association.

Burns, R. (2022, January 18). *Yes, children are being taught critical race theory in K–12 schools in the U.S.* Areo. Retrieved from https://areomagazine.com/2022/01/18/yes-children-are-being-taught-critical-race-theory-in-k-12-schools-in-the-us/

Center for American Women and Politics (CAWP). 2024. *Women officeholders by race and ethnicity.* Center for American Women and Politics, Eagleton Institute of Politics, Rutgers University-New Brunswick. https://cawp.rutgers.edu/facts/women-officeholders-race-and-ethnicity (accessed September 17, 2024)

Chaplin, J. (1999). *Feminist counselling in action*. SAGE.

Chapman, S. J., & Benis, N. (2017). Ceteris non paribus: The intersectionality of gender, race and region in the gender wage gap. *Women's Studies International Forum, 65*, 78–86. http://dx.doi.org/10.1016/j.wsif.2017.10.001

Collins, P. H. (1990). *Black feminist thought: Knowledge, consciousness, and the politics of empowerment*. Unwin Hyman.

Collins, P. H., Gonzaga da Silva, E. C., Ergun, E., Furseth, I., Bond, K. D., & Marinas-Palacios, J. (2021). Intersectionality as critical social theory. *Contemporary Political Theory, 20*, 690–725. https://doi.org/10.1057/s41296-021-00490-0

Conlin, S. E. (2017). Feminist therapy: A brief integrative review of theory, empirical support, and call for new directions. *Women's Studies International Forum, 62*, 78–82. https://psycnet.apa.org/doi/10.1016/j.wsif.2017.04.002

Crenshaw, K. W. (1989). Demarginalizing the intersection of race and sex: A Black feminist critique of anti-discrimination doctrine, feminist theory, and anti-racist politics. *University of Chicago Legal Forum, 140*, 139–167. https://scholarship.law.columbia.edu/faculty_scholarship/3007

Crenshaw, K. W. (1991). Mapping the margins: Intersectionality, identity politics and violence against women of color. *Stanford Law Review, 43*(6), 1241–1299. https://doi.org/10.2307/1229039

Cross, W. E. (1971). Negro-to-Black conversion experience: Toward a psychology of Black liberation. *Black World, 20*(9), 13–27.

DiAngelo, R. (2011). White fragility. *International Journal of Critical Pedagogy, 3*(3), 54–70.

DiAngelo, R. (2018). *White fragility*. Beacon Press

Dicker, R., & Piepmeier, A. (Eds.). (2016). *Catching a wave: Reclaiming feminism for the 21st century*. Northeastern University Press.

Disch, L., & Hawkesworth, M. (2016). *The Oxford handbook of feminist theory*. Oxford University Press.

Downing, N. E., & Roush, K. L. (1985). From passive acceptance to active commitment: A model of feminist identity development for women. *The Counseling Psychologist, 13*, 695–709.

Enns, C. Z. (2012). Feminist approaches to counseling. In E. M. Altmaier & J.-I. C. Hansen (Eds.), *The Oxford handbook of counseling psychology* (pp. 434–459). Oxford University Press.

Erikson, E. H. (1980). *Identity and the life cycle*. W. W. Norton.

Evans, K. M., Feather, K. A., Bordonada, T., & Rogers, T. (2017). Creating a more inclusive feminist identity development model. *National Cross-Cultural Counseling and Education Conference for Research, Action, and Change, 10*. https://digitalcommons.georgiasouthern.edu/ccec/2017/2017/10

Evans, K. M., Kincade, E. A., & Seems, S. R. (2011). *Introduction to feminist therapy*. SAGE.

Ford, B. Q., Green, D. J., & Gross, J. J. (2022). White fragility: An emotion regulation perspective. *American Psychologist, 77*(4), 510–524. https://doi.org/10.1037/amp0000968

Garcia, M. (2021). *We are not born submissive*. Princeton University Press.

Gase, L. N., Glenn, B. A., Gomez, L. M., Kuo, T., Inkelas, M., & Ponce, N. A. (2016). Understanding racial and ethnic disparities in arrest: The role of individual, home, school, and community characteristics. *Race Social Problems, 8*, 296–312. https://doi:10.1007/s12552-016-9183-8

Hamad, R. (2020). *White tears/brown scars: How white feminism betrays women of color*. Catapult.

Hardy, K. V. (2023). *Racial trauma: Clinical strategies and techniques for healing invisible wounds*. W. W. Norton.

Jodry, J. (2011). *The future of feminist theory in professional counseling: Reaching for a multicultural pinnacle* [Unpublished doctoral dissertation]. Argosy University, Tampa.

Johnston, O., Wildy, H., & Shand, J. (2021). "Believe in me, and I will too": A study of how teachers' expectations instill confidence in grade 10 students. *Social Psychology of Education, 24*, 1535–1556. http://doi.org/10.1007/s11218-021-09668-1

Jungert, T., Hubbard, K., Dedic, H., & Rosenfield, S. (2019). Systemizing the gender gap: Examining academic achievement and perseverance in STEM. *European Journal of Psychology Education, 34*(2), 479–500. https://doi.org/10.1007/s10212-018-0390-0

Kelly, M. (2015). Feminist identity, collective action, and individual resistance among contemporary U.S. feminists. *Women's Studies International Forum, 48*, 81–92. https://doi.org/10.1016/j.wsif.2014.10.025

Keramidas, A. M. (2021). *Protecting the self, protecting white supremacy: Exploring the relationship between psychological defense, gender, and white fragility* (Order No. 28492279). Available from ProQuest Dissertations & Theses Global. (2540712053). https://www.proquest.com/docview/2540712053?pq-origsite=gscholar&fromopenview=true

Kirylo, J. D. (2017). An overview of multicultural education in the USA: Grandest social experiment. *Social Studies Research and Practice, 12*(3), 354–357. https://doi:10.1108/SSRP-06-2017-0029

Kwate, N. O. A., & Meyer, I. H. (2010). The myth of meritocracy and African American health. *American Journal of Public Health, 100*, 1831–1834. https://doi.org/10.2105%2FAJPH.2009.186445

Maier, S. F., & Seligman, M. E. P. (2016). Learned helplessness at fifty: Insights from neuroscience. *Psychological Review, 123*(4), 349–367. http://dx.doi.org/10.1037/rev0000033

Marine, S., & Lewis, R. (2014). I'm in this for real: Revisiting young women's feminist becoming. *Women's Studies International Forum, 47*(A), 11–22.

McNamee, S. J., & Miller, Jr., R. K. (2009). *The meritocracy myth*. Rowman & Littlefield.

Moradi, B., Subich, L. M., & Phillips, J. C. (2002). Revisiting feminist identity development theory, research and practice. *The Counseling Psychologist, 30*(1), 6–43.

PBS Newshour. (2005, February). *Harvard president Summers' remarks about women in science, engineering*. https://www.pbs.org/newshour/science/science-jan-june05-summersremarks_2-22

Pew Research Center. (2019, October). *In their own words: Behind Americans' views of "socialism" and "capitalism."* https://www.pewresearch.org/politics/2019/10/07/in-their-own-words-behind-americans-views-of-socialism-and-capitalism

Pew Research Center. (2022, September 13). *How U.S. religious composition has changed in recent decades*. https://www.pewresearch.org/religion/2022/09/13/how-u-s-religious-composition-has-changed-in-recent-decades/

Pew Research Center. (2023, May). *Racial disparities persist in many U.S. jails*. https://www.pewtrusts.org/en/research-and-analysis/issue-briefs/2023/05/racial-disparities-persist-in-many-us-jails

Pew Research Center. (2023, March). *How Americans view their jobs*. https://www.pewresearch.org/social-trends/2023/03/30/how-americans-view-their-jobs

Pew Research Center. (2023, March). *The gender pay gap in the U.S. hasn't changed much in two decades*. https://www.pewresearch.org/short-reads/2023/03/01/gender-pay-gap-facts/#:~:text=While%20the%20gender%20pay%20gap,from%2035%20cents%20in%201982

Pew Research. (2023). *The changing face of Congress in 8 charts*. https://www.pewresearch.org/short-reads/2023/02/07/the-changing-face-of-congress

Piaget, J. (1968). *Six psychological studies*. Anita Tenzer (Translator). Vintage books.

Potter, D., & Morris, D. S. (2017). Family and schooling experiences in racial/ethnic academic achievement gaps: A cumulative perspective. *Sociological Perspectives*, 60(1), 132–167. https://doi:10.1177/0731121416629989

Rogers, C. R. (1995). *On becoming a person*. Houghton Mifflin. (Original work published 1961)

Seligman, M. E. P., & Maier, S. F. (1967). Failure to escape traumatic shock. *Journal of Experimental Psychology*, 74, 1–9. http://doi.org/10.1037/h0024514

Smith. G. A. (2021, December). *About three-in-ten adults are now religiously unaffiliated*. https://www.pewresearch.org/religion/2021/12/14/about-three-in-ten-u-s-adults-are-now-religiously-unaffiliated

Sorhagen, N. S. (2013). Early teacher expectations disproportionately affect poor children's high school performance. *Journal of Educational Psychology*, 105(2), 465–477. http://doi.org/10.1037/a0031754

Stevens, N. R, Heath, N. M., Lillas, T. A., McMinn, K., Tirone, V., & Sha'ini, M. (2018). Examining the effectiveness of a coordinated perinatal mental health care model using an intersectional-feminist perspective. *Journal of Behavioral Medicine*, 41, 627–640. https://doi.org/10.1007/s10865-018-9973-0

Szasz, T. S. (2010). *The myth of mental illness*. Harper Perennial. (Revised edition published 1974)

Tiefer, L. (1991). A brief history of the Association for Women in Psychology (AWP): 1969–1991. *Psychology of Women Quarterly*, 15, 1–28.

Timmermans, A. C., Boer, H., van der Werf, M. P. C. (2016). An investigation of the relationship between teachers' expectations and teacher perceptions of student attributes. *Social Psychology Education*, 19, 217–240. http://doi:10.1007/s11218-015-9326-6

Tone, J., Chelius, B., & Miller, Y. D. (2022). The effectiveness of a feminist-informed, individualized counselling intervention for the treatment of eating disorders: A case series study. *Journal of Eating Disorders*, 10, Article 70, 1–12. https://doi.org/10.1186/s40337-022-00592-z

Trahan, D. P., & Lemberger, M. E. (2014). Critical race theory as a decisional framework for the ethical counseling of African American clients. *Counseling and Values*, 59, 112–124. https://doi:10.1002/j.2161-007X.2014.00045.x

Martinez, A., & Christnacht, C. (2021). *Women are nearly half of U. S. workforce but only 27% of STEM workers*. https://www.census.gov/library/stories/2021/01/women-making-gains-in-stem-occupations-but-still-underrepresented.html

Yalom, I. D. (1980). *Existential psychotherapy*. Basic Books.

# 3

# Feminist Intersectional Theory Considerations: Ethics

## Kathleen McCleskey, Michelle Sunkel, and Barbara J. Shaya

*Ethical guidelines are attempts to ensure that professionals practicing in mental health do not harm. Who ensures that the mental health system, filled with labels, inequities, lack of access, and social stigmas, does not harm?*

All clinical helping professions are guided by codes of ethics that encode aspirational, gold-standard work practices with clients, colleagues, supervisors and supervisees, research participants, and the general public. These ethical codes aim to protect clients' safety while guiding clinicians to apply best clinical practices. Ethical codes are living documents regularly updated and evolving as professions advance, and the culture presents new and ever-changing world scenarios.

Most clinical mental health professional codes of ethics share commonalities resting on clearly stated ethical principles and values. The clinical ethical codes from various mental health disciplines include (listed alphabetically) the American Counseling Association (ACA) (2014), the American Mental Health Counseling Association (AMHCA) (2020), the American Psychological Association (APA) (2017, and the National Association of Social Workers (2021). All of these codes include a section listing core ethical principles and/or values, except for the AMHCA code. Core shared ethical principles and values identified in codes include autonomy (ACA), beneficence (ACA, APA), nonmaleficence (ACA, APA), justice (ACA, APA), fidelity (ACA, APA), veracity (ACA), and respect for the dignity of clients (APA, NASW). Some codes contain other principles and values, including integrity (APA, NASW), social justice (ACA, NASW), competency (ACA, APA, NASW), valuing human relationships (ACA, NASW), and service (NASW). It is important to note that some of these listed values are seen within standards in codes that do not list them as values or principles. Standards in ethical codes cover work with clients, colleagues, other professionals, students, supervisees, and research participants. All listed codes provide some guidance about ethical decision-making.

# Existing Feminist Ethical Decision-Making Frameworks and Models

Ethical decision-making frameworks and models provide an outline and process on how to conceptualize and understand an ethical dilemma. Ethical dilemmas are seen as problems in which there are competing values, principles, ethical standards, professional policies, and so on that suggest more than one possible ethical response (Kitchener, 1984). Ethical frameworks/models include understanding ethical principles, ethics code standards, practice behaviors, and values, and they create a process to evaluate the best outcomes of decision-making. Most models start with identifying the ethical dilemma, applying ethical principles and codes, exploring current ethical literature, consulting with other professionals, among other suggestions, and then determining the most justifiable and ethical outcome. However, complications arise as principles and values are not prioritized in the same way across all disciplines, experts, and clinicians. These differences shift the lens in how to conceptualize and prioritize the needs of the client. If one clinician is utilizing autonomy as the priority principle and another is utilizing protection of life through the principle of nonmaleficence, this can add to the complexity of addressing the ethical issue.

From a feminist perspective, clinical mental health ethical codes have lacked adequate focus on feminist values (Evans et al., 2011). Feminism has long realized that clients' problems do not arise solely from internal challenges; instead, they can be generated by, impacted by, and maintained through the experiences of living within a Eurocentric, heteronormative, patriarchal society that oppresses some social identities while privileging others (see, e.g., Brown, 2018; hooks, 2015). Feminists believe that "the personal is political," meaning that all people are impacted by societal norms, cultural expectations, and political judgments, which are also encoded implicitly or explicitly in everything from cultural expectations to institutional structures and legal systems, and even in codes of ethics; it is imperative to examine these systemic forces as part of understanding clients' problems as well as examining how those same dynamics may be replicated within the therapy relationship (Peasley, 2004). Some of the key issues that are connected to therapy include "cultural diversities and oppressions, power differentials, overlapping relationships, therapist accountability, and social change" (FTI Code of Ethics Preamble, para. 11).

## Feminist Therapy Institute Code of Ethics

In the 1980s, the Feminist Therapy Institute (FTI) was formed by a collective of experienced feminist therapists who continued to meet for over 30 years (Brown, 2018). This collective held intensive institutes that conducted much of the feminist therapy research of the late 20th century and wrote the FTI Feminist Code of Ethics in 1987, revised in 1999 (Brown, 1991, 2018). The FTI Code of Ethics was not meant to supplant other ethics codes but rather added ethical considerations and standards from a feminist perspective (Feminist Therapy Institute, 1999).

The FTI Code of Ethics (1999) begins with a preamble that asserts that feminist therapists recognize that the society in which both clients and clinicians live grants societal power to some and withholds it from others. Therefore, a feminist practitioner's client conceptualization addresses the understanding of power and its interconnections among gender, race, culture, class, physical ability, sexual orientation, age, and anti-Semitism, as well as all forms of intersectional oppression based on religion, ethnicity, and heritage. Feminist therapists also live in and are subject to those same influences and effects and consistently monitor their beliefs and behaviors as a result of those influences (p. 1, para. 3).

A complete discussion of the FTI Code of Ethics (1999) is beyond the scope of this chapter; instead, this will be a summary of the themes of the code and a discussion of how it continues to inform feminist therapy. Additionally, there will be suggestions for updating the code for contemporary feminist clinical work. The five sections of the FTI Code of Ethics cover Cultural Diversities and Oppressions, Power Differentials, Overlapping Relationships, Therapist Accountability, and Social Change.

The Cultural Diversities and Oppressions section of the code (FTI, 1999) directs feminist clinicians to be self-reflective about their own cultural identities and to gain knowledge of other cultural identities and experiences, using multiple sources for this learning. Feminist therapists are intentional about respecting other cultural values. They continually monitor themselves for bias and/or discriminatory behaviors and reflect, address, and remediate those. They also strive to work with a diverse clientele and to use a flexible therapeutic delivery method.

The Power Differentials section (FTI, 1999) addresses the dynamics of therapeutic relationships. It identifies practices that can help create and maintain an egalitarian therapeutic relationship. This section also directs clinicians to be transparent about the nature of therapeutic services, communications, and potential advocacy. Power is discussed, monitored, and negotiated throughout the therapeutic relationship. The feminist clinician also models the appropriate use of power within therapy settings and in personal relationships.

The Overlapping Relationships section (FTI, 1999) covers dual relationships as well as other overlapping relationships. Dual or multiple relationships may occur in communities or organizations to which both clinician and client belong, including in feminist organizations (Evans et al., 2011). Client confidentiality is key. Sexual dual relationships are forbidden with current and former clients. This section also covers the many stakeholders who may be part of clinical work—third-party payers, clients' caregivers, and organizations in which the therapist works. Transparency by the therapist is required so that the client is fully aware of different parties' requirements or desires in terms of information or communication. Throughout all overlapping relationships, it is the feminist therapists who must monitor power and transparency; they are accountable for preventing harm to clients.

Therapist Accountability is a large focus within the ethical code (FTI, 1999). In this section, the first standard, IV.A. is this: "A feminist therapist is accountable to herself, to colleagues, and especially to her clients." Feminist therapists work within their trained competencies, are transparent about their training and experience, continue to develop as feminist clinicians through self-reflection, continued training, supervision, and their own personal therapy, and practice regular self-care. These ethical practices help the feminist therapist to be intentional about their practice, their evolution, and their personhood.

The last section of the ethical code is Social Change (FTI, 1999). This section describes the ethical importance of advocacy for and with clients and client populations to affect change on personal and systemic levels. Feminist therapists also teach clients how to self-advocate. They look for practices or policies that harm clients, question them, and take other actions as appropriate to stop unethical practices. Feminist clinicians, educators, and researchers resist pressure to use only mainstream methods that are endorsed by the dominant culture. They also understand that technology can have many kinds of implications, including who has access to technology. Above all, as stated earlier, "[a] feminist therapist, teacher, or researcher recognizes the political is personal in a world where social change is a constant" (FTI, 1999, V.E.).

Therefore, a feminist therapist using the FTI Code of Ethics will focus on situating the client's therapeutic conceptualization within greater heteronormative, Eurocentric, patriarchal systems of the client's experiences, assessing the intersectional social identities and power of both client and clinician, monitoring how power is used and recognized in the therapeutic relationship, and exploring ethical aspects of all of these. This combination of transparency, power sharing, collaboration, connection, validation, and inclusivity reflects the foundational goals of feminist therapy to help promote client empowerment.

As part of the Association for Women in Psychology (AWP) 2024 annual conference, a working group began forming to begin to update the Feminist Therapy Code of Ethics. In this meeting, a diverse group of feminist clinicians discussed the continued relevance of the 1999 FTI Code of Ethics as well as the need to update the code to include more contemporary issues. The seed of beginning the process to collaboratively work on this project began in that meeting (O'Shaughnessy et al., 2024).

## Suggestions for the Updated Feminist Therapy Code of Ethics

One area that could be helpful to address in the next feminist code of ethics is changes in social identities and language about them. Language continues to evolve in recognition of people with a spectrum of gender identities and affectional identities. In the preamble, it is stated that "[f]eminist therapists assume a proactive stance toward the eradication of oppression in their lives and work toward empowering women and girls" (FTI Code of Ethics, 1999). It might be more inclusive if the language about intersectional identities were all acknowledged to include empowering all genders who are oppressed. It might also be helpful to consider adding language in the code identifying the range of nonbinary, transgender, and cisgender identities, and to update "sexual orientation" to something recognizing affectional orientation or naming LGBTQ+ identities. In the 1999 FTI Code of Ethics, "anti-Semitism" is specified as one of the identities for which power must be addressed, in addition to oppression related to other identities, including religions. In a contemporary reading of the FTI code, this seems to privilege the Jewish identity over other cultural or religious-based identities; it seems more inclusive to either name other cultural or religion-based oppressions or to refer to oppression based on overarching race or religion. Another suggestion for the next iteration of the feminist code of ethics is to include further guidance on technology and therapy. In the 1999 FTI Code of Ethics, there is a statement about recognizing clients' different socioeconomic access to technology, but technology has significantly developed in the last two decades. As an example, telehealth is now an established form of therapeutic work that is used at higher than pre-pandemic rates, especially by younger clients (Costa, 2024) or by both younger and older clients as well as those who hold marginalized identities (Gangamma et al., 2022). Two possible overlapping ethical areas that may need to be addressed are client privacy and client autonomy. Regarding client privacy, feminist therapists could benefit from a discussion about collaborating with clients, possibly through informed consent, regarding being in a private location for appointments. Relatedly, a feminist therapist may want to explore any potential influence from other people, directly or indirectly, in the client's environment that would impact client sessions.

Another technological development has been artificial intelligence (AI). AI is becoming present in therapy through various software programs that write notes, for example, and that require recording sessions in order to do so. This technology is too new to have a body of professional literature exploring it; see Weisman (2023) for a blog post comparing current AI platforms; this information may become outdated as platforms develop. Solely using an external program to write notes about a session would be the antithesis of feminist work that relies on a real, present therapeutic relationship; therapists using AI software are currently encouraged to edit AI-generated notes. Is this an acceptable shortcut for documentation? Or does using AI for notes lose any of the nuances of the feminist therapeutic relationship and/ or any subtleties of what clients share? As AI applications develop, there will likely be more therapy-based options than currently imagined. If, when, and how AI can ethically be used in feminist therapy is an issue that will require much thought. Additionally, specific technology-related boundary issues have developed since the 1999 revision in terms of social media. Having some guidance about professional and personal social media use may be helpful moving into the future.

## Feminist Ethical Decision-Making

Hill et al. (1995) developed a feminist ethical decision-making model in which the personhood of the therapist was brought more fully into the decision-making process. A criticism feminists make about many models is that they present ethical decision-making as a series of steps that do not examine issues of power, culture, and different interpretations of ethical principles (Evans et al., 2011). Hill et al. (1995) explain that the therapist's personal experiences with social identities, power, oppression, family background, values, countertransference, and so on, all connect to how that individual therapist will interpret and respond to an ethical dilemma. Without examining those intersectional therapist variables related to the other ethical factors, therapist factors are assumed to be inconsequential. Additionally, since consultation is standard in ethical quandaries, any consultant's personal and clinical experiences may impact the guidance. Lastly, Hill et al. (1995) discuss the need to include the client in the decision-making process as much as possible, not only because of the feminist value of sharing power in the therapeutic relationship but also because discussions with the client may uncover new material or new ways to interpret known material. Therefore, their model combines rational-evaluative and emotional-intuitive aspects and an awareness of power differentials and potential cultural biases.

The Hill et al. (1995) decision-making model begins with *recognizing a problem*. In addition to having rational-evaluative awareness of a problem, the emotional-intuitive task is for the therapist to examine their feelings to discern any way they may be blocking the exploration of the ethical issue. *Defining the problem* involves the rational-evaluative exploration of ethical codes, laws, best clinical practices, stakeholders, and so on, to outline the conflict. The emotional-intuitive task is to include the therapist's own feelings about themselves, the client, and/or the situation to add depth and nuance to understanding the issue. Collaborating with the client is an expected part of this stage as long as there are no clinically supported reasons not to include the client. After learning the client's perspective, the therapist employs a rational-evaluative framework to explore any cultural differences between the client and the therapist that may impact the problem definition. If cultural differences result in differing perspectives on the ethical problem; the therapist may want to consult with a qualified feminist clinical professional as well as to continue dialogue with the client.

In the *developing solutions* stage, the rational-evaluative process includes creating potential courses of action and evaluating these regarding benefits and harm (Hill et al., 1995). Using the emotional-intuitive perspective, the therapist, and often the client, can discuss how different options make them feel. These feelings may help to narrow down or refine choices. In the *choosing a solution* stage, thoughts and feelings are not separated while narrowing choices. The focus is on a solution that aligns with thoughts and feelings for everyone involved, including the therapist. In the *reviewing process* stage, the therapist again rationally considers the previous steps. Hill et al. (1995) recommend considering any bias the therapist may have introduced into the process. They also recommend considering if the therapist would be satisfied with the decision if the roles were reversed, if the decision would be similar for different clients, and if it would hold up to public scrutiny. Emotionally and intuitively, the therapist "sits with" the decision for a brief time, if possible, while discerning if the decision "feels right" (p. 116). The decision is then shared with the client, and the two can collaboratively process how the client receives the decision.

*Implementing and evaluation of the decision* involves not only moving ahead with the plan but also continuing to monitor how it plays out (Hill et al., 1995). Once the plan is implemented, it may uncover new aspects of the problem not previously seen. Hence, it is essential for the therapist, together with the client, when possible, to continue evaluation of the decision and address any adjustments that need to be made. The last stage is the *continuing reflection* stage. As Hill et al. (1995) say, "Every experience changes the people involved" (p. 115). It is for the therapist to be reflexive about how this process with this ethical problem has impacted them professionally and personally.

# A New Feminist Intersectional Ethical Decision-Making Model

## Feminist Therapist Education, Practice, and Reflection

Before an ethical problem arises, there are things a feminist therapist can do to build a strong, feminist, ethical practice foundation. Education is the first step, not only in terms of formal education but also in continuing education. This includes education in feminist therapy principles and practice and keeping up with the latest professional literature related to the therapist's clinical work. Feminist therapists also gain education in systems that the therapist and their clients are likely to interact with, such as insurance/managed care systems, medical systems, legal systems, educational systems, local governance, and so on. Beyond understanding how these systems might oppress people, it is also essential for feminist therapists to be grounded in how patriarchal influences intersectionally impact them. "The personal is political" (FTI Code of Ethics, 1999) is accurate in both a literal and figurative sense. It is also important for a feminist therapist to be attuned to what is occurring in the current political sphere to have context about how that can impact clients, the larger society, and themselves.

Because self-awareness is so important in feminist therapy, continuing to grow reflexive skills is imperative. It can be beneficial to find a feminist supervisor or, lacking that, other feminist practitioners to have peer consultation and peer supervision opportunities. Since feminist therapists are a smaller population within the medical model system, it is important to mentor each other, especially when ethical issues arise.

## When an Ethical Problem Arises

A feminist perspective contextualizes client issues within broader, systemic forces. When an ethical problem arises, a feminist therapist needs to understand any specific systems involved with this client and this problem, including systems that the client inhabits and the therapist does not; these may include cultural, family, social, political, and community systems. At this point, consultation with another feminist practitioner can help ensure that the feminist therapist adequately processes the problem and related systems from a feminist perspective and that they can identify how Eurocentric, heteronormative, Christian-dominant, patriarchal influences may affect the problem definition and/or exploration.

## Collaborating with the Client

In this stage, the feminist therapist and the client discuss the ethical problem. During this discussion, how each person defines the problem will be explored, including who is included in the problem, identifying any systems that may be involved, and what that involvement entails. Each will clarify their role and their responsibilities in the situation. The therapist can explain any professional, ethical, legal, and/or clinical mandates or expectations, and the client can share their role in the dilemma. Connecting the ethical problem to systems the client interacts with and is impacted by may uncover opportunities for advocacy as part of the ethical decision-making or as additional areas of therapeutic focus. This situational advocacy may be specific to this problem, in which case it would be client-centered and could be client-led. If the therapist identifies areas for broad advocacy unconnected to this specific client, the therapist can plan to do their advocacy to address systemic injustice or oppression.

## Exploring Options and Making a Decision

In examining different courses of action and talking through these together, the feminist clinician and the client will explore different options for resolving the problem. These explorations may include examinations of where and how the client is experiencing having power in the situation and how the client is experiencing oppression, including any perceived oppression from the therapist. The feminist therapist continues to share power in the exploration and decision-making process while balancing professional, ethical, legal, and/ or clinical mandates or expectations. After these explorations, the client and therapist will ultimately either agree on an ethical solution or will not. If there is agreement, this stage is concluded. Even if the therapist and the client disagree on an ethical solution, a feminist therapist can support the client's autonomy and agency in having differing perspectives on the solution. Continuing to honor the client and to share power while not in agreement is an important demonstration of the feminist egalitarian relationship. The feminist therapist ensures that the client understands the decision the therapist will be implementing and the reasons for it. If the disagreement involves the therapist needing to report to one of the social service systems or reaching for different levels of care, and so on, the client might be invited to make the reports together to signal to the reporting agency that there is a collaboration, and that the client is part of the process. It may also be possible for the client to voice their opposing views to the report.

## Implementing the Plan

If the feminist therapist and the client agree on the ethical solution, they implement that plan collaboratively. If they disagree on a common solution, the feminist therapist honors the client's agency and power while still doing what the feminist therapist is ethically or legally required to do. How this looks will vary based on the client and the situation. The feminist therapist stays on the journey with the client throughout the process, often encouraging them to advocate for themselves, even when they disagree with the client choices. In some cases, however, the feminist therapist may not be able to support the client in self-advocating to continue behaviors or practices that harm others or to themselves.

## Continuing the Work Together

After the ethical solution is implemented, the feminist therapist and the client can continue to work together with this process and outcome, becoming one part of the journey together. The results of the course of action can be monitored and adjusted as needed. Working through an ethical dilemma together may strengthen the collaborative therapeutic relationship. On the other hand, if the client chooses to stop working with the feminist therapist due to disagreements on the ethical plan or for any other reason, the feminist therapist honors the client's autonomy and behaves ethically to end the professional relationship.

# Feminist Intersectional Ethical Scenario Example

Applying a feminist intersectional lens to any client involves examining the dynamics of power, gender, intersectional identities, patriarchal influences, and embedded societal roles. Considering how societal structures and norms impact individuals based on their identities and experiences is vital. Here is one way a feminist therapist might engage this client's ethical scenario by applying the feminist intersectional ethical decision-making model.

A feminist therapist working at a community mental health center has been seeing a 72-year-old retired teacher named Robert for individual therapy sessions for the past three months. During sessions, Robert has disclosed that he has a strained relationship with his adult daughter, Maria, who lives near him and comes to see him weekly. During the last session, Robert says that he discovered that Maria stole and forged two checks, taking out large sums of money from his bank account. She had been pressuring him to give her large sums of money, but he lives on a fixed income and cannot afford to give her the money she wants. He is devastated by the loss of money and also by the betrayal by his daughter. This feminist therapist practices in a state that has adult protective services that mandate therapists report suspected elder abuse.

## Therapist Education, Practice, and Reflection

The feminist therapist has maintained currency in her feminist clinical field as well as the current community and world situations to be versed in the most updated structures and system changes in the culture society. It is vital to understand the mandatory reporting laws and expectations in the feminist therapist's state and any agency policies and procedures. As a feminist therapist, transparency about reporting requirements is critical to ensure your client's full autonomy and rights. The feminist therapist, in this case, should be curious about developmental models, attachment models, and family system models while learning more about Robert, given that he is a 72-year-old retired teacher. It will be essential to know if he is cisgender, LGBTQIA+, in a relationship, and so on, as this assists with understanding his connections, supports, conflicts, and potential experiences within the patriarchal systems.

Power dynamics and gender roles are also essential to understand in this situation. For example, what potential power imbalances are associated with Robert's vulnerabilities? Robert's position in society, as an elderly individual on a fixed income, places him in a vulnerable position. Do his daughter Maria's actions exacerbate this vulnerability? Additional considerations include gender and age expectations based on patriarchal social norms and values. The feminist therapist can collaboratively scrutinize how gendered norms contribute to Robert's feelings of helplessness or vulnerability. This might impact his overall mental health and sense of value within his family system. Intersectionality of identities is also a key to understanding the ethical issue—age, gender, and other social identities could intersect social locations that need to be viewed as such.

Elder abuse awareness is essential in the feminist clinician's education and reflection. In general, a feminist intersectional approach would advocate for raising awareness about elder abuse and the specific pressures faced by elderly individuals, especially within family dynamics. Understanding systemic issues and advocating for stronger protections for vulnerable populations is a vital part of feminist work. Additionally, the feminist intersectional lens can challenge societal norms around aging and gender, promoting discussions about the roles and expectations placed on elderly individuals and their families. This includes addressing stereotypes and working toward more equitable and supportive systems for elderly people.

## When an Ethical Problem Arises

Because, in this situation, there is a mandated reporting concern, the feminist therapist works with Robert to learn more about his family system and specifically his relationship with Maria. Robert shares that Maria has been unemployed after losing her job a year ago. Maria was closer to her mother, now deceased, and had had a turbulent relationship with Robert throughout her adult life. However, they love each other, and Maria's weekly visits, while strained, also help him feel connected to her. Therefore, this betrayal is not only financial but also deeply emotional.

## Collaboration with the Client

Within the same session, the feminist therapist asks Robert to define the problem as he sees it. He says that Maria stole from and betrayed him, leaving him in a precarious financial situation as he is no longer employed. He worries he may need to look for work to try to make some money back to have some financial cushion. He does not want to report Maria to the police. He also feels guilty; he thinks that for his child to do something like this, he has failed as a father.

The feminist therapist endorses Robert's framing of the problem except for the part of him being a failure as a father. They explain the ethical and legal reasoning behind therapists being mandated to report elder abuse and remind Robert of the exceptions to confidentiality, including this one. The therapist, therefore, needs to report suspected elder abuse. Robert is upset about this, and the therapist processes this with him.

## Exploring Options and Making a Decision

The feminist therapist asks Robert what he would like to do to respond to this situation. He says he wants to talk to Maria and see if she can return any money. He also wants to tell her how angry and hurt he is. The feminist therapist agrees with those as goals to process what happened. The feminist therapist offers a possible frame to Robert that he has been disempowered by having limited financial means and that he is now further disempowered by Maria's actions. In addition, the feminist therapist is saying they need to report this, which is another form of disempowerment.

Robert agrees. The therapist shares that they wish they could honor Robert's wishes to give him that power of choice but that, in this situation, they cannot. What they can do is invite Robert to assist in reporting the suspected elder abuse, and then they can consider what therapeutic pathways might be helpful. After some thought, Robert agrees.

## Implementing the Plan

The feminist therapist involves Robert in the process as much as possible, including discussing potential questions he will be asked, making the reporting phone call, and providing ongoing support to ensure his voice is part of the process and outcomes.

## Continuing the Work Together

Robert was very angry and hurt by this whole process. He felt betrayed by Maria, and he also felt somewhat betrayed by his therapist and by "the system" for getting other people and agencies involved. He continued coming to therapy despite these feelings. Over time, he and the feminist therapist continued to work on his goals for his financial situation. This included referring him for empowering financial and legal advice so he could understand his rights and explore options for managing and protecting his finances. Reviewing all community resources also helped to support community connection, friends, support groups, and a sense of belonging. Robert found a part-time job at a local store, which helped him feel more secure with a little money coming in. His relationship with Maria remained strained since she was questioned by social services and, ultimately, by the police.

# Special Topics in Ethical Practice

## Feminist Implications of Informed Consent

As all therapists know, informed consent refers to the process through which the therapist provides information to their clients regarding their rights and responsibilities, thus enabling clients to make an informed choice about engaging in therapy. The act of obtaining informed consent from potential clients can be fraught with tension regarding the feminist principles of egalitarian relationships and a commitment to the analysis of power differentials within the therapeutic dyad. That consent is requested by the therapist, and given by the client, superficially appearing to empower the client with autonomy and choice. However, the terms of the informed consent document are authored by the therapist (or their agency), sometimes in conjunction with legal representation, and are generally not open to negotiation. Feminist therapists look beyond informed consent as a document to be signed and, instead, view the document as the opening of a meaningful conversation about the relationship between the client and therapist that will be revisited continually throughout their work together.

The client generally completes the informed consent document along with other client intake forms. Born from the medical profession and third-party payor systems (Julesz, 2023), the filling out of forms and indicating acceptance of policies and procedures via one's signature can feel less voluntary and more compulsory than the feminist therapist probably wishes to convey. Therefore, feminist therapists can use informed consent during the intake session as an opportunity to model the collaborative and open discourse that characterizes feminist therapy.

In the first meeting, the feminist therapist sets the stage to discuss the collaborative nature of the therapeutic space with the client. This models the standards of the FTI Code of Ethics (1999) section on power differentials. The feminist therapist can inquire about any prior therapy experience the client may have, especially regarding what approaches, tools, and techniques the client found particularly helpful or unhelpful. As part of informed consent, the feminist therapist can share information such as an overview of their general approach to therapy, areas of competency, specific tools and techniques for which they are trained and/ or certified, rights of the client, how differences of opinions will be resolved, and how and where to file any grievance against the therapist. The client can be asked to articulate their reasons for pursuing therapy and their goals, considering that asking for help creates a power differential. The therapist and client discuss how they will work together to achieve their goals. These topics are revisited regularly, and adjustments are made as therapy progresses with an ongoing monitoring power in the therapeutic relationship. If the therapist is considering using a particular approach or technique, they can transparently share their thought process with the client and provide sufficient information about the proposed technique to offer an informed choice. This also models the FTI Code of Ethics (1999) Power Differentials section. The client is empowered to inform the feminist therapist when a given approach is not helpful, and there will again be a discussion about how to move forward. Where the client desires or requires treatment outside the scope of the therapist's competence, the feminist therapist will assist the client in finding a suitable alternative.

## Confidentiality and Mandatory Reporting Considerations

One of the most delicate aspects of informed consent is the limits to confidentiality and, in many states, the requirement for mandatory reporting. Mandatory reporting is a legal mandate to break confidentiality and report certain behaviors and situations to the appropriate authorities (Wheeler & Bertram, 2019). Situations, where a licensed therapist may be mandated to break confidentiality, include when a client is in imminent danger of harming themself or others or when a child or elder abuse is suspected; therapists must know and understand the mandates of the state(s) in which they practice. The fact that the feminist therapist has the power to break confidentiality and report a client to outside authorities creates a power differential in the therapeutic relationship (Brown, 2004, 2016; Darby & Weinstock, 2018; Sisti & Stramondo, 2015).

The feminist therapist reduces the tension of the power differential by clearly outlining the limits to confidentiality in the intake session, providing psychoeducation on the thresholds of making reports and the resulting processes, and then revisiting these topics as needed throughout treatment. Research suggests that clients may not, for example, report any suicidal thoughts to their therapist because they fear that any such disclosure will result in involuntary hospitalization (Blanchard & Farber, 2018). Feminist therapists can seek to maintain radical transparency about such requirements and situations.

The feminist therapist can explain a desire to work collaboratively if any need to break confidentiality arises. At the same time, they also need to be clear that to protect the safety of the clients and/or others; there may be times when the feminist therapist needs to follow legal, ethical, and policy mandates. The feminist therapist can assure the client that they will share decision-making power as much as possible if any situation arises involving a potential need to break confidentiality. Brown (2018) discusses the pull therapists may feel to take control when a client reports being suicidal and says, "The feminist therapist in that situation must instead be creative in finding ways to both empower a client to create safety and also continue to respect the client's autonomy to the degree possible while preserving life" (p. 81).

She further explains that a feminist stance invites exploration of alternative ways to assert power other than killing oneself, even if it must be reported.

Although the previous example is regarding suicide, the same process can be used for any other instances of mandated reporting, such as reporting suspected child or elder abuse or reports to the criminal justice system for clients legally mandated to therapy. The benefit of this approach is the likelihood of preserving the therapeutic relationship. Unilaterally reporting a client or a client's information to authorities not only breaches confidentiality (albeit legally) but can also break the foundation of trust between client and feminist therapist.

## Ethics Related to Diagnoses and Assessments

The process of diagnosis often creates tension within the feminist therapist since the *Diagnostic and Statistical Manual of Mental Disorders* (DSM; American Psychiatric Association, 2013) and labeling clients with a diagnosis are often counterintuitive to the principles of feminist therapy. The medical model supports third-party payors such as insurance companies who require various medical codes that label clients. Feminist therapists view the process of diagnostic labeling as potentially harmful to clients. Feminist therapists view clients as whole human beings with strengths, intersectional oppressions, and a uniqueness that cannot be minimized and marginalized by a label. In addition, feminist therapists recognize a history of bias in diagnostic categories and use, which have impacted people with marginalized identities (Evans et al., 2011; Szasz, 2010).

If a client would like to use their insurance to pay for their therapy, the feminist therapist will explain to the client the purpose and potential necessity of a DSM diagnosis, will be transparent about the various diagnoses that may be appropriate for the client's presenting symptoms, and will collaborate with the client on how to proceed. In some cases, the feminist therapist and client can read the DSM together to explore the most collaborative, accurate diagnosis. The feminist therapist will continue to discuss with the client any potential positive and negative consequences of having a specific diagnosis in one's permanent health record. For instance, a client may meet the DSM-5 TR criteria for an autism spectrum disorder; however, the client's goal may be to learn how to manage high levels of anxiety. The feminist therapist will discuss the pros and cons of listing autism spectrum disorder versus an anxiety disorder as the diagnosis while remaining within the ethical guidelines of proper diagnosing.

A similar approach is used whenever a psychological assessment instrument is considered by the client. The therapist will discuss why this particular assessment may be helpful, what it is designed to measure, and whether there are any costs or inherent risks in completing the assessment. The client and feminist therapist collaborate on deciding on using the assessment or not. Once the feminist therapist has obtained the results of any assessment, it is transparently shared with the client and thoroughly discussed until the client has had all questions answered. Then, as modeled throughout the collaborative relationship, the feminist therapist and client discuss how the assessment results may influence their therapeutic plan. Together, they can decide whether they would like this assessment to be considered moving forward in the therapeutic process.

## Clinical Practice in Areas with Discriminatory Laws or Regulations

Working in states with discriminatory laws presents significant challenges for feminist clinicians and can create ethical and legal challenges for all parties involved. Understanding how statutes and regulations can impact clients and clinical practice is essential. For example, Grzanka et al. (2020) investigated how Tennessee's "conscience clause" statute impacts potential clients. This statute allows counselors and therapists to deny services to clients because of the therapist's "sincerely held beliefs" (p. 52). This study's participants identified as sexual and gender minority individuals; they perceived their state's therapist "conscience clause" statute to be discriminatory, making therapy seem less safe and including broad enough language that many marginalized groups and individuals could be targeted. Adopting such laws can send messages that therapists can legally discriminate against groups of potential clients (Grzanka et al., 2020).

Along with Tennessee, other states have considered or enacted similar legislation. In addition to specific legislation regarding mental health care, there are also state laws and proposed state laws that impact or curtail issues, including reproductive rights and healthcare (Center for Reproductive Rights, 2024), LGBTQ+ rights (Human Rights Campaign, 2024), and medication-assisted treatment for pregnant people (Kaminski, 2019). Any law that feels discriminatory to clients may come into the therapy room as they process their lived existence or feel specifically challenged to their intersectional identities because of it.

Feminist therapists, like all therapists, are ethically required to stay within their scope of practice and cannot provide medical or legal advice. Feminist therapists can, however, help clients outline all options, connect clients to resources, provide psychoeducation about options, and help clients think through all options. Feminist clinicians must be informed of their state laws and can provide accurate information without providing legal guidance, setting and maintaining clear professional boundaries to avoid legal complications. Feminist clinicians are encouraged to provide safe resources for clients to seek legal advice and gain insight into all options. If practicing in a state that does not allow specific treatments or procedures a client wants or needs, feminist clinicians understand and may recommend out-of-state safe resources for the client. This may include alternative options such as telehealth, national resources, and funding sources, including supportive travel, housing, medical, and treatment options across the United States. As mental health clinicians, we are obligated to provide resources and support to our clients. Feminist therapists do not make decisions for our clients.

Feminist therapy has always included aspects of advocacy, as seen in the FTI Code of Ethics (1999) section on social change. In states where discriminatory laws exist or are being proposed, feminist therapists should advocate, educate, collaborate, and network to fully understand these regulations' impact and strive for change where equity is needed. Feminist therapists can participate in legislative advocacy, policy change, awareness campaigns, workshops, continuing education, and peer support. Laws, policies, and cultures change, and feminist therapists engage in social justice advocacy to create systemic change while creating a safe and inclusive space for their clients.

# Potential Pitfalls of a Feminist Intersectional Approach

The feminist intersectional ethical model aims to foster an egalitarian therapeutic environment that addresses individual concerns while also being attuned to systemic influences and impacts. However, it would be remiss not to discuss the potential pitfalls of this approach. Potential pitfalls of this feminist intersectional approach include homogeneity within feminism and missing the broad range of feminist perspectives and diversity of feminist thought. The feminist theory does not "belong" to any one founder, and there are many ways to apply feminist thought and values to ethical conceptualizations and clinical work; this model is one way to approach making ethical decisions, but there are other models and approaches and more that have not yet been designed.

To overcome these and any other pitfalls, consider the following thoughts. First, feminist therapists should continue ongoing critical reflection of their knowledge, their self-awareness, and their professional practice from a feminist standpoint. Second, feminist therapists should continue to dialogue with other feminist practitioners about bringing feminist perspectives into therapeutic work. Third, feminist therapists should commit to viewing clients and themselves through an intersectional lens to ensure they are not missing or ignoring fundamental dynamics in people's lived experiences. These suggested practices may serve to enhance the effectiveness of feminist intersectional ethical decision-making. While we offer one model of feminist decision-making here, it is essential to continuously adapt and refine models based on feedback and evolving understandings of feminist ethical, clinical, and social justice issues.

# What If?

What if therapists were able to practice clinically without the medical model guidelines of diagnosis?

What if all state regulation boards adopted the feminist inclusive ethical codes, and we treated everyone as equals?

What if all therapy was truly collaborative and there was never an "us and them" in therapy, particularly among people with conditions that make them marginalized by society (psychosis, addiction, etc.)?

# References

American Counseling Association. (2014). *2014 ACA code of ethics*. https://www.counseling.org/docs/default-source/default-document-library/ethics/2014-aca-code-of-ethics.pdf?sfvrsn=55ab73d0_1

American Mental Health Counselors Association. (2020). *AMHCA code of ethics (Rev. 2020): Ethical priorities for clinical mental health counseling*. https://www.amhca.org/viewdocument/2020-amhca-code-of-ethics?CommunityKey=88ff9fb7-8724-4717-8a7c-4cf1cd0305e9

American Psychiatric Association. (2013). *Diagnostic and statistical manual of mental disorders* (5th ed.). American Psychiatric Association.

American Psychological Association. (2017). *Ethical principles of psychologists and code of conduct*. https://www.apa.org/ethics/code

Blanchard, M., & Farber, B. A. (2018). "It is never okay to talk about suicide": Patients' reasons for concealing suicidal ideation in psychotherapy. *Psychotherapy Research, 30*(1), 124–136. https://doi.org/10.1080/10503307.2018.1543977

Brown, L. S. (1991). Ethical issues in feminist therapy: Selected topics. *Psychology of Women Quarterly, 15,* 323-336.

Brown, L. S. (2004). *Subversive dialogues: Theory in feminist therapy*. Basic Books.

Brown, L. S. (2016). *Supervision essentials for the feminist psychotherapy model of supervision*. American Psychological Association.

Brown. L. S. (2018). *Feminist therapy* (2nd ed.). American Psychological Association.

Center for Reproductive Rights. (2024). *After Roe fell: Abortion laws by state*. https://reproductiverights.org/maps/abortion-laws-by-state

Costa, M. (2024). *More teens are opting for virtual therapy*. https://reasonstobecheerful.world/teens-virtual-therapy-mental-health-crisis

Darby, W. C., & Weinstock, R. (2018). The limits of confidentiality: Informed consent and psychotherapy. *FOCUS, 16*(4), 395–401. https://doi.org/10.1176/appi.focus.20180020

Evans, K. M., Kincade, E. A., & Seem, S. R. (2011). *Introduction to feminist therapy: Strategies for social and individual change*. SAGE. https://doi.org/10.4135/9781483387109

Feminist Therapy Institute. (1999). *Feminist Therapy Institute code of ethics*. https://www.apa.org/pubs/books/supplemental/Supervision-Essentials-Feminist-Psychotherapy-Model-Supervision/Appendix_D.pdf

Gangamma, R., Walia, B., Luke, M., & Lucena, C. (2022). Continuation of teletherapy after the COVID-19 pandemic: Survey study of licensed mental health professionals. *JMIR Formative Research, 6*(6), Article e32419. https://doi.org/10.2196/32419

Grzanka, P. R., DeVore, E. N., Frantell, K. A., Miles, J. R., & Spengler, E. S. (2020). Conscience clauses and sexual and gender minority mental health care: A case study. *Journal of Counseling Psychology, 67*(5), 551–567. https://doi.org/10.1037/cou0000396

Hill, M., Glaser, K., & Harden, J. (1995). A feminist model for ethical decision making. In E. J. Rave and C. C. Larsen (Eds.), *Ethical decision making in therapy: Feminist perspectives*. Guilford Press.

hooks, b. (2015). *Feminist theory: From margin to center*. Routledge.

Human Rights Campaign. (2024). *State legislation and LGBTQ2+ rights*. https://www.hrc.org/resources/map-state-legislation-lgbtq-rights

Julesz, M. (2023). The legal history of informed consent. *Journal on European History of Law, 14*(1), 161–171. Central & Eastern European Academic Source.

Kaminski, A. C. (2019). No-win situation: Pregnant mothers in medication assisted therapy programs face discrimination for following doctors orders. *Hastings Women's Law Journal, 30*, 143–166. https://repository.uclawsf.edu/hwlj/vol30/iss1/7

Kitchener, K. S. (1984). Intuition, critical evaluation and ethical principles: The foundation for ethical decisions in counseling psychology. *The Counseling Psychologist, 12*(3-4), 43–55. https://doi.org/10.1177/0011000084123005

National Association of Social Workers. (2021). *Code of ethics of the National Association of Social Workers*. https://www.socialworkers.org/About/Ethics/Code-of-Ethics/Code-of-Ethics-English

O'Shaughnessy, T., Tao, K., & Pitts, C. (2024, March 8–10). *Creating a working group to revise the feminist therapy code of ethics* [Roundtable]. AWP 2024: Decolonizing Feminist Psychology: Resilience, Healing and Embodiment, Virtual. https://www.awpsych.org/2024_conference.php

Peasley, E. M. (2004). *Therapists' experiences of power in feminist therapy: An exploratory study* [Unpublished master's thesis]. University of Toronto.

Sisti, D., & Stramondo, J. (2015). Competence, voluntariness, and oppressive socialization: A feminist critique of the threshold elements of informed consent. *IJFAB: International Journal of Feminist Approaches to Bioethics, 8*(1), 67–85. https://doi.org/10.3138/ijfab.8.1.0067

Weisman, H. (2023). *Making therapy documentation easier: A comparison of AI note automation tools for private practice therapists*. https://www.linkedin.com/pulse/making-therapy-documentation-easier-comparison-ai-hannah-weisman-phd

Wheeler, A. M., & Bertram, B. (2019). *The counselor and the law* (8th ed.). American Counseling Association.

# 4

# Feminist Intersectional Theory and Human Development

## Kathleen McCleskey, Mariah Moran, Ronee Rice, and Joanne Jodry

*As people move through life tasks or stages of growth from birth to death, many assimilate to social, cultural, and political norms established by the dominant patriarchy without critical examination of these constructs or how their intersectional identities evolve in patriarchal hierarchies.*

Lifespan development models have long been used in therapeutic work as a foundation for understanding stages of the human experience. Developmental frameworks allow therapists to recognize common human experiences of growth and change throughout life. Developmental models serve several clinical purposes. They can help therapists have a developmental underpinning about the client's level of function, which may be physical, psychological, or intellectual. They also may serve to help therapists as a guide to consider what a client may be experiencing at different points in life (e.g., a client in midlife having aging parents). Lastly, developmental models can provide a template against which to examine any experiences that contrast with traditional developmental stages in a client's life (e.g., a child experiencing the death of a parent). Many existing models of human development, particularly of lifespan development, have been conceptualized through an androcentric lens, influenced by Eurocentric, heteronormative, Christian-dominant, patriarchal culture.

## Traditional Developmental Models

Traditional models of human development are either holistically built or focus on aspects of development such as intellectual, social, sexual, spiritual, bioecological, and so on, of the "self." (Adler, 2009; Bronfenbrenner, 2005; Erikson, 1980; Fowler, 1981; Freud, 1905/1949; Piaget,1968). Many of these groundbreaking theories reflected the historical, social, cultural, and political norms of the times they were developed. Some of these developmental theories, often with modern additions, have remained underpinnings for therapists to conceptualize helping people through their suffering.

Adler's theory of individual psychology moved the psychological development focus away from the unconscious sexual conflicts of Freudian perspectives to the more conscious early childhood physical, cultural, and social positioning as a more significant contributor to influencing human development (Adler, 2009). Adler theorized a more holistic view of social development of the self and suggested that childhood factors, such as parenting styles, physical appearance, health, birth order, socioeconomic factors, and so forth, shaped a child's early years and contributed to their future "attitudes" and perspectives of the self (Adler, 2009). This is a step closer to feminist perspectives of development, which suggests that the self develops within an interpersonal context, with some scholars even labeling this the feminist developmental concept of "self-in-relation" (Surrey, 1991; Miller & Stiver, 1997).

Erikson theorized the human ego development through his conceptualization of psychosocial stages throughout the lifespan from birth to death (Erikson, 1963, 1982). During each stage, a person grapples with the "crisis" between two opposing needs or expectations and attempts to find a healthy balance; doing so leads to "ego virtue/ego strength." Erikson's (1963, 1980) eight stages include *trust v. mistrust* (infancy), *autonomy v. shame and doubt* (early childhood), *initiative v. guilt* (play age), *industry v. inferiority* (school age), *identity v. role confusion* (adolescence), *intimacy v. isolation* (young adulthood), *generativity v. stagnation* (adulthood), and *ego integrity v. despair* (old age). The theory postulates that biological changes propel a person into each stage, building upon the psychological ego-building experience of the previous stages with any unresolved conflicts being carried forward. Later stages of life can incorporate psychological work from earlier stages so the resolution of crisis tasks can be a lifelong experience as life events and maturation can bring previous stages to the foreground (Orenstein & Lewis, 2022). Syed and Fish (2018) suggested that Erikson, although not known for his developmental model being associated with cultural race and ethnicity, did have these multicultural factors figured prominently in his theorizing. They also suggested that the developmental model is "quite consistent with contemporary theory and research in cultural and ethnic minority psychology" (p. 8). This also suggests that Erikson's developmental model (1980) has elements aligned with feminist clinical philosophies.

# Female/Feminist Models

Borysenko's feminine life cycle model (1996) is one model of lifespan development that is consistent with the second wave of feminist theory. Borysenko (1996) focuses entirely on females and examines how they develop over the lifespan in 7-year intervals holistically, considering biology, psychology, and spirituality; she also places emphasis on how females develop wisdom throughout life. She conceptualized these intervals into four life quadrants: maiden (0–21 years), mother (21–42 years), guardian (42–63 years), and crone (63 years and older). The maiden quadrant includes childhood and adolescent development, and a balance emerges that will continue throughout the lifespan—questioning how someone gets her own needs met without rejecting others' needs? In this stage, females' brains develop receptiveness to being in relation with others, centering that as a way of being. Females are reinforced in right-brain focus through physical experiences such as menstruation that have been culturally framed as negative but which highlight females' intuitive wisdom. The mother, young adult quadrant, is the most stressful, including romantic relationships, nurturing children, and/or nurturing careers. Sexuality and reproduction are key foci of this quadrant; later, women will try to find balance among guilt, resentment, and burnout. As women begin the midlife transition, they seek new meaning (Borysenko, 1996).

In midlife, in the guardian quadrant, females come into a new sense of self if they have benefited from healing in the previous stage (Borysenko, 1996). Borysenko (2013) describes this stage as women being "faced more clearly with those parts of you that cover over your wisdom" (p. 33). Hormones are shifting, and this can result in women becoming more assertive and taking charge. Women may become change agents in this period; this is a quadrant where females can come into a new sense of power and connectedness with people, communities, and the world. In the crone quadrant, the last quadrant of life, significant benefits can be seen from healing work in the previous stage (Borysenko, 1996). Borysenko also suggests that from age 63 until death, women continue investing in connection with others. They lose some socially imposed filters and dare to speak the truth. Although their physical development may decline over this stage, they continue to grow spiritually and psychologically. Borysenko's model is a specific female counterpoint to Erikson, highlighting the potential differences in development based on the biology and culture of gender.

Another second-wave alignment is Conarton and Kreger-Silverman's (1988) feminist model of development, which also describes the lifelong development of females. It is built upon the concept of the self as integrated, multifaceted, dynamic, and emotional, which develops at multiple social levels: individual relationships and wider societal contexts. Attachment is also included as a critical concept that influences development. For all eight stages, areas of focus for counseling are suggested.

In the first phase of the model, bonding, the interconnected bond with the mother creates a template for relationships with attachment as a central issue (Conarton & Kreger-Silverman, 1988). In the orientation to others stage, a female creates relationships that may or may not be balanced; potential concerns include self-nurturing skills and not being overly dependent in relationships. In the cultural adaptation stage, females may conform to Western expectations and emulate masculine ideals, losing their "voice." Concerns in this stage are regaining lost values and skills, such as valuing intuition. In the fourth stage, awakening, and separation, women pull away from patriarchal expectations, which is seen as akin to separation anxiety; women should be supported through this.

In the development of the feminine stage, women explore the struggle to reject patriarchal norms and to be true to their values; therapists can help them process the feelings that this brings up (Conarton & Kreger-Silverman, 1988). In the empowerment stage, women learn to retain their power and defend it from being taken by others. They can be empowered to trust themselves and reach their goals. Power is deeply explored in the spiritual development stage, and younger (less powerful ways of being) are set aside. Potential concerns might include mourning the previous self. In the last stage, integration, women are at midlife or beyond. Though still interconnected to families, they may turn toward others as teachers to pass on gained wisdom. This challenging stage can be supported in therapy to help people self-reflect and create new connections.

Both Borysenko's (1996) and Conarton and Kreger-Silverman's (1988) models of female development broaden lifespan development beyond androgenic models, and both include feminine wisdom and intuition as a legitimate way of knowing. However, they both center females and their development within dominant, masculine cultures. Neither model integrates the wide range of genders or intersectional social identities.

# Multicultural Identity Development Models

In addition to lifespan development models, other developmental models explore specific areas of development. Two of these areas that are salient to feminist theory are racial, cultural, and ethnic identity development and affectional identity development. Identity development models arose, in part, as a reaction to developmental models rooted in patriarchal norms. Cross (1971) created a model of Black identity development, which was followed by models about Chicano/Latino identity development (Ruiz, 1990), Asian identity development (Kim, 1981), White identity development (Helms, 1984), biracial identity development (Poston, 1990), and multiethnic models that applied to minority identity development (see, e.g., Atkinson et al.,1998; Phinney, 1993). These models generally follow a pattern of development whereby a person begins in a stage of conforming to the dominant majority culture, has an experience that creates dissonance about the conformity, reacts by becoming immersed in the person's minority culture, and ultimately comes to find values in both the minority and majority cultures.

Similar models were also created for minority sexual identity development. Cass (1979) created a model of homosexual identity formation followed by models for lesbian identity development (see, e.g., Chapman & Brannock, 1987) and bisexual identity development (see, e.g., Fox, 2003). These and other models typically follow stages in which a person feels confusion and often shame when realizing they are not heterosexual and may try to deny their orientation. They later become comfortable enough to experiment with their orientation but may still hide it from others. Coming out openly may occur over time and only with certain people. Individuals typically seek out others who are similar, work to accept their orientation, and ultimately develop pride in their orientation.

Many developmental models discussed have had a global androcentric or femicentric genesis. Some theorists have widened general development to highlight specific social identities and their impacts on lifespan development. Intersectionality, coined by Crenshaw (1989), refers to the inextricably connected nature of two or more social locations, such as gender and race, such that examining them singly is too reductionist. This trajectory of developmental theory highlights the need for greater attention to social contexts that exist at multiple levels within ecosystems and impact social locations including, but not limited to, gender, age, race, ethnicity, ability, affectional orientation, religion, spirituality, and intersections of any of these. Further, relationships are shaped by social, cultural, political, and economic structures that exert power in different ways to different oppressed individuals. A Black female and a White female can have differing experiences of sexism, not only because of the addition of racism for the Black female, but because misogynoir creates a particular type of bias against Black females (Bailey & Trudy, 2018). This complex intersectional dynamic can challenge, facilitate, or stunt human development. For fourth-wave feminist theorists, considering intersectional identities, acknowledging all genders, and all aspects of privilege and oppression should be considered as part of future feminist development. This allows for a more holistic, unique, realistic understanding of each person.

# A Feminist Intersectional Model of Lifespan Development

Feminist intersectional clinicians can explore what promotes optimal development as well as what oppressive barriers are hindering optimal development for their clients. This may include systemic barriers related to how problems are defined, experienced, and resolved.

This feminist intersectional model of development, inspired by previously discussed developmental models, offers an examination of the impact on human development that matures and progresses in a Eurocentric, heteronormative, Christian-dominant, patriarchal culture throughout the lifespan. This model is designed to spark inquiry with clients of all intersectional genders and identities. This feminist intersectional development model contains seven stages: Infant and Toddler, Early Childhood, Middle and Late Childhood, Adolescence, Early Adulthood, Middle Adulthood, and Older Adulthood.

## Infant and Toddler

In this first stage, even before an infant is born, societal influences are present. Parents-to-be may learn the sex of their child, may decorate a nursery based on that information, with gendered colors, bedding, clothing, accessories, and so forth. They may also have a "gender reveal" event to announce their gender to family and friends. All of this often begins the process of gendered expectations from parents. These gendered expectations are influenced by and are usually replicated in cultural and societal expectations. Once the infant is born, they are assigned a sex, likely to be female or male. Intersex babies are estimated to make up around 1.7% of births and are not always recognized at birth (InterACT, 2021). Parents may decide to have surgical procedures done to "correct" intersex variations; often these are done before age 2. The United Nations interprets these surgeries as human rights violations if they are done without the person's consent (InterACT, 2021).

Assignment of sex, coupled with parental expectations, often solidifies many gender expectations. In therapeutic work, parents' dreams and expectations for their child could be explored related to the desire for alignment with patriarchal expectations or resistance to them. If a child is assigned intersex, potential topics could include interpretations of being intersex (a defect or a human variation), exploring ways to respond to that (medical treatment, or no treatment until the child is older and can participate in such decisions), and societal influences on both.

As the child ages into toddlerhood, toy selection and clothing selection may reinforce gendered norms (Mesman & Groeneveld, 2018). Even attachment can include a gendered component. Although attachment theory is presented as being gender neutral, parents have their own conscious and unconscious gendered socialization, and they bring that into their relationships with their gendered infants (Orbach, 2013). As Orbach (2013) points out, it is rare to discuss a new baby without referencing the baby's gender. While there may not be as many societally endorsed, gendered parenting choices as there once were, there are many observable explicit and implicit differences in how infants and toddlers are cared for (Mesman & Groeneveld, 2018). These can include aforementioned differences in choices of toys, books, and clothing (explicit choices), stereotypical reinforcement of gendered behaviors (explicit) as well as more subtle examples such as how parents discuss gender while reading books to their children (implicit), and role modeling gendered activities (indirect). These topics can all be an area for exploration from an intersectional clinical feminist perspective.

In terms of intersecting identities, impacts regarding these in this stage may focus more on parents than on children. Several questions could be helpful to explore. Was there any aspect of racism, sexism, ableism, ageism, and so on, and any intersections of those for parents as they planned for, prepared for, and experienced pregnancy, delivery, and new parenthood? Was there adequate and available prenatal, delivery, and postnatal care? Were/are family resources adequate? Any oppressive dynamics that impact parents' abilities to provide optimal care to the baby and to themselves can be identified and worked on.

## Early Childhood

In early childhood, some of the same trends from the earlier stage often continue. Preschoolers are often exposed to and endorse gender stereotypes due to their natural assimilation into patriarchal environments. Developmentally, as they socialize in early childhood such as playgroups, they learn each other's norms and the system's expectations. These early experiences often become embedded in their psyche throughout future stages. For example, preschoolers may display no gender-based ability differences in scientific activities, but despite this, girls report less interest in STEM work (Master, 2021). Both girl and boy preschoolers have also been found to implicitly endorse boys as being more suitable for toys used in spatial play, and boys also explicitly endorsed this (Ebert et al., 2024).

As children in this stage start socializing with a broader range of peers, it is possible that gendered and other stereotypes could become more reinforced by others or could be more rejected or refined by others. Children may become more aware of social locations beyond gender, such as race, abilities, and differences in socioeconomic status (SES; Sullivan et al., 2020). Interacting with more families and peers could reinforce or challenge Eurocentric, heteronormative, Christian-dominant, patriarchal messaging. As in every stage, an oppressive childhood or family experience can impact the child, including a lack of resources, external experiences of bias, or accepting "isms" as normal. Concerns that may be helpful to consider include how parents handle stereotypical and nonstereotypical behaviors—what gets reinforced? From a relational standpoint, how are independence vs. interdependence endorsed? How much do the parents encourage assimilation, following social norms, and so forth?

## Middle and Late Childhood

When children start school, they usually enter one of the Eurocentric, heteronormative, Christian-based, patriarchal systems that can impact all forms of social identities with privilege and oppression based on the child's intersectional identities. Children will start being assessed in terms of academic and other abilities. Comparisons of the self in relation to others increase because education systems are set up with hierarchical norms. By late childhood, self-esteem drops, more so for girls than boys, and this trend remains throughout much of life (Helwig & Ruprecht, 2017).

Gendered stereotypes develop further during the stage of late childhood/early adolescence and have been shown to be present in diverse populations around the world (Blum et al., 2017) Children 10–14 years old and their parents were surveyed in the Global Early Adolescence Study (Blum et al., 2017); themes emerged of (1) systemically reinforced norms that girls are vulnerable and that boys are independent and strong; (2) girls in puberty are seen as potential sexual victims and boys as predators; girls' receive messages about having less power while also having the responsibility to not be tempting; (3) girls' mobility is negatively impacted by needing to stay safe; (4) boys are seen as problematic because of sexual concerns and this impacts preexisting cross-gender friendships that cannot continue; and (5) all groups knew peers who were gender nonbinary or nonconforming in some way, and these peers were pressured to conform to the gender binary; boys were especially intolerant of these nonconforming peers. Because this study included worldwide participants, it illustrated the salience of gender stereotypes among diverse cultures.

As illustrated by the Global Early Adolescence Study (Blum et al., 2017), systemic, patriarchal pressures are felt by children in this stage and are reinforced in multiple ways through media, families, friends, schools and organizations, and so on. Social media use is rising over childhood and can connect children to positive and negative people and experiences (Bozzola et al., 2022). Whether in person or online, children may be bullied. Johnston (2015) discusses bullying as disrupting relational affirmative feedback loops, which help children see themselves positively through others' direct or indirect affirmations of their identities and traits. Bullies are seen as reinforcing their own positive affirmations loops through gaining power from bullying, while victims are cut off from receiving positive affirmations and may be given negative affirmations; this can impact victims' trajectories of developing positive identities and causes them to become disempowered. Bullying can target children for different reasons, one of which is perceived differences, including in social locations (Johnston, 2015). Transgender children have not only been impacted by bullying (Kosciw et al., 2022) but can also be impacted by legislation that denies their gender identities (Translegislation, 2024).

Concerns that may emerge in feminist intersectional therapy might include parent's concerns about any intersectional developmental issues and the meanings related to them. For example, if a child has a learning challenge, how do parents, peers, the school, and the child interpret that? How are children's problems impacted by often-oppressive patriarchal norms, messages, and expectations (e.g., boys will be boys)? Do parents endorse those or reject the messages? As in any stage, any oppression the family and/or child are experiencing in terms of bias or discrimination is important to know as those will impact presenting problems or may even be the cause of presenting problems.

## Adolescence

In the adolescent stage of development, individuals encounter a wide variety of societal expectations and pressures that are intertwined with their intersectional identities and judged by social, cultural, and political patriarchal norms. Experiences that are particularly relevant and impactful at this stage of development often include body image and sexuality (Kaestle et al., 2021), socialization and peer pressure (Cook et al., 2019), education and career aspirations (Super, 1963), family dynamics (Prioste et al., 2020), and identity exploration (Erikson, 1980). Examining these areas through a feminist intersectional lens can help feminist clinicians to better understand the challenges, privileges and oppressions faced by adolescents as they navigate this developmental stage in Western patriarchal society.

In the adolescent stage, the impact of societal patriarchal structures often becomes more evident as they begin to internalize and become more aware of gender roles, which are often emphasized during the physical changes associated with puberty. Societal expectations regarding body image often begin to intensify during this stage. Adolescent girls may feel immense pressure to conform to societal beauty standards that prioritize thinness (Johnson & Engeln, 2021), while boys are compelled to develop muscular physiques (Obeid et al., 2018), with social media amplifying these expectations (Burnell et al., 2024).

As adolescents begin to explore their sexuality and gender identity, patriarchal norms can also shape these experiences (Reiss, 1960; Lyons et al., 2014). Girls experience heightened scrutiny, shame, and judgment surrounding their sexual behavior and often face archaic societal pressure to conform to ideals of purity and modesty while simultaneously being objectified and sexualized in the media and popular culture. This mixed messaging often causes girls to feel judged harshly based on both expressing and repressing their sexuality. Girls may experience labels such as "prude" or "slut." This reinforces a binary view, perhaps born in Christianity's archetypes of "virgin" or "prostitute" defining women (Attwood, 2007). This establishes social norms of female sexuality, where autonomy and self-expression are limited and often oppressed. The labels can have lasting internalized effects on girls' self-esteem, mental health, and their perceptions of their bodies.

Adolescents are highly influenced by their peer groups, which also often enforce gender norms (Crockett et al., 2003; Kornienko et al., 2016). While there are some strides being made, girls might experience pressure to prioritize relationships and physical appearance, adhering to societal ideals of femininity. At the same time, boys might feel compelled to suppress emotions and exhibit toughness as markers of masculinity. These peer dynamics can be further complicated by the intersectional identities of adolescents and the role of social media, which often amplifies these gendered expectations and creates an environment where constant comparison and validation based on patriarchal standards are the norm.

As adolescents start considering their futures, patriarchal influences can subtly steer their educational and career aspirations. Although some progress has been made, gendered expectations often channel girls toward professions emphasizing nurturing roles, such as teaching or nursing. According to the Bureau of Labor Statistics (2021), women comprise 87.4% of registered nurses and 79.6% of elementary and middle school teachers. At the same time, boys may be encouraged to pursue leadership positions or careers in STEM fields (Reinking & Martin, 2018).

Within the family, expectations around gender roles may also become more pronounced during adolescence. Teens might be expected to take on responsibilities that align with traditional gender norms, such as caregiving tasks for girls and physical labor for boys. These patriarchal expectations are frequently unspoken yet deeply ingrained, shaping how adolescents see their roles currently and in the future within the family and society. Discussions around autonomy, curfews, and dating can also reveal underlying patriarchal biases. For instance, girls may be more closely monitored or have stricter rules compared to boys, reflecting societal concerns about preserving their "purity," controlling their sexuality, or implying weakness or a lack of ability to care for herself. These dynamics not only reflect social and cultural patriarchal family values but also serve to reinforce the social beliefs.

Intersectional identity exploration may occur during this stage in terms of not only gender but also culture, race, affectional orientation, and/or ability, and so on. Whatever salient identities an adolescent recognizes is where exploration is more likely to happen. With more abstract thought available to them, adolescents may be developing a more nuanced understanding of their intersectional identities of the self. Feminist therapists can assist adolescents in all of these identity explorations and associated social privileges and oppressions.

## Early Adulthood

As individuals transition from the adolescent stage to early adulthood, they face significant life changes and milestones that are often greatly influenced by societal norms. The pursuit of career goals marks early adulthood, the formation of long-term relationships, and the possibility of starting a family (Few-Demo & Allen, 2020). Patriarchal structures and systems influence these significant life choices and impact professional careers and personal relationships remembering that many of these critical life choices are not made independent of external influences. These choices are shaped by a variety of factors, including, but not limited to, societal norms, cultural expectations, economic conditions, and social structures such as patriarchy.

Patriarchal structures also influence career trajectory and economic independence. The gender wage gap is a significant issue that often places women at a disadvantage, and wage gaps remain between White people and Brown and Black people (Hegewisch & Mefferd, 2021). Women are often restricted by glass ceilings that limit their advancement into leadership roles. Minorities are also underrepresented in leadership roles in many fields (Buttner et al., 2009). Women may also be expected to navigate the dual expectations of excelling in their careers while also fulfilling societal expectations around family life. Women often find themselves in a balancing act that creates a double burden to be successful in both areas of their lives. Men, on the other hand, are often expected to prioritize their careers, which can serve to reinforce traditional gender norms that may connect economic success and masculinity. In households, there may be expectations of traditional gender roles regardless of work outside the home (Dunn et al., 2013).

Another consideration is the role of heteronormativity, which marginalizes gender-nonconforming or gender-expansive individuals as well as affectional orientations other than heterosexual. In terms of relationship structure, monogamy is the norm and other relational structures or arrangements are often marginalized and pathologized (see, e.g., Trexler, 2021). A feminist clinician who utilizes an intersectional perspective can help deconstruct these oppressive norms and encourage equitable relationships that include shared responsibility and mutual support.

Lastly, the transition to parenthood may be a significant milestone in early adulthood that is heavily influenced by patriarchal norms. Women face immense pressure to have children and prioritize their families over their careers, which is often at the expense of their professional aspirations. Many working mothers put immense pressure on themselves to be both a perfect employee and mother, often at the cost of their well-being (Forbes et al., 2020). Issues surrounding reproductive rights, including access to contraception and reproductive autonomy, are also shaped by Western patriarchal norms. In addition, since this period is the traditional time to marry and start a family, anyone who does not do either or both of those may feel pressure to conform or feel "othered" by remaining single and/or child-free (Graham et al., 2019).

## Middle Adulthood

Middle adulthood is a lengthy period within the lifespan in which many transitions occur. This is the stage of life where production and career are typically important. For women in middle adulthood, the tension between career advancement and family responsibilities often becomes more pronounced (Lee & Tang, 2015). The "double burden" of work and home life can lead to burnout and limit opportunities for career growth. Patriarchal expectations may also dictate that men in this stage should be at the peak of their careers, facing pressure to provide financially while potentially neglecting personal well-being and relationships (Marks, 1977; Marks & MacDermid, 1996). Exploring how these expectations vary across different cultures and intersecting identities can reveal additional layers of patriarchal influence.

Gendered and other intersectionally experienced expectations continue to influence parenting styles and the division of labor in households, even as children reach adulthood. Women might still be expected to provide emotional support and caregiving, while men might be seen as providers. The concept of "sandwich generation," is where middle-aged adults care for their children and aging parents. As of 2022, more than half of Americans in their 40s fall into this category (Horowitz, 2022). This can be explored from a feminist perspective, highlighting how these responsibilities are often unequally distributed based on gender.

Patriarchal society often devalues people as they age, complicated by other intersectional identities, often leading to issues with self-esteem and body image (Williams et al., 2024).

The emphasis on youth and beauty in women can result in a fear of aging and pressure to maintain a youthful appearance. Men may also face societal expectations around aging. These often center on maintaining power and virility, which can lead to issues such as age-related anxiety or a possible midlife crisis (Robbins et al., 2016). The role of social media and cultural narratives that reflect patriarchal social values play such a large role in shaping these perceptions and can be critically examined with the feminist therapist.

The impact of patriarchal stressors on physical and mental health in middle adulthood is a critical area of exploration. Women might experience health issues related to chronic stress, caregiving burdens (Allen et al., 2017), or the long-term effects of gender-based discrimination (Kahsay et al., 2020). Men might face challenges related to suppressing emotions or dealing with the pressures of maintaining their role as providers, which can result in mental health issues that are often stigmatized (McKenzie et al., 2022). Access to healthcare and how it is influenced by gender and intersecting identities might also be an important topic of discussion particularly for more oppressed populations.

## Older Adulthood

Older or later adulthood continues to evolve as many people live longer, so this stage of life, once brief, is now potentially the longest stage of life. Similar to the idea of emerging adulthood, it has been suggested to consider a new stage of emerging elderhood (Skerrett et al., 2022) that would mark the transition from midlife to older adulthood. However it is conceived, this last part of the life cycle typically includes a new set of challenges due to aging, loss, and approaching death still normed in the patriarchal social context and impacted by their intersectional identities.

Many losses can occur during older adulthood, including systemic losses such as retirement or job loss, loss of friends and family members through death or inability to remain in touch, and personal losses in health, mobility, and independence (Erikson, 1980; Moon, 2023). With patriarchal capitalistic pressures, careers may have mandatory retirement ages, or older people may feel pushed out of their workplaces. There may be oppression through financial insecurity, fear for safety, and/or experiencing ageism. As in other stages of life, any other intersectional oppressions can occur or can continue to be a factor, such as misogynoir. Gender and racial/ethnic differences in lifespan projections and accumulated income can impact the quality of this stage of life (Brown, 2012). The dominant culture of the West values youth over age in most areas, and so elders may experience a loss of visibility in society and become seen as less attractive and vital individuals. All of these experiences can impact an elder's sense of agency and autonomy. In addition, patriarchal messages about being elderly are more negative than positive, and they may even be more stereotypical than accurate when it comes to what younger people think of as common experiences of being older (Pew Research Center, 2009).

In this stage, dealing with losses and potentially facing more losses will likely be clinical concerns for a feminist therapist understanding how oppressive social systems may continue to challenge the client's autonomy and agency. It is vital to empower people losing agency through loss or illness to be able to exercise agency wherever possible. This can be a time of reflection including the patriarchal context surrounding their lives. As the end-of-life approaches, feminist clinicians can help elders assess, based on their intersectional identities, which decisions they are facing and what they want to happen. Perhaps no time is more important for people to have agency than in planning or experiencing end-of-life decisions. Given that death is often a challenging topic for many to talk about, feminist therapists are well positioned to discuss approaching death with elders, both in terms of meaning-making and as a way to continue monitoring power over available choices.

Planning for the end of life may include financial decisions, wills and legacies, evaluating or reevaluating important relationships (reconciliations, giving gifts, saying goodbye, etc.), and making plans for end-of-life medical decisions. While feminist therapists are not in a position to give medical or financial advice, they can have a trusted network of referrals for these needs. What can be addressed therapeutically is power and autonomy and ensuring that, as much as possible, an elder has power over such things as what care they receive, when/if they wish care to be discontinued, what funeral arrangements they want, if any, what setting they wish to die in, and so forth. There may be no greater time to help empower a person than when facing death.

TABLE 4.1  *Feminist Intersectional Model of Lifespan Development*

| Feminist Model of Lifespan Development | Potential Patriarchal Influences | Potential Challenges | Potential Areas of Client Exploration |
|---|---|---|---|
| Infant and Toddler | Gender assigned at birth. Gendered expectations from parents, family may influence parenting. How is role of relationships conveyed and reinforced? | Any impacts of intersectional oppression on family resources. Racism, sexism, ableism, etc., including any impacts on maternal prenatal, and postnatal health care. | Parents can consider dreams and goals for children. Are they conveying patriarchal expectations in terms of any/all/intersecting social identities? |
| Early Childhood | Increasing interactions with other children bring race, gender, ability, religion, etc. into more focus. Comparisons with others may increase awareness of privilege and oppression. Relational messages may start to convey differences by gender. | Interacting with other families' cultural expectations may reinforce patriarchal influences. Any impacts of oppression on resources. Racism, sexism, ableism, etc. | Parents seeing any behaviors or statements by children that do not conform to patriarchal expectations (or their own expectations). This can include independence vs interdependence. |
| Middle and Late Childhood | School aged–expectations to conform to educational settings. Comparisons with others increase in terms of academic and social expectations. Social media use may increase. Gendered messages in education and at home can reinforce dominant views on gender, relationships. | Reinforcement of patriarchal norms by schools and other institutions or by parents, or by social media. Gender non-conforming or transgender expression could be problems based on patriarchal expectations or systems/policies. Any impacts of oppression on resources. Racism, sexism, ableism, etc. | Parent concerns about children's development; any children's issues that are impacted by norms, expectations, social justice issues (resources, acknowledgment of problem, policies, etc.). |

| Adolescence | Peer network, school, and family all contribute to comparisons to others and to the greater patriarchal expectations. Great pressure to decide life map. Social media likely an influence. Implicit and explicit messages about gender, identity, sexuality. Transition to adulthood with adult expectations. Gender and relationship messages likely. | Peer pressure that reinforces patriarchal influences. Social media can be disempowering and can include misinformation. Families may or may not respect attempts to develop identities. Any impacts of oppression on resources. Racism, sexism, ableism, etc. | Identity exploration can include psychoeducation about patriarchal systems and helping clients see where they do/do not fit and want/do not want to fit. Intersecting identities can be explored and hopes/dreams can be projected into future, then brought back to here-and-now in terms of mapping out how to achieve dreams, or how to modify dreams to fit current needs and systems. |
| --- | --- | --- | --- |
| Early adulthood | People seen as adults. Finding a mate, establishing a career, having children are all patriarchal expectations of this stage. Any one off-track of expected schedules may feel pressure to conform. Each sphere of life can be heavily influenced by expectations and comparisons to others. Relational messages, expectations of marriage, monogamy and having children could all be reinforced. | Any challenges related to patriarchal expectations. Any impacts of oppression on resources. Racism, sexism, ableism, etc. Definitions of success are still tied to the patriarchy—how to find balance. Potentially gendered division of labor. | Career issues, relational issues, financial issues, emerging adulthood, lack of opportunities or resources, pressures to be successful as defined by patriarchy, rejection of patriarchal expectations, friendships and meanings derived from those. |
| Middle Adulthood | Mastery of career and life spheres is expected to be gained. Launching children into successful adulthood is expected. Comparison to patriarchal expectations may be tempered with gained wisdom and flexibility. | Patriarchal definitions of middle-aged people. Career change or loss. Health problems. Loss of partner through divorce or death. Dating. Any impacts of oppression on resources. Racism, sexism, ableism, ageism, etc. | Various ways that people can feel disempowered—agism, health issues, loss or change of career, changing identities with retirement, launching children, meaning-making about moving. |

|  |  |  |  |
|---|---|---|---|
|  | Waning attractiveness and social worth is conveyed, particularly to females. Youth-oriented culture. Caretaking responsibilities and patriarchal influences/ messages. Biological and hormonal changes. Sexuality impacted. | Caretaking responsibilities and patriarchal influences/messages. Readying for older adulthood. | toward being elders, may be more sense of androgyny in this stage, resources in this stage may be tied to lifelong or situational oppression or privilege. |
| Older Adulthood | Many life transitions in this stage including possible loss of career (retirement), loss of people, and loss of aspects of independence over this lengthy stage. Patriarchal messages are mostly negative with a few positive ones. Life options may be reduced. Meaning-making is critical. | Patriarchal definitions of elders. Many kinds of loss— health, independence, relationships, people. Any impacts of oppression on resources. Racism, sexism, ableism, etc. | Dealing with loss of power in multiple life areas. Meaning-making in the face of loss of power. Readying for death. Making final meaning of intersectional identities. |

# Strengths of a Feminist Intersectional Developmental Approach

A feminist intersectional approach to development can add more social, cultural, and political contexts than other approaches. By trying to contextualize the development of the self within Western patriarchal impacts and expectations, this model can help connect a client and their concerns to potentially embedded oppressive, marginalizing, or privileging messages that may be experienced within most interactive ecosystems. Feminist therapists can use this developmental approach as a guide to explore power, autonomy, agency, and authenticity with clients. It is anticipated that with more research on intersectional identities throughout the lifespan, the model can become even more robust. Clients may find it helpful to examine seen and unseen forces and structures that impact them, their families, their communities, and the greater society.

# What If?

What if there were no gender expectations associated with sex identification? How might gender expression change?

What if sexuality could be equally and freely expressed by all genders with no social, cultural, or political norms embedded in them? What would sexuality be like?

What if the majority religion was not Christianity in the United States? How might development be different?

What if there were no social hierarchies permitted in school systems? What if we have no grading systems and only comments about what has been learned and what will be learned next? How would that impact development?

What if all stages of life were equally celebrated and seen as growth-enhancing opportunities?

# References

Adler, A. (2009). *Understanding human nature*. Oneworld.

Allen, A. P., Curran, E. A., Duggan, A., Cryan, J. F., Chorcorain, A. N., Dinan, T. G., Molloy, D. W., Kearney, P. M., & Clarke, G. (2017). A systematic review of the psychobiological burden of informal caregiving for patients with dementia: Focus on cognitive and biological markers of chronic stress. *Neuroscience & Biobehavioral Reviews, 73*, 123–164. https://doi.org/10.1016/j.neubiorev.2016.12.006

Atkinson, D. R., Morten, G., & Sue, D. W. (1989). *Counseling American minorities: A cross-cultural perspective* (5th ed.). W. C. Brown.

Attwood, F. (2007). Sluts and riot grrrls: Female identity and sexual agency. *Journal of Gender Studies, 16*(3), 233–247. https://doi.org/10.1080/09589230701562921

Bailey, M., & Trudy. (2018). On misogynoir: Citation, erasure, and plagiarism. *Feminist Media Studies, 18*(4), 762–768. https://doi.org/10.1080/14680777.2018.1447395

Blum, R. W., Mmari, K., & Moreau, C. (2017). It begins at 10: How gender expectations shape early adolescence around the world. *Journal of Adolescent Health, 61*(4 Suppl), S3-S4. doi: 10.1016/j.jadohealth.2017.07.009

Borysenko, J. (1996). *A woman's book of life: The biology, psychology, and spirituality of the feminine life cycle*. Riverhead Trade.

Borysenko, J. (2013). On spirituality, sustainability, and the great soul wound. *Spirituality & Health*, 32–33.

Bozzola, E., Spina, G., Agostiniani, R., Barni, S., Russo, R., Scarpato, E., Di Mauro, A., Di Stefano, A. V., Caruso, C., Corsello, G., & Staiano, A. (2022). The use of social media in children and adolescents: Scoping review on the potential risks. *International Journal of Environmental Research and Public Health, 19*(16), 9960. doi: 10.3390/ijerph19169960

Brown, T. (2012). The intersection and accumulation of racial and gender inequality: Black women's wealth trajectories. *The Review of Black Political Economy, 39*(2), 239–258. https://doi.org/10.1007/s12114-011-9100-8

Burnell, K., Trekels, J., Prinstein, M. J., & Telzer, E. H. (2024). Adolescents' social comparison on social media: Links with momentary self-evaluations. *Affective Science.* https://doi.org/10.1007/s42761-024-00240-6

Buttner, E. H., Lowe, K. B., & Billings-Harris, L. (2009). The challenge of increasing minority-group professional representation in the United States: Intriguing findings. *The International Journal of Human Resource Management, 20*(4), 771–789. https://doi.org/10.1080/09585190902770604

Cass, V. C. (1979). Homosexual identity formation: A theoretical model. *Journal of Homosexuality, 4*(3), 219–235.

Chapman, B. E., & Brannock, J. C. (1987). Proposed model of lesbian identity development: An empirical examination. *Journal of Homosexuality*, *14*(3–4), 69–80. https://doi.org/10.1300/J082v14n03_05

Conarton, S., & Silverman, L. K. (1988). Feminine development through the life cycle. In M. A. Dutton-Douglas & L. E. A. Walker (Eds.), *Feminist psychotherapies: Integration of therapeutic and feminist systems* (pp. 37–67). Ablex Publishing.

Cook, R. E., Nielson, M. G., Martin, C. L., & DeLay, D. (2019). Early adolescent gender development: The differential effects of felt pressure from parents, peers, and the self. *Journal of Youth & Adolescence*, *48*(10), 1912–1923. https://doi.org/10.1007/s10964-019-01122-y

Crockett, L. J., Raffaelli, M., & Moilanen, K. L. (2003). Adolescent sexuality: Behavior and meaning. In G. R. Adams & M. D. Berzonsky (Eds.), *Blackwell handbook of adolescence* (pp. 371–392). Blackwell Publishing.

Cross, W. E. (1971). Negro-to-Black conversion experience: Toward a psychology of Black liberation. *Black World*, *20*(9), 13–27.

Crenshaw, K. (1989). Demarginalizing the intersection of race and sex: A Black feminist critique of antidiscrimination doctrine, feminist theory and antiracist politics. *University of Chicago Legal Forum*, *1989*(8). https://chicagounbound.uchicago.edu/uclf/vol1989/iss1/8

Dunn, M. G., Rochlen, A. B., & O'Brien, K. M. (2013). Employee, mother, and partner: An exploratory investigation of working women with stay-at-home fathers. *Journal of Career Development*, *40*(1), 3–22. https://doi.org/10.1177/0894845311401744

Ebert, W. M., Jost, L., & Jansen, P. (2024). Gender stereotypes in preschoolers' mental rotation. *Frontiers in Psychology*, *15*, 1-13. https://doi.org/10.3389/fpsyg.2024.1284314

Erikson, E. H. (1980). *Identity and the life cycle*. W. W. Norton.

Few-Demo, A. L., & Allen, K. R. (2020). Gender, feminist, and intersectional perspectives on families: A decade in review. *Journal of Marriage and Family*, *82*(1), 326–345. https://doi.org/https://doi.org/10.1111/jomf.12638

Forbes, L. K., Lamar, M. R., & Bornstein, R. S. (2020). Working mothers' experiences in an intensive mothering culture: A phenomenological qualitative study. *Journal of Feminist Family Therapy*, *33*(3), 270–294. https://doi.org/10.1080/08952833.2020.1798200

Fowler, J. W. (1981). *Stages of faith*. Harper Collins.

Freud, S. (1949). *Three essays on the theory of sexuality*. (J. Strachey, Trans.). Martino Fine Books. (Original work published 1905)

Fox, R. C. (2003). Bisexual identities. In L. Garnets and D. Kimmel (Eds.), *Psychological perspectives on lesbian, gay, and bisexual experiences* (2nd ed.), 86–129. Columbia University Press.

Graham, M., McKenzie, H., Turnbull, B., & Taket, A. (2019). "Them and Us": The experiences of social exclusion among women without children in their post-reproductive years. *Journal of Research in Gender Studies*, *9*(1), 71–104. https://doi.org/10.22381/jrgs9120193

Hegewisch, A., & Mefferd, E. (2021). *The gender wage gap by occupation, race, and ethnicity 2020*. Institute for Women's Policy Research. http://www.jstor.org/stable/resrep32127

Helms, J. E. (1984). Toward a theoretical explanation of the effects of race on counseling: A Black and White model. *The Counseling Psychologist*, *12*(3-4), 153–165. https://doi.org/10.1177/0011000084124013

Helwig, N. E., & Ruprecht, M. R. (2017). Age, gender, and self-esteem: A sociocultural look through a nonparametric lens. *Archives of Scientific Psychology*, *5*(1), 19–31. https://doi.org/10.1037/arc0000032

Horowitz, J. (2022). *More than half of Americans in their 40s are "sandwiched" between an aging parent and their children*. Pew Research Center. https://www.pewresearch.org/short-reads/2022/04/08/more-than-half-of-americans-in-their-40s-are-sandwiched-between-an-aging-parent-and-their-own-children

InterACT Advocates for Intersex Youth. (2021). *What is intersex?* https://interactadvocates.org/faq/

Johnson, S. N., & Engeln, R. (2021). Gender discrepancies in perceptions of the bodies of female fashion models. *Sex Roles*, *84*, 299–311. https://doi.org/10.1007/s11199-020-01167-5

Johnston, T. R. (2015). Affirmation and care: A feminist account of bullying and bullying prevention. *Hypatia, 30*(2), 403–417. https://www-jstor-org.proxy.longwood.edu/stable/pdf/24542163. pdf?refreqid=fastly-default%3Ac17fc864cf90ac73b4a8d40d9228b18c&ab_segments=&origin=& initiator=&acceptTC=1

Kaestle, C. E., Allen, K. R., Wesche, R., & Grafsky, E. L. (2021). Adolescent sexual development: A family perspective. *The Journal of Sex Research, 58*(7), 874–890. https://doi.org/10.1080/0022449 9.2021.1924605

Kahsay, W. G., Negarandeh, R., Nayeri, N. D., & Hasanpour, M. (2020). Sexual harassment against female nurses: A systematic review. *B.M.C. Nursing, 19*(1), 1–12. https://doi.org/10.1186/s12912-020-00450-w

Kim, J. (1981). *Processes of Asian American identity development: A study of Japanese American women's perceptions of their struggle to achieve positive identities as Americans of Asian ancestry* [Doctoral dissertation]. University of Massachusetts Amherst.

Kornienko, O., Santos, C. E., Martin, C. L., & Granger, K. L. (2016). Peer influence on gender identity development in adolescence. *Developmental psychology, 52*(10), 1578–1592. https://doi.org/10.1037/dev0000200

Kosciw, J. G., Clark, C. M., & Menard, L. (2022). *The 2021 National School Climate Survey: The experiences of LGBTQ+ youth in our nation's schools.* GLSEN. https://www.glsen.org/sites/ default/files/2022-10/NSCS-2021-Full-Report.pdf

Lee, Y., & Tang, F. (2015). More caregiving, less working: Caregiving roles and gender difference. *Journal of Applied Gerontology, 34*(4), 465–483. https://doi.org/10.1177/0733464813508649

Lyons, H., Giordano, P. C., Manning, W. D., & Longmore, M. A. (2011). Identity, peer relationships, and adolescent girls' sexual behavior: An exploration of the contemporary double standard. *The Journal of Sex Research, 48*(5), 437–449. https://doi.org/10.1080/00224499.2010.506679

Marks, S. R. (1977). Multiple roles and role strain: Some notes on human energy, time, and commitment. *American Sociological Review, 42*(6), 921–936. https://doi.org/10.2307/2094577

Marks, S. R., & MacDermid, S. M. (1996). Multiple roles and the self: A theory of role balance. *Journal of Marriage and Family, 58*(2), 417–432. https://doi.org/10.2307/353506

Master, A. (2021), Gender stereotypes influence children's STEM Motivation. *Child Development Perspectives, 15*, 203–210. https://doi.org/10.1111/cdep.12424

McKenzie, S. K., Oliffe, J. L., Black, A., & Collings, S. (2022). Men's experiences of mental illness stigma across the lifespan: A scoping review. *American Journal of Men's Health, 16*(1). https://doi.org/10.1177/15579883221074789

Mesman, J., & Groeneveld, M. G. (2018). Gendered parenting in early childhood: Subtle but unmistakable if you know where to look. *Child Development Perspectives, 12*(1), 22–27. https://doi.org/10.1111/cdep.12250

Moon, P. J. (2023). Revisiting a time of study: Older adults learning through grieving. *Journal of Social Work in End-of-Life & Palliative Care, 19*(2), 88–92. https://doi.org/10.1080/15524256.20 23.2198674

Obeid, N., Norris, M. L., Buchholz, A., Henderson, K. A., Goldfield, G., Bedford, S., & Flament, M. F. (2018). Socioemotional predictors of body esteem in adolescent males. *Psychology of Men & Masculinity, 19*(3), 439–445. https://doi.org/10.1037/men0000109

Orbach, S. (2013). Bringing a gendered perspective to attachment theory in therapy. In N. A. Danquah & K. Berry (Eds.), *Attachment theory in adult mental health* (pp. 161–169). Routledge.

Orenstein, G. A., & Lewis, L. (2022). Eriksons stages psychosocial development. In *StatPearls [Internet].* StatPearls Publishing.

Pew Research Center (2009) *Growing old in America: Expectations versus reality. Pew Research Center Report.* https://www.pewresearch.org/social-trends/2009/06/29/growing-old-in-america-expectations-vs-reality

Piaget, J. (1968). *Six psychological studies* (A. Tenzer, Trans.). Vintage books.

Phinney, J. S. (1993). A three-stage model of ethnic identity development in adolescence. In M. E. Bernal & G. P. Knight (Eds.), *Ethnic identity: Formation and transmission among Hispanics and other minorities* (pp. 61–79). State University of New York Press.

Poston, W. C. (1990). The biracial identity development model: A needed addition. *Journal of Counseling & Development*, 69(2), 152–155.

Prioste, A., Tavares, P., Silva, C. S., & Magalhães, E. (2020). The relationship between family climate and identity development processes: The moderating role of developmental stages and outcomes. *Journal of Child & Family Studies*, 29(6), 1525–1536. https://doi.org/10.1007/s10826-019-01600-8

Reinking, A., & Martin, B. (2018). The gender gap in STEM fields: Theories, movements, and ideas to engage girls in STEM. *Journal of New Approaches in Educational. Research*, 7, 148–153. https://doi.org/10.7821/naer.2018.7.271

Reiss, I. (1960). *Premarital sexual standards in America*. Free Press.

Robbins, M. J., Wester, S. R., & McKean, N. B. (2016). Masculinity across the life span: Implications for older men. In Y. J. Wong & S. R. Wester (Eds.), *APA handbook of men and masculinities* (pp. 389–409). American Psychological Association. https://doi.org/10.1037/14594-018

Ruiz, A. S. (1990). Ethnic identity: Crisis and resolution. *Journal of Multicultural Counseling & Development*, 18(1), 29–40.

Skerrett, K., Spira, M., & Chandy, J. (2022). Emerging elderhood: Transitions from midlife. *Clinical Social Work Journal*, 50(4), 377–386. doi: 10.1007/s10615-021-00791-2. Epub February 16, 2021.

Sullivan, J., Wilton, L., & Apfelbaum, E. P. (2020). Adults delay conversations about race because they underestimate children's processing of race. *Journal of Experimental Psychology, General*, 395–400. https://doi.org/10.1037/xge0000851

Super, D. E. (1963). Vocational development in adolescence and early adulthood: Tasks and behaviors. In D. E. Super (Ed.), *Career development: Self-concept theory* (pp. 17–32). New York: College Entrance Board.

Surrey, J. L. (1991). The "self-in-relation": A theory of women's development. In J. V. Jordan et al. (Eds.), *Women's growth and connection: Writings from the Stone Center*. Guilford.

Syed, M., & Fish, J. (2018). Revisiting Erik Erikson's legacy on culture, race, and ethnicity, identity. *Identity: An International Journal of Theory and Research*, 18, http://doi:10.1080/15283488.2018.1523729

Trexler, B. (2021). When two is too few: Addressing polyamorous clients in therapy. *Sexual and Relationship Therapy*, 39(3), 644–659. https://doi.org/10.1080/14681994.2021.1998424

U.S. Bureau of Labor Statistics. (2021). *Women in the labor force: A databook* (Report 1095). https://www.bls.gov/opub/reports/womens-databook/202/

Williams, L., Gurung, J., Persons, P., & Kilpela, L. (2024). Body image and eating issues in midlife: A narrative review with clinical question recommendations. *Maturitas*, 188, 108068. https://doi.org/10.1016/j.maturitas.2024.108068

# PART TWO

# Feminist Intersectional Therapy Clinical Modalities

# 5

# Fourth-Wave Feminist Intersectional Applications: The Personal Is Political

## *Joanne Jodry and Kathleen McCleskey*

*Eurocentric, Christian-dominant, heteronormative, and patriarchal norms have been established in society. Those with intersectional identities that reflect views of "good," "successful," or "right" often have more power and opportunities than those who do not. Oppressed people frequently blame themselves for their failures instead of blaming the impact of the marginalization.*

One way feminist theory can continue to evolve into a more utilized clinical conception and stand-alone theory is to help clinicians with ease of use. Much like existential theory (Yalom, 1980) and person-centered theory (Rogers, 1961/1995), feminist theory may have traditionally been considered an underpinning or addendum theory to other clinical theories considered more complete that include specific models and techniques. *Feminist Intersectional Therapy: Fourth-wave Clinical Applications* will add more possibilities for a potentially fuller theoretical conceptualization and clinical applications of feminist theory to contribute to the feminist theorists' implementation ideas. These models, conceptualizations, and applications are not perceived as the one or only way to do feminist therapy but as one way to apply fourth-wave feminist therapy. It would defeat the point of feminist thinking by making it more like traditional theories that are born from structured patriarchy. The uniqueness and healing factors in feminist theory are the creativity within the therapeutic relationship and application, as well as honoring the clients' contextualized intersectional experiences.

One unique position of feminist intersectional theory is that it moves beyond other traditional theories that focus on the person's behavior, perceptions, thoughts, or family systems or relations as the main etiology of psychological suffering. Feminist theory adds social, cultural, and political contexts as a clinical underpinning to the therapeutic process through a lens of intersectional power, privilege, and oppression. This theory views the client's suffering as a result of, or at least with a great contribution from, attempts to assimilate into an unequal, oppressive Eurocentric, heteronormative, Christian-dominant, patriarchal society (Brown, 2018; Evans et al., 2011; Collins, 2000). The patriarchal legacy favors the privileged who fit into the social, cultural, and political norms and ideals that have historically been passed down through the dominant majority or, in some cases, just the most powerful due to position. These norms and ideals have become directly embedded in social and cultural constructs and systems (e.g., laws and education) and have also been influential in setting and maintaining social standards based on patriarchy. Anyone who does not fit into these systems or norms is marginalized and/or oppressed by society and often punished through a lack of opportunity afforded to the privileged. Those who reject or rebel against the norms or systems risk being marginalized, ostracized, or rejected. Additionally, the patriarchal concept of meritocracy—that anyone can work hard and become successful—places the sole blame for lack of success on any individual who is oppressed by society (Hardy, 2023). At a minimum, this contributes to psychopathology; at a maximum, it causes it (Brown, 2018; Hardy, 2023). Feminist intersectional therapy does not help the client fit into the oppressive systems and constructs of society; instead, it helps the client to analyze them critically, navigate them where necessary, reject them where possible, and even advocate to change the systems (if consistent with the client's desires). These responses to the patriarchal system may help the client to live the most empowered, best possible life.

For many people seeking therapy, it may be helpful for them to understand how culture and society reflect embedded Eurocentric, heteronormative, Christian-dominant, patriarchal values and have created subsequent hierarchical systems that favor the privileged in society and oppress the people who do not fit in or hold the same traditional values (Brown, 2018; Evans et al., 2011). Feminist intersectional theory may help the client to dissect their personal beliefs and perhaps contextualize their values or beliefs that have been consciously or unconsciously embedded in them since birth. This may lead to discussing how that may contribute to their current suffering and how they can navigate some of the marginalization and oppression. In feminist intersectional theory, the personal is political; it is fruitless to consider an individual's issues without considering how patriarchal systemic influences may have created or contributed to them. This feminist examination might allow the client to raise their consciousness, feel empowered, and make future decisions with freedom from the pulls of oppression, hierarchies, and social judgment. Raised consciousness, freedom of choices free of embedded norms, and empowerment are goals of feminist theory.

# Basic Therapeutic Underpinnings for Feminist Intersectional Therapy

## Power and Empower

Power is related to autonomy—a person holds power in spaces and in relationships where they are seen, heard, and valued; where they can make decisions singly or in collaboration with others; and when they can have control over what they do and do not do. This power is not meant to be absolute or to include power over others—rather, it is individual power to move through the world without barriers. Power can be thought of as being present in many spheres of life, including those related to the physical body, the internal mind and psyche, in relationships with others, and in terms of spirituality and meaning-making (Brown, 2018). Evans et al. (2011) discuss different types of power, including coercive, legitimate, informational, expert, and referent. How power is defined, given, taken, perceived, and used is also deeply impacted by greater Western patriarchal norms, contracts, and systems.

Power is present in all relationships. People may seek power to define themselves, to gain their position, and even to protect their consciousness/ego/truth. All relationships have power dynamics at every level within a person's ecosystem. Often, the person who seems to care the least or has the least need in a relationship is the one who holds the power. This may be seen when people are navigating romantic relationships and one person acts aloof. The aloof position may be trying to feel powerful through passive-aggressive means, purposefully keeping distance to maintain power, struggling internally to create a real connection, or genuinely uninterested. Whatever the cause, a goal of feminist therapy is to help the client (whichever person that is) to examine the relational situation through an intersectional identity lens, monitor how power is used or experienced within the relationship, and move toward a more empowered existence where power can be recognized and shared intentionally. In feminist intersectional therapy, examining this relational power dynamic begins within the therapeutic relationship with the transparent feminist therapist, creating a partnership of shared power. The person seeking therapeutic help typically experiences some loss of power connected to the presenting problem. It is the feminist therapist's goal to help them find or regain their power and to be able to generalize it to other relationships.

Patriarchal social and cultural systems oppress individuals whose intersectional identities are vulnerable and not part of the perceived collective privileged "good" people (Brown, 2018; Hardy, 2023; Sue, 2015). Examples can be seen in school achievement gaps, racial inequality in the legal system, and so on. As part of the clinical therapeutic process, the client might examine how society interacts with them, the people they love, and their community. This is one reason social justice and advocacy have traditionally been grounded in clinical feminist theory. The client must learn to become empowered and navigate these oppressive systems for themselves (and others if they desire). It is important to note that many clients feel helpless, and the reality is that they may continue to be oppressed by the patriarchal system. The feminist intersectional clinical goal is for the client to resist internalizing the oppression and recognize its external origins in the quest for social and cultural empowerment.

## Therapeutic Transparency

Clients often enter therapy believing there is a mystical process of analyzing them and giving them a cure. Media frequently shows therapists doing just that and, therefore, does not help clients understand the actual therapeutic process. The feminist therapist demystifies the therapeutic process and the concept of therapy itself. This can be thought of as a deeper form of role induction. The feminist therapist does not want the client to feel manipulated or to worry about what the therapist is thinking or how they may be judged. The therapeutic alliance becomes a true collaborative partnership between therapist and client, and the relationship is one striving for shared power. Using psychoeducation and immediacy, for example, a therapist can explain the therapeutic process and be responsive and open to a client's questions at any point in the therapy. From this stance, while the feminist therapist is educated on psychological theories and techniques, the client is educated on their life, perceptions, and lived realities. Both are seen as equal and equally important and valued as such. This can be a difficult transition for any therapist who likes to be seen as an expert. If not done skillfully, a client could mistake transparency and shared power for incompetence. When done authentically, this feminist therapeutic alliance can create a deep investment by the client in the therapeutic work.

## Social and Cultural Context for Suffering

Feminist intersectional theory frames suffering in a context of historically, socially, culturally, and politically embedded messages of oppression and privilege. Although each client must take full responsibility for themselves, a goal of the therapeutic work is to examine how they came to their beliefs connected to their therapeutic issues, to examine if those beliefs make sense to them, to provide social and cultural context, and to empower them to decide future choices based on a raised consciousness of these frameworks. Feminist therapists may also help clients contextualize the oppression and bias of the mental health systems, including diagnosing based on the norms of society (Brown, 2018; Hardy, 2023; Mullan, 2023). The classifications of mental disorders themselves are often oppressive and limiting to the whole of human existence and diagnosing labels clients that may contribute to their issues. For example, once someone is labeled with a significant disorder such as psychosis, social constructs and norms impact the difficulties and challenges they may face such as true freedom of choice in their treatment or lifestyles, ability to obtain their dream careers, or opportunities for a desired social relationship. Most labels, diagnostic or not, place boundaries and limitations around roles and possibilities.

Additionally, social constructs born from Eurocentric, heteronormative, Christian-dominant, patriarchal legacies collectively define successful living, proper expressions of "respect," acceptable sexual behaviors or gender expressions, when a personality is "disordered," and so forth. Social norms often promote obtaining a successful life that is underpinned by financial success. This often creates competitive goals of hierarchies between people, financial gains at the base of career considerations, educational gains as a tool for future financial success, and so on. Western social norms promote this success associated with financial gain as being equally accessible for all, "the American dream." In reality, this itself can be a source of suffering for people who, due to inequity, can never reach these socially collective definitions (Hardy, 2023). These social, cultural, and political embedded constructs reward privileged individuals with social positionality that can easily assimilate into the norms. Conversely, for individuals who do not have intersectional identities or values that are congruent with these Western patriarchal norms, devaluation, marginalization, and oppression occur. The concept of "learned helplessness" (Peterson et al., 1993) describes a situation where a person begins to give up hope through consistent social or cultural obstacles. Additionally, if an individual believes the "anyone can do it" social mantra, and they are not able to become "successful," internalized oppression may set into the person (Brown, 2018; Hardy, 2023). Moreover, this may contribute to or even cause what society and the medical model deem psychopathology (Brown, 2018; Evans et al., 2011).

## Equality

Feminist theory sees all people as equal, with everyone having strengths and social value. This can become challenging when a feminist clinician must fight their own embedded messages and are working with people who are often social outcasts, like individuals who have committed crimes, women who have lost custody of their children, people who have done sexual offenses, and others. These examples are chosen because these are often people who are more socially acceptable to dislike as a group and to be judgmental toward, which leads to acceptable marginalization and oppression. Feminist intersectional therapy honors each person by their human existence. It recognizes cognitive and emotional shaping by family and society rooted in Western patriarchal constructs forming the embedded perceptions and behaviors that individuals display as adults. These adaptations and reactions to society can be conceptualized and respected as each person's journey to survive their unique intersectional circumstances. As part of this strength-based view of equality among all people, the mental health medical model is rejected and replaced with an individual intersectional narrative experience of contextualizing problems and navigating through them with empowerment.

## Raising Consciousness to Intersectional Identities and Associated Privileges and Oppressions

One main goal of feminist intersectional therapy is to collaboratively raise the client's consciousness so that they have conscious, as opposed to unconscious reactions, and the ability to make clearer decisions and embrace the responsibility of those decisions. Many people assimilate and automatically adhere to embedded patriarchal social constructs without questioning them. They often blame themselves for perceived individual shortcomings in reaching the happiness they desire within these constructs (Hardy, 2023). This theory helps the client deconstruct social, cultural, political, and social positionality norms and allows the client to examine, evaluate, and make decisions on a conscious level.

## Advocacy for Self and Others

Part of the historical feminist movement that feminist therapy has evolved from is the fight for equality of women's rights. When feminist therapy evolved, advocacy was a natural marriage to the theory. Therapeutically, advocacy has many benefits. Adler (1927/2009) suggested that social interest had curative properties. Adler (1956/1964) also suggested, "When social interest has been from the first installed into the upward strivings of the psyche, it acts as automatic certainty, coloring every thought and action" (p. 155). Adler's (1927/2009) early theory supports the feminist views of advocacy work as therapeutic healing. Social interest and advocacy may also benefit individuals by connecting people and expanding personal support systems in a healthy community while working for a common cause. However, it must be made clear that clients choosing advocacy as part of their therapy must make a conscious choice themselves. Feminist intersectional therapy promotes clients being free from coercion, including and particularly from their feminist therapists. Advocacy (especially beyond self-advocacy) should never be a pressured or expected part of the therapeutic process, consciously or unconsciously. Self-advocacy through assertiveness is organic to the concepts of feminist therapy, but what it may look like is different for each individual. It often becomes a natural occurrence in the therapeutic process due to the client's raised consciousness. The client has the free choice of whether and how to do this advocacy, whether exclusively for themselves or if they would like to advocate for others. Likewise, it must be noted that advocacy takes many forms, such as standing up for oneself in quiet ways, publicly protesting, or running for political office. Advocacy can also happen in private ways, such as within families where parenting practices, divisions of labor, or relational needs could be addressed. What can never happen is that the feminist therapist pushes their agenda on a client. This is contraindicated to feminist intersectional therapy as it mimics the power, hierarchies, and oppressive systems of the patriarchy.

## Feminist Intersectional Therapeutic Relationship

The feminist intersectional therapeutic relationship differs from other theories due to a few unique, transparent, egalitarian dimensions. Full transparency during the entire therapeutic process is a necessity. The therapeutic work needs to be demystified entirely and understood by the client in order for the client to participate fully as an equal collaborator. Part of this transparency is the clarity with the client that no magical analytical powers wield the "truth," the "right" way, or "techniques" of trickery. This relationship is simply a collaborative exploratory process, and clients explore and consider their thoughts and contexts for their issues.

Transparency sets the stage for another key factor in the feminist therapeutic relationship: acknowledging and monitoring the power dynamic within the relationship. It is organically implied that the clinician holds more power. When one person seeks help from another person, the neediest person is usually the most disempowered. In feminist intersectional therapy, it is critical to acknowledge these power differentials and work to break those traditional hierarchical constructs of relationships. Both people bring expertise to the process—the clinician brings training (often embedded in patriarchal systems) and therapeutic experience, and the client brings their strengths from developing and navigating their lived experiences. Neither of these is more important than the other. However, this can be challenging for both parties—sometimes therapists want to be more in control (for example, danger must be addressed), and sometimes clients want therapists to take control (for example, to make a difficult choice for them). Transparency and immediacy can help explore who holds the power in the therapeutic dynamic at any given time. It is the feminist clinician's responsibility to monitor this power dynamic and to explore and navigate any imbalance of therapeutic power.

One way power sharing might be achieved could be by measuring therapeutic self-disclosure. From a feminist perspective, self-disclosure can serve several purposes in creating and maintaining a therapeutic relationship. Saying "that happened to me, too" as a self-disclosure is not traditionally considered helpful and could serve just to marginalize the client's experience that they just revealed. However, a feminist intersectional therapist might share a common experience of disempowerment in the patriarchal society, which could be validating. Therapeutic self-disclosure might also include stories or reference experiences of the therapist being human, with similar struggles. However, it is essential to remember that everyone is unique in their intersectional identities, and any "that happened to me, too" could shift the focus to the therapist and could also discount the client's disclosure and create alienation. Any disclosure must be carefully thought through and have a therapeutic purpose.

Another key to the feminist therapeutic relationship is that role induction may also differ from traditional theories. As part of this process, the feminist clinician may acknowledge social positionality that may be different from or similar to their clients. The client can physically see things in the feminist clinician: race, age, sex, gender, clothes, office, and so on. Additionally, the client might assume perspectives related to more implicit embedded social associations about the feminist clinician: being educated, wealthy, and even having values that align with society and perhaps a local area. With technology, clients have often searched for the therapist's name. If "feminist" is associated with them, there may also be presumptions about that. Lastly, there are characteristics or values that the client might place on a feminist clinician unique to their own unconscious transference needs. The feminist clinician needs to be aware of all of these potential ways that the client may use to disempower themselves and place the therapist in a hierarchical, superior, powerful position.

# Feminist Intersectional Therapy: A Clinical Process Model

## Before Client Contact

Like all therapists, feminists must continue on a lifelong journey of self-awareness. They must remain current in their respective mental health fields and recognize the continued oppressive systems (including mental health) in the ever-changing social, cultural, and political environments and how that impacts their sense of self. Feminist therapists are not immune from biases, fears, and unacknowledged assimilations to oppressive systems. It is essential to do regular self-inventories, particularly when their ecosystemic experiences change. Lastly, many of these feminist conceptualizations challenge existing power, hierarchies, and oppressive systems; it may be beneficial to have a feminist tribe for support when navigating these rough waters.

## Transparency: The First Contact

The feminist intersectional therapist demystifies the therapeutic process from the first contact. This is an opportunity to discuss the collaborative process and the issues the client is presenting. As part of informed consent, egalitarian roles are explained, and the therapeutic concept of sharing power in the collaborative journey to navigate the client's suffering is also discussed. During this time, demographic information is exchanged. The informed consent must be transparent and discussed, not just read and signed as if it were a medical office. The main goal of feminist introductions is for the client to clearly express their perspective about their cause of suffering and feel supported by the clinician. The initial meeting aims to allow the client's narrative to be heard and intersectional experience to be understood from their perspective, not from the judgments that society might place on them. Moreover, perhaps most importantly, the client should feel honored by the feminist therapist for their strength of adaptation and survival.

## Honor Unique Narrative: After the First Meeting

After the initial meeting, it is important to begin by understanding how the client experienced the first meeting and to ask for feedback. Looking for power differentials, the feminist therapist can seek information about whether there was anything the client had wished the therapist did or asked in the first meeting. The therapist can also ask if any new information needs to be added or if any information provided initially should be changed. Many clients are not confrontational or are very polite, so it is crucial that the therapist remains open and genuinely seeks the information holistically. The feminist therapist's ego must be in check, and any information given must be received nondefensively, or the client may know and respond to that. This early stage of feminist intersectional therapy is the time to listen more deeply to the client's narrative and to identify the strengths, power, self-insights, and the like. This is the stage to fully engage with the client's perspective without judging it from the feminist therapist's personally, culturally, or socially embedded experiences. Even if the feminist therapist moves to an anxious state hearing the narratives and perspectives, they must remain nonjudgmental. They must remain aware that most therapist's judgments are also rooted in Eurocentric, heteronormative, Christian-dominant, patriarchal societal norms.

## Contextualize the Suffering: Expand Consciousness

In this phase of a feminist intersectional model of helping, the feminist therapist collaborates with the client to contextualize their suffering within their ecosystem, personal intersectionality, perceptions of power, actual power, oppression in society, and embedded messages using social, cultural, and political frames. This is where the therapist may collaborate with the client and choose different feminist clinical applications to explore their psyche and potential injuries further. Options may include an intersectional power analysis, social atom, imposter no more exercise, and so on.

Clients can identify new thoughts, ideas, or feelings that emerge through this exploration process, and those new conceptions can be discussed related to the presenting problem or etiologies of suffering. This clinical process of intersectional identity exploration attempts to create a deeper self-understanding by examining the client's values, thoughts, behaviors, and problems within the hierarchies of privilege and oppression within their social and cultural systems. In this phase, clients may recognize that problems they have interpreted as internal and individual may stem from or be impacted by greater social systemic messages, values, and expectations. Before leaving this phase of therapy, it is helpful to collaborate with clients to ensure they have thoroughly explored all relevant intersectional areas. Are there any existing beliefs that they still do not understand or whose genesis is still mysterious? It is important to examine any existing "I just do that" or "that's the way it is" beliefs or behaviors that may inhibit therapeutic healing.

## Empowerment: Responsibility for the Future

After the consciousness-raising intersectional examination of ecosystems, beliefs, behaviors, and so on, the feminist intersectional therapist can collaboratively work with the client to examine how the client has, thus far, been privileged and/or oppressed by society. Helping clients identify specific social positionality empowers them to navigate society from that position awareness. The client can examine how they have been accepted or rejected in their experiences and how they have navigated systems through adaptations, functional or not, to survive and adapt to the ecosystem. These therapeutic examinations are centered on any pain these experiences, beliefs, and possible adaptations may or may not cause, as well as their current and overall human suffering. It is essential that the client does not become stuck in a "victim of society" spot. Although, in many cases, oppressed clients are indeed victimized, the goal of feminist intersectional therapy promotes "victim" as a descriptive adjective, not a noun identity. Exploring new decisions and behaviors that offer navigation tools to oppressive systems based on empowerment will be helpful. It is also important to note that it is perhaps naive to think that all clients can advocate for change in their circumstances. The oppression within constructs and systems is sometimes so great that changing the systems is not currently an option and the client must learn to deal with such systems remaining in place. Empowerment does not solely depend on outcomes; it comes from an internal process of recognizing one's voice, continuing to use it, and not internalizing oppressive messages as learned helplessness, trauma, or hopelessness.

Not all patriarchal systems in the client ecosystem need to be challenged, dismantled, or rejected; some may need to be embraced. Clients will identify and explore the parts of the social/cultural/political systems that work for them, which they would like to keep "as is," and which offer the most significant challenges to their potential problems or suffering. This exploration could include a systemic review of relevant systems impacting the client's life, embracing or rejecting systemic beliefs or behaviors related to any part of their intersectional identity and self-defined problems. What new values or social, cultural, or political constructs about themselves are helpful to healing and creating a more meaningful existence? Recognizing intersectional privilege, how do they want to handle those areas of their life where they are given advantages over others? What new thoughts can they identify that allow them to remain in current conditions, if necessary or desired, but which reduce the suffering they previously had experienced? Are there beliefs or behaviors that they want to reject or reframe?

## Advocacy and Assertiveness: Self and Others

In the final phase of the feminist intersectional therapeutic process, the client's assertiveness training and empowerment can dictate how they would like to move forward with their new thoughts, beliefs, and navigation skills, perhaps connecting those to actions and behaviors. Advocacy can have healing properties associated with it; however, it is vital for the clinical practitioner not to impose advocacy values on the client. It is important to remember that advocacy ranges from assertively standing up for oneself in situations (or deciding not to) to fighting for the rights of others. There might be situations when it is counterintuitive to be assertive or self-advocate if safety is in question or if the client, after consciousness raising, has chosen to leave their circumstances unaltered. The client must fully decide with no influence from the feminist clinician what kinds of advocacy or assertiveness they would like to engage in to further their personal healing.

# Feminist Intersectional Clinical Applications

## Feminist Power Analysis

One of the most central techniques associated with the legacy of feminist theory is a power analysis (Ballou et al., 2008). This traditional clinical feminist application entails helping the client identify members in their systems (family, work, friends, or even constructs like society or culture) and examining who holds power within each relationship. This can be done in written form or orally, usually using a Likert-type or other scale (such as a range of 1–10, where 1 connotes the least power and 10 is the most power). Clarity and acknowledgment are sought regarding the realities of who holds the power within their relevant relationships, not the idealism of who should hold it. How is power determined? Power may be culturally informed in terms of traditionally hierarchical relationships (gendered relationships, or adult children/parents); structurally set such as in working relationships (boss/employee), practically in terms of relationships with differing ages and abilities (children/parents), or in some other way as defined by the client. When exploring who holds power, a feminist intersectional therapist explores the intersectional identities and power, understanding all aspects of the complications of relationships, privilege, and oppressive social positioning, and neediness toward or from the other. Power may be held by the person who appears less emotionally invested in the relationship, who has more financial resources, or someone who has an impact on one's future. There may also be a pattern the client has been taught in the family or by society to give away power to others or to maintain power with all others. The goal of examining the client's relationships from a power lens allows the client to raise their consciousness about where they hold or do not have personal power, if there are any patterns to the type of people or relationships that impact the client being more or less empowered, and whether or not they would like to change any of those dynamics.

## Therapeutic Relationship Power Monitoring

As stated earlier, the therapeutic relationship is essential to feminist intersectional therapy. It is also essential that the power dynamic within this relationship be monitored throughout the process. The goal is to create an authentic relationship with the client that collaboratively shares power while modeling empowerment for the client. This can be challenging because the feminist clinician must remain genuine, therapeutic, and focused on collaboration and honoring the client's preferences and desires. Complications might arise. Collaboratively, the differential power must be addressed with immediacy, transparency, and integrity. It is important to note that shared power does not mean there is always agreement. There may be situations involving danger or mandated reporting when the client disagrees. The feminist therapist must navigate that process by empowering the client to collaborate to ensure safety. For example, this could look like reporting to mandated reporters together. As stated, social hierarchies are also deconstructed in the therapeutic relationship and self-disclosure may aid in that process, remembering any self-disclosure must still remain therapeutic. People who are used to being socially oppressed may be more vulnerable to self-deprecation to assimilate to situations. This dynamic should be noticed and avoided by both the feminist therapist and the client. When the client puts the feminist therapist in an elevated status above their own, that needs to be acknowledged and addressed with the goal of remediation of the power differential.

## Feminist Intersectional Analysis

Although Crenshaw (1991) introduced the concept of intersectionality in a non-clinical modality, there are strong implications and applications for clinical use of this concept for psychological analysis, social exploration, and healing wounds of oppression. A feminist therapist can use an intersectional lens to help clients explore their social identities and positionality related to the patriarchally imbued privilege or oppression between and among aspects of the self, contextualizing that analysis to their problems and suffering. There are various structures that a feminist clinician can introduce to an intersectional analysis, discussion, or activity. For a less-structured method, verbally exploring specific intersections of identities through open-ended questions could prompt a fruitful discussion. Identity discussions might include which identity intersections the client feels strongest about and may believe are most prevalent in society. Does the client feel congruent with their identities and with the way society may perceive them? How could potential complications or even conflicting segments of their intersectionality be difficult to navigate within society?

For a more structured approach, two frames of exploration might be considered; while not yet found in the literature of clinical applications, each may offer a more structured way to explore intersectional identities. The first, the Matrix of Domination, was developed by Collins (1990) in the context of Black feminist thought. This model has since been widely explored as a model of intersectionality. In Collins's model, four domains describe how oppressive power is organized. The Structural domain includes laws and policies that codify dominant norms. This ensures that oppression continues on structural levels. The Disciplinary domain is the level that ensures that laws and policies from the Structural domain are upheld. It reinforces compliance and also promotes surveillance; both of these serve to strengthen dominant, oppressive structures. The Hegemonic level touches all other levels. It presents the oppression as being true, normal, and the like, and includes ideologies, values, and norms. It can result in internal as well as external oppression. Lastly, the Interpersonal domain is the personal domain where each person lives their daily life, experiencing privilege, oppression, and/or marginalization. According to Collins (1990), no one is totally oppressed or totally privileged. Intersectional identities are experienced on this level; this is also where relationships may help honor intersectional identities and encourage resistance of oppressive messages and norms.

Using Collins's (1990) model, a feminist intersectional clinician could begin by asking a client to identify their social identities (race, gender, class, ability, socioeconomic status [SES], religion, age, spirituality, etc.) and to identify how they intersect. In other words, which combinations of identities cannot be reduced to single constructs? Next, the therapist could briefly explain the four levels of domination to the client and ask them to reflect and map out how their identities interact on each level. For example, at the Structural level, are there laws and policies that oppress or privilege the client? Are these privileges or oppressions reinforced at the Disciplinary level by intense oversight or by turning a blind eye? Are there Hegemonic messages that explain oppression or privilege and reinforce it? Has the client internalized any messages of oppression? Finally, how can any individual experiences be contextualized within these definitions of oppression or privilege?

A second structured model that might be applied clinically to explore intersecting identities can be adapted from Fuller's (2020) model of autoethnographic feminist reflection, titled the "7 Up Intersectionality Life Grid" (p. 1). Fuller (2020) developed a process, with a nod to the "7 Up" documentary series, to examine her lived experiences in 7-year intervals beginning at birth, exploring her personal life, professional life, and scholarship. This examination resulted in a rich grid with her chosen identities of education, race, class, and gender across the top of the grid and two categories of "personal, family and community factors" and "educational policy context, sociocultural and geopolitical factors" (p. 6). Taken together, these two categories helped contextualize and position her individual experiences. She further interpreted the information through three lenses: complacency, discomfort, and transformation.

A feminist intersectional therapist could work with a client to create a similar grid that was salient to the client's identities. The client could identify identities to examine in 7-year intervals using the same personal/family/community and sociocultural/geopolitical categories, adding a professional category if that was desired, or any other frames that would be helpful. Intersectional identities could initially be charted as combinations or as single identities; in the latter case, intersections of identities could be clarified as part of the clinical exploration and the client's interpretation of their individual grid. As with other graphic representations, it would be vital for the client and therapist to collaborate on meanings and interpretations as well as how those may have changed over the years or how the client may want them to change in the future.

## Feminist Social Atom

The social atom is a technique developed in psychodrama by Moreno (1943). It is a graphic representation of a moment in time regarding relationships to people, entities, or even constructs. As an adaptation for feminist individual therapy, a clinician could ask clients to draw a circle or other symbol to represent themselves on a piece of paper. Next, the client who wanted to identify relational power could draw symbols to represent other people, entities, or constructs (such as patriarchal society) and each of these symbols could show by their relative size and proximity to the client's symbol how much power the client is experiencing them to have. For example, a spouse may be placed close to the client and have the same size symbol if power is shared. Alternatively, a workplace could be placed close to the client but could be large if the client is disempowered at work. The feminist intersectional therapist and client collaboratively examine this snapshot of proximity, power, and possible oppressions for consciousness raising. This kind of exercise can be used creatively to get a snapshot of the significant issues or concerns of the moment and inform any possible patterns where the client had not previously accessed awareness.

## Feminist Genogram

Genograms, initially developed by Bowen (1966), have a long history of use in family therapy. Genograms typically show three generations of a family tree using specific symbols and connecting lines to illustrate gender, relationships to each other, and even emotional closeness or distance (Bowen, 1966). Although feminist genograms can use traditional symbols, they can also be adapted to examine patterns or issues of power, oppression, and privilege in a family. For example, a feminist intersectional therapist could ask a client to create a genogram in session, with therapist assistance as needed, and then to identify in each generation or relationship who had power in the family dynamic. Was/is power connected to gender, age, race, career, or the intersection of any of the identities? How did the client learn about power in relationships? How did family relationships model the use of relational power? Genograms can be an excellent impetus for rich discussions around power and empowerment.

## Patriarchal Differentiation

Also, in family therapy (Bowen, 1966), the concept of differentiation of self allows the clients to individuate and become fully responsible for their decisions, free of their current or generational family influence. Bowen (1966) stated, "The terms *defining a self* or *working toward individuation* are essentially synonymous with *differentiation*" (p. 539). Józefczyk (2023) later added, "The degree to which human functioning depends on the convictions and expectations of others is represented by the constructs defined as *differentiation of self*" (p. 635). Differentiation does not mean rejecting the family (or societal) influence. Instead, it allows the client to deeply examine the embedded messages, power dynamics, and hierarchical roles that a client plays in their ecosystems.

This feminist intersectional theory application of differentiation shifts the focus from family differentiation to differentiating from the Eurocentric, heteronormative, Christian-dominant patriarchal constructs and norms that dominate society, cultures, and political systems. This allows the client a similar differentiation process through an examination of their (1) intersectional identities and their subsequent social positionality and determine satisfaction within the hierarchy of the world; (2) examining specifics of their privileges and oppressions within the dynamics of social and cultural norms; (3) experiences of being influenced to assimilate and or passively unconsciously assimilating to accept painful social and cultural norms through embedded messages; (4) beliefs to recognize if any destructive or oppressive social, cultural, or political messages have become internalized; and (5) limits that have been placed on their intersectional identities that may hinder their potential due to the larger ecosystems that dictate norms in society.

The goal of this feminist intersectional examination of the client's cultural and social norms is to empower the client to take ownership and responsibility for their own beliefs and differentiate from society the same way a healthy differentiation might take place from a family of origin as described by Bowen (1966). The beliefs or guidelines the client chooses in the future are fully conscious and fully responsible instead of being embedded into them unconsciously throughout the developmental process. This raised consciousness, and subsequent new context is now the client's to accept or reject.

## Reframe Problems as Related to the Patriarchy

As clients discuss their etiology of suffering, the feminist intersectional therapist can help the client reframe the issue to contextualize the role society has played in the formation of their views or explain how that may be contributing to the pain. The client is invited to examine the potential perception of society based on their intersectional identities, how the client may be viewed by society related to privilege and oppression, and whether these views have been internalized. For example, a client who may be having extramarital sexual relations may feel guilty about that fact or may feel that people will look poorly on them due to society's norms or both. Helping the client tease through which beliefs are their beliefs versus the larger social norms may help the client in decision-making. Does this client believe an open relationship may be better but is too afraid to examine this because of society's stigma?

## Assertiveness Experiments

The feminist theory grew from gender inequalities and oppression, particularly toward women. Historically, Western patriarchal norms have traditionally accomplished having women and other oppressed groups forced to be submissive and hide or restrict their expressions of self. This legacy lingers. Often, those embedded messages result in a need to become more assertive for oppressed people, while society does not necessarily encourage the oppressed to do so. Hence, many people in society lack assertiveness skills. Some people may react to oppression with aggression rather than with assertion. Once aggression is seen, they can become further dismissed and even rejected by society as behaving poorly or being damaged (particularly for people of color). One technique of feminist intersectional therapy is helping clients to unlearn skills of submission and learn skills to become more assertive. Assertiveness is defined here as advocating for oneself, a positional view, or others with intention and diligence. Assertive people are able to clearly state their ideas, desires, needs, opinions, and hopes in a situation, even if it is through tears, fears, or shaking body parts. Assertiveness has often been interpreted by the patriarchy as not feminine by nature, and so females who are assertive have often been labeled as "bitchy" "pushy," or even "nasty." A vital place where clients can gain assertiveness skills is within the therapy relationship where they can safely experience things like disagreeing with the feminist clinician and stating their own needs. The client needs to decide whether, how, and when they would like to generalize these skills to their larger environment. It is important to note that although women have traditionally been taught to not be assertive, there are many factors that contribute to oppressive voices. This is not just a women's issue; the intersectionality of oppressed identities will also interact with abilities and perceptions of assertiveness.

## Imposter No More

Clance and Imes (1978) coined the term "imposter phenomenon" to describe people who believe they have others fooled about their efficacy. This concept has become widespread throughout social, educational, and workplace settings, often called "imposter syndrome." "The impostor 'syndrome' refers to the notion that some individuals feel as if they ended up in esteemed roles and positions not because of their competencies, but because of some oversight or stroke of luck" (Feenstra et al., 2020, p. 1). To be an "imposter," one must feel like they are "faking" the competencies expected from a particular situation. The projected or real expectations are born in a patriarchal context with privileges and oppressions. In feminist intersectional therapy, the client and therapist collaboratively examine the social, cultural, and political constructs that underpin a client's "imposter syndrome." Once that examination happens, the client decides whether they would like to remain with those perceptions.

## Bibliotherapy/Cinema/Video Therapy

Feminist therapy has a tradition of using bibliotherapy with clients to help them raise consciousness (Worell & Remer, 2003). Later, films and videos began to be used similarly. Books and films can be used as psychoeducation or to spur discussions with clients about various issues. A feminist intersectional therapist could use books or films to examine patriarchal messages and influences, intersectional identities, relational or family issues, career possibilities, social justice, advocacy, losing and gaining power, and other relevant topics. Using bibliotherapy is also a feminist process as it shares information with clients, creating a more egalitarian foundation for discussion. Of course, feminist therapists would want to be familiar with a resource before referring it to a client. After reading or watching material, the client and clinician could have an organic discussion about the resource, or there could be a more structured approach with prepared questions, or clients could even journal about reactions and responses and then share those in sessions.

## Advocacy: Client-Centered

Advocacy has long been a part of feminist therapy. There is therapeutic value and power in helping others. Adler (1927/2009) suggested that "[n]ext to the striving for power, it is social feelings that plays the next most important role in the development of character" (p. 139). Since its beginning, advocacy has been an underpinning to feminist philosophy, feminist movements, and hence, feminist therapy. Feminist therapy aims to educate about social injustice and change systems of oppression to help the client engage in a healing process of social interest, community engagement, and creating support networks. Feminist advocacy must also not do harm. Many people who engage in feminist concepts, feminist therapy, advocacy, and empathy care greatly for others and become emotional when they see injustice and/or oppression that causes undue suffering. It is vitally important that the feminist therapist remains in the client's moments and does not place undue influence, verbally or nonverbally, on the client to take any particular action in response to any oppression they may be suffering. Clients must have autonomy to decide what sort of advocacy, if any, they want to engage in. For some clients, it may be dangerous to advocate for themselves in particular ways, which needs to be acknowledged and validated.

Feminist advocacy is often an organic outcome of therapy due to the nature of the process of examination, differentiation, and empowerment. What advocacy means must be defined solely by the client. Standing up for oneself in a difficult situation can be considered advocacy, as can fighting to change legislation, or making intentional parenting choices. There are many ways to resist patriarchal influences and challenge unjust systems. Deciding how and whether to be involved with advocacy efforts must always be the client's choice. If therapists coerce clients to engage in any particular advocacy efforts, they replicate the same patriarchal systems they seek to challenge. Any feminist clinician who influences a client, consciously or unconsciously, is abandoning the principles of feminist theory based on autonomy, freedom, and decisions free from social influence.

# Special Considerations with Feminist Intersectional Therapy

## Difficult Dialogues

As part of feminist intersectional therapy, topics that have traditionally been overlooked or left out are brought to the forefront. In early feminist therapy, this involved bringing gender into conversations and examining how gender is both impacted by and impacts client experiences. As stated earlier, intersectionality is now a focus of fourth-wave feminist therapy (acknowledging it began in the third wave) to bring multiple, overlapping, and dynamic social identities and locations into therapeutic work (Brown, 2018). Additionally, calls to decolonize therapy and therapeutic training point to the deeply embedded White supremacist past in which therapy was developed and in which it still functions today (Mullan, 2023).

This means that one of the things a feminist intersectional therapist has to be comfortable with is facilitating potentially difficult dialogues involving explorations of race, ethnicity, gender, ability, age, and so forth, and offering clients a way to examine these through lenses of privilege, oppression, and marginalization. In describing talking about race, Sue (2015) notes that this can churn up many emotions and defensiveness. That same can be said for consciousness-raising discussions around other social locations. A feminist intersectional therapist needs to continue to reflect on their own social identities and their comfort and discomfort in providing psychoeducation and facilitating discussions that may be challenging for them.

## Black Feminism, Womanist, and Mujerista Approaches

In the second wave of feminism, gender was the primary focus explored and was the stated focus of resistance toward patriarchal norms, rules/laws, and expectations as seen in the second-wave literature. Centering gender by White, middle-class, feminist therapists has disregarded how the gendered experience has been experienced in both similar and different ways depending on race (Brown, 2018; Collins, 2000; hooks, 1984/2015; Mullan, 2023). In her writings, hooks (1984/2015) discusses how the feminist movement long remained racist and focused on White women achieving more parity with White men within a maintained oppressive system that did not lift up Black women.

One of the responses to this exclusion was the development of womanist psychology. The term "womanist" was coined by Walker (1983), who defined it in part as follows:

> From Womanish. (Opp. of "girlish," i.e., frivolous, irresponsible, not serious.) A black feminist or feminist of color. From the black folk expression of mothers to female children, "You acting womanish," i.e., like a woman. Usually referring to outrageous, audacious, courageous or willful behavior. . . . A woman who loves other women, sexually and/ or nonsexually. Appreciates and prefers women's culture, women's emotional flexibility. . . . Loves the Folk. Loves herself. Regardless. . . . Womanist is to feminist as purple to lavender. (pp. xi–xii)

Womanist approaches are intersectional, respecting the multiple identities of Black women; they draw on survival strategies that are empowering, communal, and celebratory (Williams, 2005). Mujerista psychology is a womanist perspective developed by Latina women (Bryant-Davis & Comas-Díaz, 2016). For some Black clients, Latina clients, or clients from other minoritized groups, a womanist or mujerista approach may be consistent with their experiences. For therapists who have White privilege, it is recommended that they approach working from or teaching from these perspectives with humility, mindful of their privilege and focused on ending intersectional oppression for all (Bryant-Davis & Comas-Díaz, 2016).

## Working with Men

Historically, second-wave feminist therapy was focused on working with people who identified as female. This is no longer the case. People across the gender spectrum can be feminist therapists or clients of feminist therapists. This is because third-wave feminist theorists recognized that we are all impacted by living in the restrictive Eurocentric, heteronormative, Christian-dominant, patriarchal systems that oppress people intersectionally at different levels of privilege and oppression. People who identify as male, while traditionally thought of as being at the pinnacle of power in the patriarchy, are also oppressed within these systems and can, therefore, benefit from a feminist lens. Males have traditionally been socialized to repress many human feelings, such as fear or vulnerability, and have also been pressured to fulfill specific roles as providers and defenders. "Boys don't cry" has a long legacy in patriarchal systems. Feminist intersectional therapy can help male clients contextualize their development and its impact on their issues and life trajectories. This can help them decide, which values, beliefs, and roles they wish to intentionally retain and which they reject or need to alter to connect to their true selves.

# Feminist Intersectional Therapy Example

The client is a 53-year-old heterosexual, cisgender, Jewish, White woman who has owned a successful business for 22 years. The business manufactures medical equipment and employs approximately 250 people. The client owns a four-bedroom home in an affluent area and is able to financially afford anything she desires. She has never been married and has no children. She has a sister who has one child who is on the pervasive developmental spectrum and whom she often helps financially. She presents for therapy because she has been "down for the last year" and cannot seem to "get her groove back" when she felt happy. She thought she would try therapy because someone recommended it to her as a possible solution. She is a solution-focused person.

*First Contact:* The client called and left a message inquiring about the time commitment it would take to be involved in therapy. When the client was called back; the question of time commitment was left up to the client to decide. The client explained vaguely on the phone that she was just "off" and was not as productive as she normally had been in the past and wanted some "coaching" to become more productive and to enjoy work like she used to do when she was younger. The client made an appointment to come to the office, and at the first meeting, it was evident that the client was sad. She cried within minutes of entering the office. She apologized for crying and said that she did not know why this happened. In discussion, the client was told that this process is collaborative and that there was no magic; what we could do is sit and examine different thoughts and ideas together and see if any of them were helpful to her. Although she was clearly a boss to many people, in the therapy office she seemed to not hold any power at all. She was asked about how she felt and her answer was "vulnerable." In an attempt to flatten the power, the clinician truthfully said that she felt impressed and a bit intimidated by her accomplishments and status she had attained in the world.

*Honor Unique Narrative:* In the next session, the therapist asked for input about the first session. The client said that she felt understood but was also a little surprised that the therapist did not begin to tell her what she needed to do to "fix the problem." The therapist thanked her for her honesty and discussed more about the collaborative nature of the work. The therapist then asked her to share more about her situation. Over the next few sessions, the client expressed regret over not having had a relationship that produced a committed marriage and children. She was so focused on her career that she thought she did not want children. She recently experienced menopause and began to question her life choices of not having a spouse. When she goes out socially, people consistently question if she is married and has children, as if that is the model of success for a woman. Although she has friends, her friendships have been challenging to maintain. Because she works so many hours, her friends are often employees, so those friendships come with boundaries and barriers. She asked if she was having a "mid-life crisis," and together they explored what she meant by. She decided that this unhappy feeling actually has been with her longer than she realized. It has just more recently in the last year become unmanageable. She reported thoughts around meaninglessness and a lack of purpose.

*Contextualize and Expand Consciousness:* The client examined her life through her intersectional identities. She defined herself as a middle-aged woman who was heterosexual, able-bodied, not very attractive, not religious but raised Jewish, White, and financially secure. When asked to put a value on how she was most seen by society, she stated as a "middle aged unattractive woman." She said that each time someone asked her about her marital status or children, it reinforced that her biggest value to society was a wife and mother. While considering her Jewish heritage, when jokes are made about her not being able to get married so she had to marry a business, she experiences these comments as stereotypes about Jewish people and money. She acknowledged that when she reached menopause, she lost hope of ever "getting to" the part of her life that included marriage and children. Together with the therapist, she examined society's "scripts" about gender and age expectations. She realized that she had felt pressure throughout her adolescence and adulthood to try to be more physically attractive and to conform to social expectations of marrying and being a mother. She had sometimes felt like an outsider while she focused on her business but was also enormously proud of what she had built. When examining her intersectional identities of being Jewish and being female, she realized that although her family had not been outwardly religious, there had still been pressure from them for her to marry that was tied to their Jewish values about Jewish women. As she examined these perspectives, she realized that she had felt successful in her career but not in her identity as a woman. She thought she had failed in some aspects.

*Empower:* The client examined her beliefs by differentiating society's values from hers. She examined if she made choices around relationships and children or believed she had no choice. She acknowledged that she made choices because there were many avenues she did not pursue or investigate. The client shifted from having been too unattractive to find a partner and decided she made the choices to not have children. She had never said that before because she was afraid of how that would make her seem. Women who did not want to have children—what is wrong with them? She also decided to redefine what attractive meant. Instead of the word "attractive" (meaning to attract another) she replaced it with "beauty." Defining beauty from an existential perspective rather than a social perspective created a shift for her around her self-image. The image that she had from social beauty was tied to a Jewish cultural view of what a woman's role and beauty should entail. The existential view of beauty was about creation and meaning. Making medical equipment for disabled people and empowering and helping many families make a good living and thrive all seemed beautiful.

*Advocacy/Assertiveness:* The client decided to no longer entertain questions from people that made her feel less than others. When anyone asked about relationships, she and her therapist came up with ways to respond that quickly shut down those questions. Also, when people asked about children, she said she had 250 of them that she supports. She decided to start a small scholarship program to help fund higher education expenses for workers and/or their families. This program allowed her to "pay it forward" in a meaningful way in terms of financially helping others and demonstrating her care for them.

# Strengths and Challenges of Feminist Intersectional Therapy

There can be great strength in using a feminist intersectional therapy approach. This perspective adds rich context to clients' presenting issues and explores who clients are intersectionally, the ecosystems they inhabit, and their privileged and oppressed experiences. Adding this social, cultural and political context brings a holistic lens to therapeutic conceptualization and work. Striving for an egalitarian, power-sharing therapeutic relationship helps clients become more empowered within therapy and learn how to share power in other relationships.

There are also challenges in using a feminist approach. One example is the negative perception of "feminists" and of people who identify as feminists. Research has shown that there are still both positive and negative stereotypes of what "feminist" means. In Implicit Association Tests, participants have more quickly paired negative words with "feminist" over "traditionalist" (Jenen et al., 2008). Negative stereotypes, in particular, may keep people from identifying as feminists even when they endorse feminist values (McLaughlin & Aikman, 2020). Stigma against identified feminists has been found to lessen the desire to be friends with or date someone, though not to hire someone for a job (Anastosopoulos & Desmarais, 2015). In looking at the body of research on the stigma against feminists, many of the definitions of "feminist" align more with second-wave gender binaries and focus on only women's/girls' issues. What could this mean for therapists who openly identify as feminists? It could mean some clients self-select to come to them, and others do not. It could mean that feminist therapists can educate clients about how they define feminist and feminist therapy. It could also mean that feminist therapists could use much of what is offered in this book without explicitly identifying it as feminist; some clients may embrace the concepts without embracing the term. Of course, if clients do not embrace the approach or the term, feminist therapists will not force it onto them.

Another challenge to a feminist intersectional approach could be that clients identify with systemic pressures and influences and use that to exclude personal responsibility. Feminist intersectional therapists do not serve clients well when they only focus on oppressive systemic factors without empowering clients to resist systemic pressures, seek to change systems where possible, and consider advocacy for systems they cannot alter alone. Only focusing on blaming patriarchal influences could be quite disempowering for clients, which is the opposite of what feminist therapy aims to do.

Self-disclosure is another area that could be challenging for a feminist intersectional therapist. Wanting to "flatten the hierarchy," sharing more of ourselves with the client may be tempting. Feminist intersectional therapists must be mindful of self-disclosures; they must carefully, and with discernment, not shift the focus onto them and away from the client.

Lastly, some clients may not be looking for power sharing, therapist self-disclosure, or an egalitarian therapeutic relationship. Sometimes, a client wants the therapist to tell them what is wrong and what they must do to fix it. Such a client may even perceive the feminist intersectional therapist as less skillful or qualified if they do not have such an expert orientation. This may feel challenging for a feminist therapist who does not want to operate from that stance. In this situation, a feminist therapist could use education to explain their approach and highlight the work's collaborative nature and the reasons why that is valued. Ultimately, if a client does not want that therapeutic approach, and the therapist does not want to work without it, then the therapist facilitating referral options to other therapists may be the most empowering option for that client.

# What If?

What if the Western mental health system embraced the narrative lived experience of all people and held everyone in high esteem? Instead of "assessments and evaluations," mental health professionals could learn the client's lived experience without looking for the category (and codes) to assign to them.

What if an "intake" really meant getting to know someone and understanding their suffering rather than evaluating what the system thinks is wrong with them? What if the intake was just helping the client create safety and hold the pain together?

What if therapists never had to diagnose someone? How would therapy be different?

What if therapists all used words in describing suffering that did not have diagnostic implications? Instead of depression, they could use the term deep sadness. Alternatively, instead of borderline personality disorder, they could say "when your heart panics." How would this change the therapy?

# References

Adler, A. (1964). *The individual psychology of Alfred Adler*. HarperPerennial. (Original work published 1956)

Adler, A. (2009). *Understanding human nature*. Oneworld. (Original work published 1927)

Anastosopoulos, V., & Desmarais, S. (2015). By name or by deed? Identifying the source of the feminist stigma. *Journal of Applied Social Psychology, 45*, 226–242. https://doi.org/10.1111/jasp.12290

Ballou, M., Hill, M., & West, C. (2008). *Feminist therapy: Theory and practice*. Springer Publishing Company, LLC.

Bowen, M. (1966). The use of family theory in clinical practice. *Comprehensive Psychiatry, 7*(5), 345–374. https://doi.org/10.1016/S0010-440X(66)80065-2

Brown, L. S. (2018). *Feminist therapy* (2nd ed.). American Psychological Association.

Bryant-Davis, T., & Comas-Díaz, L. (2016). Introduction: Womanist and mujerista psychologies. In T. Bryant-Davis & L. Comas-Díaz (Eds.), *Womanist and mujerista psychologies: Voices of fire, acts of courage* (pp. 3–25). American Psychological Association.

Clance, P. R., & Imes, S. A. (1978). The imposter phenomenon in high achieving women: Dynamics and therapeutic intervention. *Psychotherapy Theory Research & Practice, 15*, 241–247. https://doi.org/10.1037/h0086006

Collins, P. H. (1990). Black feminist thought in the matrix of domination. In P. H. Collins, *Black feminist thought: Knowledge, consciousness, and the politics of empowerment* (pp. 221–238). Unwin Hyman.

Collins, P. H. (2000). *Black feminist thought*. Routledge

Crenshaw, K. W. (1991). Mapping the margins. *Stanford Law Review*, *43*(6), 1241–1299.

Evans, K. M., Kincade, E. A., & Seem, S. R. (2011). *Introduction to feminist therapy*. SAGE.

Feenstra, S., Begeny C. T., Ryan, M. K., Rink, F. A., Stoker, J. I., & Jordan, J. (2020, November). Contextualizing the impostor "syndrome." *Frontiers in Psychology*, *11*. https://doi:10.3389/fpsyg.2020.575024

Fuller, K. (2020). The "7 Up" intersectionality life grid: A tool for reflexive practice. *Frontiers in Education*, *5*(77), 1–15.

Hardy, K. V. (2023). *Racial trauma*. W. W. Norton.

hooks, b. (2015). *Feminist theory: From margin to center*. Routledge. (Original work published 1984)

Jankowski, P. J., & Hooper, L. M. (2012, September). Differentiation of self: A validation study of the Bowen theory construct. *Couple and Family Psychology: Research and Practice*, *1*(3), 226–243.

Jenen, J., Winquist, J., Arkkelin, D., & Schuster, K. (2008, July). Implicit attitudes towards feminism. *Sex Roles*, *60*, 14–20. https://doi.org/10.1007/s11199-008-9514-3

Józefczyk, A. (2023). Multigenerational transmission of differentiation of self: Toward a more in-depth understanding of Bowen's theory concept. *Journal of Marital and Family Therapy*, *49*, 634–653. https://doi.org:10.1111/jmft.12645

McLaughlin, K., & Aikman, S. N. (2020). That is what a feminist looks like: Identification and exploration of the factors underlying the concept of feminism and predicting the endorsement of traditional gender roles. *Gender Issues*, *37*, 91–124. https://doi.org/10.1007/s12147-019-09240-4

Moreno, J. L. (1943). Sociometry and the cultural order. *Sociometry*, *6*(3), 299–344.

Mullan, J. (2023). *Decolonizing therapy: Oppression, historical trauma, and politicizing your practice*. W. W. Norton.

Peterson, C., Maier, S. F., & Seligman, M. E. (1993). *Learned helplessness*. Oxford.

Rogers, C. R. (1995). *On becoming a person*. Houghton Mifflin. (Original work published 1961)

Sue, D. W. (2015). *Race talk*. Wiley.

Walker, A. (1983). *In search of our mothers' gardens: Prose*. Open Road Media.

Williams, C. B. (2005). Counseling African-American women: Multiple identities – multiple constraints. *Journal of Counseling and Development*, *83*, 278–283.

Worell, J., & Remer, P. (2003). *Feminist perspectives in therapy* (2nd ed.). Wiley & Sons.

Yalom, I. D. (1980). *Existential psychotherapy*. Basic Books.

# 6

# Feminist Intersectional Group Therapy

## *Kathleen McCleskey, Joanne Jodry, and Nicole Jackson Walker*

*Group dynamics, content, and process often reflect people attempting
to fit into social norms, comparing themselves to cultural standards,
and striving for significance in patriarchal hierarchies.*

Feminist theory's goals of consciousness raising, empowerment, intentional self-examination, and movement toward freedom from oppressive constructs can all be examined within the group therapy modality. Feminist intersectional therapy groups may offer specific benefits to clients that other theories may not include. Each group member brings their unique intersectional identity, personality, privileged and oppressed experiences, expectations, perceptions of power, and other personal factors into the group setting. Examining these feminist intersectional conceptualizations not only promotes self-awareness and empowerment but also creates an environment for empathy and understanding other unique experiences. Feminist therapy groups have the unique ability to help each member understand the self and the "other" through the lens of oppression, privilege, and power; group members can experience and examine complicated intersectional individual narratives. Feminist intersectional group therapy also aligns with equity and equality from an economic standpoint. Feminist group clinicians can provide services to more clients, often with a lower financial burden, which may create access for underserved, oppressed populations.

As with traditional group therapy underpinnings, the basic building blocks of feminist intersectional group work can be conceptualized in two broad areas: group content and group process (Jacobs et al., 2016). The uniqueness of feminist group theory is that content will include consciousness-raising discussions and activities around the Eurocentric, patriarchal, Christian-dominant, heteronormative messaging that each person has been conditioned to understand as "normal" or even "good." Content might also include discussions of individual power and empowerment, assertiveness, and advocacy to help the group members become empowered individually and relationally, including moving toward freedom from the chains of social, cultural, political, and developmental conditioning.

Feminist intersectional group process can be thought of as how group members react to the feminist content, the conscious and unconscious thoughts and emotions that result, and how those are enacted in group interactions. It includes all the unspoken dynamics of how group members interact with the group leader, the other members, and the content. Feminist group therapists want to be attuned to how power is being held in the group, including any overtones of bias toward the leader or other members, particularly in terms of Western patriarchal messages, norms, and so on. As with all group leaders, feminist group therapists need to be aware of both content and process and need to be able to respond to them "in the moment."

It is important to note not only what is discussed but also who is speaking, not speaking, engaged or not, connecting with whom, and so forth, and how that develops over time. In the initial stages of the group, a feminist group therapist might consider focusing on questions such as these: Who speaks more/most in group sessions? Is that related to feeling power? How do other members react to more dominant members? Does this have anything to do with privilege or oppression histories? Since members who talk more are, in effect, dominating the sessions more, are they aware of that potential impact on others in the group? Are others aware of that impact? How could dominant patriarchal messages be playing out in this? Are patterns of oppression, privilege, or marginalization repeated in group dynamics? Who is not talking? Who is not being listened to by other members, or by the therapist(s)? Is this a pattern of not being heard for that group member? Tracking and responding to such dynamics are important at every group stage but may be most important in early stages as this is when behaviors become normalized. Any member feeling lost or marginalized may feel less invested and have less desire to engage, especially if patterns of oppression experienced outside of group sessions are being repeated inside them. Any members feeling privileged or empowered to speak and also may examine why and how that has developed.

## Feminist Intersectional Stages and Healing Factors: Building on Yalom's Theory

As we know from traditional group theories, groups tend to develop through stages from the beginning stages, through the middle stages, and the ending stages (Corey et al., 2022; Jacobs et al., 2016; Yalom, 1985; Yalom & Leszcz, 2020). Much of modern group practice is still derived from Yalom's group concepts with existential undertones. Yalom (1985) discusses the initial stage of hesitancy when members try to find their roles and identities in the group. A feminist intersectional group therapist might use this stage to discuss concepts around intersectional identities and how the Eurocentric, heteronormative, Christian-dominant, patriarchal, cultural, social, and political ecosystems may impact their identities and views of themselves. In Yalom's (1985) second stage, conflict and rebellion can arise when group members strive to create a "social pecking order" (p. 304). Feminist group therapists have an opportunity in this stage to help the group understand itself as a microcosm for the larger society. There can be an opportunity to discuss ideas of social hierarchies, embedded developmental messages, and cultural values decided by the historically privileged people. The third of Yalom's (1985) stages is when groups, after experiencing previous conflicts, can create group cohesion and become profoundly productive. At this stage, the feminist therapist should ensure that cohesion does not come at the expense of losing individual voices or members feeling pressure to assimilate. The feminist therapist might use this stage to address intersectional identity concepts around individual and group empowerment.

Yalom also proposed "therapeutic factors" (Yalom & Leszcz, 2020, p. 10) that many group members experience in group therapies (p. 3,4). A feminist group therapist might consider some of the following feminist overlays, adaptations, rejections, and acceptances of some of Yalom's group therapeutic factors (Yalom, 1985; Yalom & Leszcz, 2020). Yalom's (1985) therapeutic group factors include "1) Instillation of hope, 2) Universality, 3) Imparting Information, 4) Altruism, 5) The corrective recapitulation of the primary family group, 6) Developing of socializing techniques, 7) Imitative behavior, 8) Interpersonal learning, 9) Group cohesiveness, 10), Catharsis, 11) Existential factors" (p. 1).

## Patriarchal Injuries Are *Universal*

Although many clients may not recognize injuries caused by social, cultural, and political constructs, all people have intersectional identities that result in combinations of privilege and oppression. People in much of the Western hemisphere have developed in a Eurocentric, Christian-dominant, heteronormative, patriarchal social and cultural setting, with connected norms, values, and expectations. These commonalities of social assimilation and embedded conditioning can be explored in groups, and members can support each other in recognizing individuals all being equal when hierarchical norms are removed. The universal recognition and acknowledgment of oppressive injuries from ecosystems, coupled with validation and support from group members, could have healing therapeutic properties.

## *Catharsis* of Embedded Passive Accepted Messages from Society

The feminist group therapist might facilitate discussions of cultural and social norms that are embedded and accepted as normal. Group discussions of whether norms are healthy, unhealthy, oppressive, or functional may help clients raise consciousness. The feminist group therapist might help group members collectively explore where embedded messages are rooted culturally and socially; these messages often turn into deeply held beliefs. Examining these beliefs and then consciously accepting them, rejecting them, or modifying them may help clients intentionally form future decisions. Having this new awareness can be powerful and discussions could potentially lead to catharsis for members of the group as they release emotions that have been tied to patriarchal norms and expectations.

## Recognizing Voices That *Recapitulate* Early Social Injuries of Oppression

Recapitulation of early injuries often appears in groups, among members and between members and leaders. Unlike Yalom's (1985) suggestion of focusing the recapitulation on the family of origin, the feminist group therapist might focus on processing oppressive injuries from the Western patriarchal cultural/social norms and constructs that may have been internalized and caused personal suffering. Feminist group leaders can help members explore these injuries and track if/how those same dynamics may play out in the group. If they do, group leaders can use immediacy to notice that out loud, ultimately allowing for recapitulative work. One of the most powerful group work experiences can be facilitating members to have a new understanding of a previous injury that results in wholeness and/or some sense of peace going forward. This work can help empower members to expand their abilities to face similar injuries in the future.

## *Imparting Information*

Feminist group leaders can share information about patriarchal norms, messages, and expectations and invite members to reflect on their own experiences of those. They also impart information about how intersectional identities and social locations create unique experiences for people. Group members can also impart information through their own stories of oppressions and privileges they have experienced and how that impacts them. Information imparted by either the leader or members can vary based on the group's purpose. For example, in a group for anger management, the leader can both share and ask for information regarding gendered or racial responses to being angry that are endorsed and reinforced by patriarchal norms.

## Development of *Socializing Techniques* and *Imitative Behavior* from an Egalitarian Frame

The feminist intersectional therapist uses the group as a microcosm to help clients learn empowered socialization and realize new choices of how to relate to people free of social judgments, false hierarchies, and privileged or oppressive dynamics. Group members can identify where they learned social behaviors and who they model them on, consciously and unconsciously. Feminist group leaders can help clients make decisions about how they would or would not like to imitate people now, including specific traits to emulate or not.

## Relating to Others *Interpersonally* free from Oppression and Restrictions

The feminist therapist helps facilitate an atmosphere of healing in many ways. One way is allowing clients to share experiences of social and cultural oppression and how those injuries or internalized messages may have impeded their growth. Members will have differing levels of intersectional power, privilege, and oppression; some may have guilt for having privilege, or anger toward oppressive systems; neither of these is a goal, although either/both might need to be addressed. For all group members, interpersonal empowerment is the goal. Members can determine if any of their interpersonal behaviors rest on or incorporate oppressive social dynamics. Feminist group leaders foster authentic, egalitarian interpersonal group interactions. This lets members "try on" new ways of interacting with others with full awareness of how privilege and oppression can mar interpersonal exchanges and restrict people from authentically sharing themselves and receiving from others. After learning these skills, clients can be more empowered to authentically interact with others free from oppression and restrictions.

## *Group Cohesion* without Patriarchal Constraints

The feminist clinician can help group members gain insights and learn new behaviors around goals of equality versus hierarchies, empowerment versus the need for power, empathy versus sympathy, and ego realities versus the unknown. Members can be encouraged to take risks by genuinely sharing thoughts, feelings, and experiences, being open to others' sharing, and supporting each other in this vulnerability and authenticity. The group might develop cohesiveness through members supporting each other's intersectional identities, individual power, self-advocacy, freedom to question everything, and freedom to make choices without unconscious, embedded messages.

## *Altruism* and Social Justice

Advocacy and social justice are some of the historical roots of feminist group theory. As Adler (1927/2009) suggested, social interest in others can be curative: "Community spirit, or social feeling, is influenced both by a person's feelings of inferiority and by the compensatory striving for power" (p. 139). The feminist group therapist encourages members to explore external altruism/advocacy as healing factors; however, the feminist group leader must not impose these. Social justice and advocacy have an extensive range (e.g., self-care, parenting decisions, or marching in protests) and it is important to not expect members to embrace these.

## *Hope Is Instilled* for Empowerment and *Existential Factors*

One goal for feminist group therapy is to help each group member find hope through empowerment and choices free of automatic, embedded messages. When group members have a chance to analyze their embedded beliefs and raise their consciousness, it allows more existential freedom of choices to be available. This might help add to hope and meaning for the group and group members. At the same time, group members may be more sensitized to oppressive patriarchal systems and their active or passive participation in those. The feminist group leader can strive to help group members navigate oppressive systems while also taking ownership of how they can resist perpetuating systems that marginalize and oppress people. This resistance can lead to hope that change will ripple beyond the self.

# Feminist Intersectional Group Possible Counterintuitive Therapeutic Factors

## Co"we"siveness

The notion of fitting in and being accepted by a group may be complicated by feminist values of individual examination and possible rejection of the Western patriarchal oppressive systems. It is important that the group facilitator skillfully promotes cohesion around members accepting each other's intersectional identities rather than based on assumptions or oppressive ecosystems. Group cohesion is encouraged through common respect for the equality of all, supporting intersectional identity explorations, respecting the examination of ecosystems, and not needing to conform to any oppressive norms.

## Un-universality

The concept of universality in groups helps clients realize that they are not "[u]nique in their wretchedness, that they alone have certain frightening or unacceptable problems, thoughts, impulses and fantasies" (Yalom, 1985, p. 7). In fourth-wave feminist intersectional therapy, this concept might be confusing. If people have different intersectional identities, and all people experience society differently, where is the universality in feminist group therapy? The feminist group facilitator must help the group distinguish between common human conditions that most people share and the intersectional differences in their psychological impacts, social reactions, and levels of oppression. If not aware of this, the feminist group therapist could alienate people by not recognizing these nuances.

## "No"-norming

Yalom (1985) suggested that the construction of norms in the group, "[a]re created reactively early in the life of the group, and once established, are difficult to change" (p. 118). In feminist intersectional group work, co-constructing norms for a group will be a collaborative process. This allows the feminist group leader to notice if members are endorsing rules or norms that may replicate any oppressive dynamics of external systems. For example, some groups traditionally have rigid rules about late-arriving members potentially not being allowed into the group. There is therapeutic reasoning for starting and ending sessions on time; might there also be room to collaborate on such a policy? If some members, for example, rely on public transportation and cannot easily get to the group until 15 minutes after the start time, perhaps the group can collaboratively decide to change the start time to support those members. Norms can be developed that are not simply directives of what to do or not, but also how to create and support an environment of respect and growth with considerations for privilege and oppression.

## "All"truism

In therapeutic groups, clients "[r]eceive from giving, not only as part of the reciprocal giving receiving sequence but also from the intrinsic act of giving" (Yalom, 1985, p. 14). Through a feminist group, members can understand intersectional experiences different from theirs. This deepens members' sense of empathy and could potentially lead each member to connect and want to help each other. The skillful feminist group therapist must continue to monitor the power dynamics, defensiveness, and oppressive expressions to allow each member to explore their intersectional privilege and oppression with respect and support from all. Members sharing themselves authentically and honestly can be a gift to other members, who can better understand commonalities and differences among them.

# A Feminist Intersectional Group Model

## Egalitarian Transparency Stage

In this orientation stage, transparency of the group process is critical. The feminist group therapist will explain the intersectional feminist approach being used to facilitate the group and will encourage clients to voice fears, concerns, or other inquiries about any part of that process. Feminist theory concepts of empowerment, societal context, and so on, should be explained. The egalitarian nature of the therapeutic relationship is explained and discussed. The goal is to assist members in being conscious of the expectations of exploration and make fully informed consent.

It is important from the beginning of the group process that the clients understand the egalitarian nature of the group process and that every member is valued equally, including the therapist. As group members begin role induction and building trust, the therapist can facilitate discussion topics using a social contextual frame, setting the tone for the feminist intersectional approach. Creating group rules and norms is a collaborative experience rooted in respect for each other and in honoring commonalities and differences.

Power is a central focus of feminist therapy and members may initially see the therapist as the expert. This power differential needs to be addressed with transparency to redistribute power in the group. One strategy is to demystify the experience and image of the therapist. The feminist therapist has expertise through training and experience, and members are each the experts in their own lives and experiences. Neither of these kinds of expertise is valued more than the other. The therapist might also use self-disclosure to help flatten the hierarchy. Self-disclosure is a double-edged sword and must be used with precision. However, it is important that self-disclosure does not unintentionally take the power in the group. For example, if a feminist therapist shares all their degrees and expertise, which is truthful, it may further intimidate some members. Helpful self-disclosure can provide members with a human connection to the feminist therapist. As with any therapeutic self-disclosure, it is important not to shift the attention to the therapist.

In this initial stage, an introduction to ecological systems and to the historical Eurocentric, Christian-dominant, heteronormative, patriarchal cultural, social, and political constructs can begin. This can be introduced as a context around some of the group's issues. When doing any psychoeducation, the power is again shifted to the "teacher." If psychoeducation is possible as a group discussion rather than as a lecture, allowing different members to become leaders with prompters might serve the group's power dynamic better.

## Patriarchal Differentiation Stage

In this transitioning stage, concepts of differentiation from societal norms and systems begin. Bowen (1985/2004) introduced the concept of differentiation from the family of origin and defined differentiation as "[t]he degree to which one fuses or merges into another self in a close emotional relationship" (p. 200). Concepts of differentiation and individuation can also apply to the interactions between a person and their society of origin based on their intersectional identity. This stage of patriarchal differentiation includes group members deeply examining their values, thoughts and behaviors and how they arrived at them.

In this phase, the group members will learn to fully identify their examined values versus unexamined automatic embedded social and cultural messages. The feminist group therapist might offer insights and techniques around the differentiation process with society's cultural, social, and political norms. This can include psychoeducation about societal oppressing and privileging messages, values, norms, and expectations. Members can evaluate how their values and beliefs formed within the context of society, which may include unexamined patriarchal assumptions. Deconstructing these can free the members to refine their beliefs and values. This does not mean rejecting cultural or societal norms, only examining and being fully conscious of them. This group stage leaves much room for intersectional identity discussions, internal and external conflicts, internalized oppression or privilege, healthy or unhealthy transference, and whether there is a desire for shifting of individual roles. In a changing world, group members may be feeling new emotions based on new experiences within collective ecosystems. For some, parts of the ecological system that may have been less important in the past may have moved to the forefront based on individual experiences.

Sociological conceptual topics (cultural divide, politics, race, etc.) might either connect to psychological topics causing distress or conversely, may influence group members to ignore or disengage from the larger macrosystems.

One focus for these discussions during the transitioning differentiation stage is the importance of developing the empathetic ability to understand that someone else's intersectional experience is different from one's own and is also equally important and valued. Therapists may view this stage as an expansion of everyone's understanding of many ways of being and how that may help in the differentiation process with the Western patriarchal constructs that limit people.

The goal in this stage is ultimately to come to a deeper understanding of oneself and of others, recognizing how Western patriarchal messages, norms, and expectations have impacted all. It is hoped that members can believe in the equal value of each member's individual intersectional experience. If emotional responses and defensive stances emerge, a full understanding of the other is no longer possible. The group leader can help group members understand that the defense of personal positions is often based on a desire for the particular construct they are defending to remain in place. Sometimes it can be fearful to challenge thoughts if their previous life choices have been based on existing constructs where they feel a sense of "knowing" or safety in them. Fromm (1969) postulated,

> Once the stage of complete individuation is reached and the individual is free from these primary ties, he is confronted with a new task; to orient and root himself in the world and to find security in other ways other than those which were characteristic of his preindividualistic existence. (p. 24)

The patriarchal differentiation process involves helping the group member to fully understand their own and others' experience while knowing they can still choose to keep their previous beliefs and positions. If a group member has newly raised consciousness about a topic and has fully examined it, it is a patriarchal differentiated experience. They can then decide to keep their position, values, and beliefs, or change them, having deeper awareness of conscious and unconscious embedded thoughts and taking full responsibility for current stances.

## Collective and Individual Empowerment Stage

In this phase, group members become more aware and empathetic to intersectional identity oppressions and experiences of self and others and can begin to decide on corrective experiences internally and externally. Members have begun to be more personally aware, supportive, and empowered. The group can put individual and collective issues and concepts in a raised consciousness context, remembering that all values are equal. Group discussions can be grounded in members feeling more interpersonal freedom from oppressive social constraints, labels, and expectations. Members can encourage each other to embrace their uniqueness and not allow Western patriarchal social expectations to create personal suffering; they can likewise be freer from imposing those expectations onto others. Members can be encouraged to notice and give feedback on positive and nonhelpful expressions of expectations, norms, and beliefs. A greater sense of empathy and less need for defensiveness may expand the clients' possible ways of being and allow them a fuller life, freer from social constraints.

Also, in this stage, members can embrace conscious or unconscious recapitulation of previous societal experiences. Whether trying on new beliefs or embracing old beliefs with conscious understanding, this phase of the group will allow clients a safe place to explore the relationships they would like to enhance or create with the external world. Clients can process the benefits and challenges of implementing new freedoms from oppressive norms regarding thoughts and behaviors.

## Advocacy and Social Justice Stage

During this last stage of feminist intersectional group therapy, it is important to reflect on members' developments both individually and collectively. The group can discuss new consciousness of thoughts and recognize what each member has experienced as well as what support they have given each other as a collective group. Clients can plan for how to continue evolving in self-exploration and empowerment.

As with most groups, the ending phase can become painful due to the loss of the group. To help the transition, the feminist intersectional group leader can assist members in considering how to keep growth momentum going. This might include sharing their experiences through mentorship of others or through social justice work, or in practicing new behaviors of self-empowerment. It is important to note that advocacy and social justice come in many forms. Feminist group leaders can facilitate discussions of advocacy and social justice work, but they do not impose any expectations or requirements. Personal empowerment and self-advocacy are essential for each member of the group, but that means different things to different people. If a member would like to commit to social justice or social action to create social change, that can also become part of their continued growth. However, no one should be judged based on whether they are more vocal and active in making personal or social changes. All decisions are equal when made with full consciousness.

# Feminist Intersectional Group Therapy Activities or Tools

Historically, by design, second-wave feminist therapy is loosely constructed and lacks specific applications and edicts that must be followed. Fourth-wave feminist intersectional therapy seeks to add possible applications to spark creative usage of the therapy. There is no one correct method to apply it. Several possible feminist intersectional therapeutic tools can be used during different stages of the feminist intersectional group process model. To promote egalitarian empowerment, a feminist group leader might discuss possible applications with the group and encourage group members to decide whether and when one of these tools may be helpful. Each possible activity can be done creatively based on the group's desire. They can be creatively facilitated through many modalities such as written, oral, or action methods. This is up to the group. All choices are honored. Some existing techniques that are rooted in feminist therapy can easily be adapted to group work. Additionally, more traditional clinical techniques can be adapted using a feminist intersectional lens and applied to group therapy.

## Power Analysis (Adapted from Second-Wave Feminist Therapy)

Group members identify where they have power in their lives, where they feel disempowered, where they may give their power away to others, and what the deciding factors for each might include. Each group member can identify the different people in their lives and examine who is more or less powerful in their interactions. Often, themes begin to emerge by gender, race, emotional responses, desires, authoritarian hierarchies, and the like, that uncover patterns of power or disempowerment. This gives group members information to consider in potentially making changes. If they consciously understand when they feel empowered, they can build on that; when they feel disempowered, they can examine how they are denied power or how they give power away. The group can then help each other find ways to gain power in situations or leave things as they are. All choices are equal.

## Gender Analysis (Adapted and Updated from Second-Wave Feminist Theory)

Group members might consider the constraints that focus on their gender role and how that may have created opportunities and limits in all aspects of their lives. It may be difficult for some members to not include other intersecting identities, so each person may customize their gender identities as they most feel appropriate. Discussions may center on social expectations of their gender in terms of family/relational roles, career choices, hobbies, self-efficacies around fixing things or solving problems, education, emotional restrictions, gender identity, gender expression, and experiences of privilege and oppression. Members can examine how they may have constricted experiences because of these societal expectations. Ultimately, members can decide if they are aligned with the Western patriarchal constructs that were embedded in their development or if they would like to alter or reject them. Members can discuss what positive and/or negative feedback they may get from society, friends, or family if they reject patriarchal expectations and make individual decisions about what to do.

## Feminist Intersectionality Explorations and Analysis

It can be helpful for group members to explore their intersecting identities. The concept of intersectionality came from Black feminist thought, and the term "intersectionality" was coined by Crenshaw (1989, 1991) to describe the overlapping, interlocking, irreducible dynamics of oppression that were sustained by the criminal justice system toward Black females such that racism and sexism, taken as independent effects, could not explain the gendered racism or racial sexism they experienced.

Intersectional identities can be identified and reflected upon by each group member. There are several ways in which intersectionality of group members can be explored in groups. As with other techniques, this could be done within group sessions, or it could be done privately and then processed together in group sessions. This work could be done for the sake of exploring intersectionality as consciousness-raising and for empowerment, or it could be done more specifically in connection with the topic of the group.

The feminist group facilitator might begin by explaining the many identities that each person may hold. Each member would deeply explore all social identities (race, gender, affectional orientation, religion, ability/disability, age, etc.). Group members might consider all the multiple identities they embody and do a snapshot of how these identities are weighed in importance for them in the present moment. Identities might have more weight at different times throughout life and in certain situations, so clients might also want to focus on their identities with this therapeutic group. There could be a discussion or exercise exploring which identities cannot be seen in isolation or reduced to one construct—what are the intersections, from an internal "felt" level, and from an external "treated as" level. Collins and Bilge (2020) suggest, "For many individuals, this focus on the social construction of intersecting identities that can be differently performed from one setting to the next has been a space of individual empowerment" (p. 167). Group members might be encouraged to discuss how they embrace, hide, or ignore each of their identities in society. Once identities are established and discussed, the group may want to discuss how their identities might incite privilege or oppression in the larger social and cultural norms. This is a complicated task, because each identity might have both privilege and oppression in different situations. Ideally, group members should be able to deeply understand each other's full experience in the world and build empathy for other struggles.

Another way to examine intersectional identities in groups could be to explore them through the Matrix of Domination (Allan, 2006; Collins, 2009). In the Matrix of Domination (Allan, 2006; Collins, 2009), four domains describe how oppressive power is organized. The Structural domain encompasses laws and policies that reflect dominant norms. On this level, interconnected systems can keep reproducing oppression through laws and policies. The Disciplinary domain is the level that reinforces the laws and policies from the Structural domain and any changes made to them. It encourages surveillance and compliance with the dominant, oppressive structure. The Hegemonic level interacts with all other levels. It includes ideologies, values, and norms that reinforce or "explain" oppression. It can result in internal as well as external oppression. Lastly, the Interpersonal domain is the domain that each person lives in, where daily experiences of oppression, privilege, and marginalization occur. Collins (2009) states no one is totally oppressed or privileged. This level is where intersectional identities are lived out through experiences. The interpersonal level is also where a person connects to others in healing and empowering ways, finding ways to resist oppression and domination from other levels.

Using this Matrix of Domination (Collins, 2009), the feminist therapist might explore each level and how members and the collective group are oppressed or privileged. If the group is focused on a specific topic (anxiety, stress, interpersonal issues, career work, etc.), how are the levels of domination connected to intersectional identities?

## Definitions of Success

Success is often defined in the West in a Eurocentric, Christian-dominant, patriarchal, capitalistic frame. Western school systems hierarchies reward college-bound students who are academically higher-achieving. Some values are celebrated in the workplace (ambition, motivation, and having a future orientation) while others may be less valued (creativity, empathy, or having a present orientation). Standardized tests, common to public schools, send messages about what is successful in society: math and English.

This feminist intersectional group therapy activity allows the group to redefine what it means to live a successful life without the constraints of society's definitions. Group members can first generate a list of what is perceived as successful and what are societal messages about success. Members can then, individually or collaboratively, generate a list of alternative definitions of success. The group leader can help members compare and contrast the two lists. Members can decide if their lives are successful the way they are at present or if changes can be made based on any new definitions of success. No action needs to be taken; the goal is to create a higher consciousness of awareness around the self and others.

This might be a chance for a feminist group leader to add discussions about existential issues of meaning looking at the larger realities of life such as Yalom's (1980) universally shared concerns of meaning, death, isolation and freedom and responsibility. Often, considering these existential issues moves people from the daily transactions and stresses of life to other realms of existence where different perspectives of success can be found.

## Challenges to Patriarchal Power and Disempowered Images

Embedded images of patriarchal values become so normalized that clients are often unaware of their potential impact. Clients may think in imagery, which may affect self-empowerment or other self-assigned roles. For example, when clients think of "power," is it gendered? Is "nurturing" gendered? What does a "boss" look like? Another potential example is the image of God. For Westerners, the image of God is often a White male. Chaplin (1999) wrote, "Ideas about a male god with ultimate power over everything have a profound effect on our unconscious feelings about men and women, and about fathers and male authority figures in particular" (p. 10). How does the White male image affect a woman of color's sense of empowerment? These are all individual experiences that can be explored. Harmful images to the self or the collective might be identified by the group. Certain conscious and unconscious images about bosses, kindness, empathy, leaders, scientists, and others can be given as examples to help the group identify their own potentially oppressive images. Consciously replacing harmful images could be an individual or group goal.

## Assertiveness (Adapted from Second-Wave Feminist Theory)

Assertiveness is a behavior of empowerment. Group members can discuss times when they were assertive, aggressive, or passive, define the difference between these types of responses, and analyze whether they were happy with each outcome. The group might discuss scenarios currently affecting them and what these scenarios might look like with assertive actions. This could include role plays, discussions, and/or self-reflection. If the group has previously completed a power analysis (mentioned previously), they might discuss how to be assertive with people they feel have power over them. A collective discussion might be beneficial generally and individually of how different people become less assertive or more assertive based on social roles, cultural expectations, and/or learned helplessness.

## Ecological Analysis

Bronfenbrenner (2005) created the ecological systems model with a "systematic understanding of the processes of human development as a joint function between the person and environment" (p. 107). In the feminist ecological analysis, after an explanation about the different layers of the ecosystems as conceived by Bronfenbrenner (1979) or an adaptation of that model, each group member can personalize their intersectional experiences within the microsystem, mesosystem, exosystem, and macrosystem (Bronfenbrenner, 1979; Bronfenbrenner & Evans, 2000; Rosa & Tudge, 2013). This will allow group members to understand how cultural, community, and world problems have interacted with their psyche. Discussions can include the differences in the systems per member, areas of privilege and areas of oppression, areas of power and areas of having little or no power; these will potentially help members to understand how much suffering may be caused by social and cultural norms, world events, community issues, social injustices, and so on. Additional intentional examinations might help clients understand an evolving world and how there may be a desire to adjust power, perceptions, and behaviors as the ecosystem changes.

## Labels Analysis

Each group member may want to discuss their use of categories and labels to define themselves and others. Beginning with the self, each member can discuss names they call themselves (internally and/or externally). They might also discuss the ways that other people label them, including doctors, teachers, judges, family members, friends, and so on. These names can range from pathologies to indications of skills or intellect to jokes about incompetence or gender. This exercise may work best in a written format so that the depth of label consideration can be comprehensive. Each group member can discuss with the group how labels might impact people's possibilities. Each client decides whether they want to keep labels or discard them for the future. There can be a ceremony for labels to be put down, released, or rejected and a discussion about how to resist taking them on in life.

## Exploring Embedded Messages and Oppressive Schemas

Each group member might look at their intersectional identities (see earlier exercise) and examine what social messages were embedded in their experiences based on their gender, sexuality, race, nationality, socioeconomic status, and so forth, by their immediate communities and by the larger Western patriarchal culture. Following Downing and Roush's (1985) concept of embedded messages happening as a "passive acceptance" (p. 698), group members will analyze, perhaps prompted by the feminist group therapist, if they have accepted things that they actually think are oppressive messages. Examples might include "boys will be boys," "Black men are dangerous," "women who are sexually open and free are sluts," "poor people are lazy," and so on. The group can examine the impacts of such messages and decide how to respond to them.

## Group Power Monitoring

The entire group should become mindful of when individual members might be gaining or losing power in the group. Collectively, solutions to maintain the equality of the power in the group should be decided. It might be natural for people who do not feel empowered to slip into roles of disempowerment as a comfort zone, or for people used to being in power to dominate the group. Group members should learn to recognize when they feel their power is low or when they may be taking power from other members. Simple group check-ins around "How powerful do you feel today?" or "Is anything taking your power from you today?" might set the tone for this recognition and monitoring.

## Bibliotherapy and Cinematherapy

The group may collectively decide to read a book or watch a movie to focus discussions on social differentiation or empowerment. As a group, all members need to embrace the activities and not be pushed into them to please others. If all of members would like to make this part of the therapy, each member should have an opportunity to nominate a book or movie for discussion. Group members can collaboratively decide on one to employ. This activity can be empowering because it can potentially be a form of self-care for members. Importantly, not all clients can read, can read well, have time to read, can afford to read, or even like to read. Likewise, not all clients can afford television, paid movies, streaming services, or other forms of nonessentials. These all need to be considered. With films, collective decisions can be made about watching in session or outside group meetings. Discussions of books or films can include societal and cultural themes, portrayals of power, and patriarchal messaging. Group members can discuss these in terms of ones they have experienced, endorse, want to refine or reject, and so on.

## Social Justice and Action

The group can discuss topics of social justice on all ecosystem levels. This range spans from individual empowerment to a social justice movement. Discussions can explore how social justice and/or advocacy can be healing or therapeutic. Importantly, each member decides how they want to engage or not, and there should be no judgment of any choices. All decisions are equal if they are made on the basis of a higher consciousness and freedom to choose. It is important that clients do not pressure or belittle other members who do not embrace the same levels of passion for the same topics. Existential journeys are different for all people, and that tone needs to be set early in the group process. Social justice and advocacy are important aspects of feminist work, but we do not use pressure to force people to participate in it.

## Feminist Intersectional Genograms

The feminist group can create their family genograms. This is a technique borrowed from family systems theory (Bowen, 1985/2004) where at least three generations of a family are depicted graphically and then information about members' relationships is indicated. A feminist genogram might use a specific lens by exploring power in family dynamics and relationships—who has/had power and who did not, including the group member; exploring family patterns of oppressive or privileged messages in terms of career, relationships, parenting, and so forth; investigating supportive and healing people in the family network; or identifying those family figures that clients wish to emulate and why. In a deeper exploration, group members may discuss how their linage of power dynamics and oppressive or privileging messages impact them today.

## Social Atom

The group members might explore their individual lives, relationships and perceptions through the use of a social atom, a technique borrowed from psychodrama (see, e.g., Dayton, 2005). Traditionally, a social atom maps a person's social and other relationships in terms of emotional closeness at the time of the exercise, in the past, or in an ideal future. One way to create a social atom is as follows: the member draws a symbol on a sheet of paper and adds symbols for other people, institutions, and the like, with symbol proximity and size indicating closeness or distance as well as importance or impact. A feminist therapist can adapt the use of social atoms to depict social and cultural interactions and/or power. Members can include not only people, but also environments (work, school) as well as oppressions and privileges—racism, sexism, ageism, cissexism, religious intolerance, ableism, and so on—represented in terms of their presence, size, closeness, intersections, and impact. Power in relationships can also be depicted using proximity and size dimensions. Discussion can then process members' social atoms.

## Narratives with Patriarchal Frames and Early Childhood Patriarchal Injuries

As group members share their individual experiences with other members, it may be helpful to reframe some of the experiences with a feminist lens. A feminist group leader can listen for and point out themes of where the power lies in childhood situations, whether members express guilt or feelings of self-doubt for not fitting into society, and any overall fears about being different from patriarchal norms and expectations that they were exposed to. These potentially oppressive and limiting norms may have been assumed as truth and been internalized by members, who may then have developed self-doubt, self-hate, or a lack of self-efficacy based on notions that all people are equal, and everyone has the same opportunities (Hardy, 2023). Reframing self-messages from earlier development may be helpful for members' empowerment.

## Internalizing Interpersonal Consciousness Turned into New Behaviors . . . or Not

This is a process whereby a group member has cognitively learned something about their privileges and/or oppressions. They may have a corrective emotional experience in an interpersonal context. If new thoughts, "aha" moments, or higher awareness happen, the member might be asked what they would like to do with this new awareness behaviorally . . . or not. Members are not pressured or rushed to make behavioral changes but can be asked to reflect on any new awareness.

# Feminist Intersectional Group Process Example

## Stage 1 Egalitarian Transparency Stage

A primary goal for the feminist therapist is to *demystify the experience and image of the therapist.* The White, male, heterosexual, middle-class, married, feminist clinician acknowledges the privileges that exist for him in society but disavows them in the group, encouraging members by reminding them that this is "their group." He makes a clear distinction between the terms "leader" and *"facilitator."* He recognizes that as the group forms, members may be hesitant to participate. He explains that while he may be more active in this initial stage, he wants to share power with members from the beginning. *Development of Socializing and Imitative Behavior* begins with the feminist therapist and then extends to some group members, then the entire group. He utilizes appropriate *self-disclosure*, sharing with the group that he is also hesitant to open up when meeting new people. He considers *"un"-universality*, and where it might impact cohesiveness with group members. He points out that while all members of this group are here to treat addiction to alcohol, there is a level of un-universality in that each member's unique intersectional experience, cultural and social reactions, and privilege and oppression with addiction are different. For example, there are members of the group who do not perceive themselves to have a problem with alcohol. Traditional approaches to drug and alcohol treatment might label these persons as resistant or in denial. Instead, the feminist group leader might encourage the group to refrain from such categorizations and labels.

The therapist makes note of times where there is only "one." Whenever this is the case, the therapist is acutely aware of the possible impact this has on group co"we"siveness. The feminist therapist makes note of times where "one" person who person stands out. For example, in a group comprising mostly cisgender persons, a transgender person may feel alone. The therapist emphasizes the concept of "no-norming" by encouraging group members to pay attention to natural patterns that emerge in group participation. As the group's "regular" ways of behaving emerge, the therapist takes time in the group to explore if patriarchal concepts influence norms. For example, if it becomes apparent that males in a group typically speak first, feminist therapists might consider changing this dynamic by encouraging a female to speak instead.

## Stage 2 Patriarchal Differentiation Stage

In this stage, the feminist therapist used various techniques to encourage members to consciously consider patriarchal differentiation. The feminist therapist monitored how, for example, a client's privilege showed itself in the group as well as outside of the group. The group examined how power and oppression appeared in the group. The feminist therapist considered clients' unique intersectionality, completed a *power analysis* with each member, and utilized *"un"-universality* to help members see the unique impact of each of their identities on the development of their current drinking behavior. Specifically, the feminist therapist could aim to help members examine, through their unique intersectional identities and roles, how society's expectations, personal privileges and oppressions influence their drinking behavior. An additional benefit is that clients might experience increased empathy for one another and behave in an *"all"truistic* manner. *Imparting of information* may be used to inform members about their addiction while taking precautions not to appear as the authority on the subject. The feminist therapist encourages that all suggestions be made tentatively, including modeling language such as "Might it be ok with you for me to share some thoughts?" The feminist therapist can use *label analysis* to help clients gain a deeper understanding of how words like "addict" might be harmful. The group *explored embedded messages and oppressive shcemas* such as "once an addict, always an addict" for a similar impact. They noted that it was these very concerns that prevented some members from taking a more in-depth look at their drinking behavior for fear of stigma. The feminist therapist encouraged *challenges to images* by exploring images that conjured up by "addict" stereotypes that are embedded in patriarchal oppressive messages. This was intended to allow clients to decide if they would like to differentiate from the patriarchal constructs that did not serve their recovery.

## Stage 3 Collective and Individual Empowerment Stage

After the group had explored each of its members' unique experiences with privileges and oppression, the therapist offered *consciousness raising* for empowerment. The ultimate goal being that each member understood how society has impacted their development and contributed to their self-reported concerns about alcohol use. As part of this examination, the feminist therapist was more acutely aware of this stage's *recapitulation of social injuries*. For example, the feminist therapist noted microaggressions occurring in the group with a member telling a Hispanic female to calm down. The feminist therapist encouraged that member to notice and examine the impact of such a statement on the group member and the group as a whole. This experience of *catharsis* was relieving to the targeted member as well as other members. This experience of catharsis was relieving to the targeted member as well as other members. The micro aggressive member was compassionately invited to share their experience of having patriarchal rooted behavior acknowledged by the group. The feminist therapist requested that such statements are acknowledged by the group as an ongoing empowerment. In this way, the members moved toward *advocacy* for themselves.

## Stage 4 Advocacy and Social Justice Stage

Throughout the process, the feminist therapist continued to discuss intersectional marginalization, privileged, and oppressive disparities that existed between members, consciously or unconsciously. The feminist therapist may provided *assertiveness* activities for the members to learn and practice self-advocacy and advocacy for others, if desired. In this group, the feminist therapist pointed out that there may be intersectional social reasons why some members have legal issues and others do not. When members attributed differences to circumstance, the feminist therapist encouraged further exploration of social positioning.

The feminist therapist went on to explain that patriarchal injuries are universal in that the oppressive structures and systems in this culture truly benefit very few seeking to live a fully conscious life of freedom. The feminist therapist encouraged the members to consider ways current systems have hurt them and explore opportunities for self-advocacy or social advocacy. Where advocacy was not possible, the feminist therapist considered the *instillation of hope* by pointing out that there is the possibility of freedom from patriarchal chains of thought. This feminist existential perspective might challenge the traditional concept of success. What was the "true" goal of this group? Was it only abstinence from alcohol? The group decided that one goal for each client was to gain an understanding of *all* the influences on their drinking behavior, including their desire to continue to drink. In gaining an understanding, each member was free to choose for themselves. Lastly, *social justice* served as the ultimate curative factor for some. Directing their energies outside of themselves and toward aiding others became their means of transcending patriarchy. These group members may ultimately find themselves wanting to give back to others after receiving benefits from their group members.

# Challenges of a Feminist Intersectional Group Approach

One of the biggest challenges to be wary of in feminist intersectional group counseling theory is the negative association many have with the word *feminist*, which can include assumptions that feminists are all anti-male, biased toward women, and seeking immediate radical social change. While it is true that feminists do seek social change, feminist therapists do not require their clients to endorse this position; rather, they seek to help all clients become more aware and more empowered. Clients need to clearly understand that there is no agenda except to help the client fully understand the social constructs that may have affected their development. For this to happen, the feminist therapist must closely monitor that all choices are equal, and the group cannot develop an agenda that privileges some and marginalizes others. This would become another example of a patriarchal hierarchy in a different setting. The feminist group leader needs to remain self-aware so they do not unintentionally sway clients in a direction that might impose values on them.

Some people might incorrectly view feminist intersectional theory as an excuse for a client's pathology or unhealthy behaviors. Remember that this theory focuses on the client's empowerment, which moves the onus toward an internal locus of control and taking responsibility for oneself. The client may not recognize oppressive norms and messages and may give up. Instead, the client must decide whether they are going to continue the perception that allowed them to compare themselves to Western patriarchal standards. Advocacy toward self or others can also be empowering if the client chooses that path.

# What If?

What if all group therapy questioned social systems that oppress the clients?

What if people exposed to feminist intersectional group therapy all created a ripple effect to the larger ecosystems?

What if feminist intersectional group principles were applied in nontherapeutic groups such as task groups, political committees, business and so on?

What if feminist group theory could be used to narrow the divisiveness of conservative and liberal views?

What if people exposed to feminist intersectional group therapy all created a ripple effect to the larger ecosystems?

# References

Adler, A. (2009). *Understanding human nature*. OneWorld. (Original work published 1927)

Allan, K. (2006). Patricia Hill Collins: Intersecting oppressions. *Contemporary Social and Sociological Theory: Visualizing Social Worlds*, 1–11.

Bowen, M. (2004). *Family therapy in clinical practice*. Aronson. (Original work published 1985)

Bronfenbrenner, U. (1979). *The ecology of human development: Experiments by nature and design*. Harvard University Press.

Bronfenbrenner, U. (2005). *Making human beings human: Bioecological perspectives on human development*. SAGE.

Bronfenbrenner, U., & Evans, G. W. (2000). Developmental science in the 21st century: Emerging questions, theoretical models, research designs and empirical findings. *Social Development*, 9(1), 115–125.

Chaplin, J. (1999). *Feminist counseling in action*. SAGE.

Collins, P. H. (2009). *Black feminist thought*. Routledge.

Collins, P. H., & Bilge, S. (2020). *Intersectionality* (2nd ed.). Polity Press.

Corey, M. S., Corey, G., & Corey, C. (2022). *Groups: Process and practice*. Cengage. (10th ed. published in 2018)

Crenshaw, K. W. (1989). Demarginalizing the intersection of race and sex: A Black feminist critique of anti-discrimination doctrine, feminist theory, and antiracist politics. *University of Chicago Legal Forum*, *140*, 139–167. https://scholarship.law.columbia.edu/faculty_scholarship/3007

Crenshaw, K. W. (1991). Mapping the margins: Intersectionality, identity politics and violence against women of color. *Stanford Law Review*, *43*(6) 1241–1299. https://doi.org/10.2307/1229039

Dayton, T. (2005). *Trauma and addiction: Ending the cycle of pain through emotional literacy*. Health Communications, Inc.

Downing, N. E., & Roush, K. L. (1985). From passive acceptance to active commitment: A model of feminist identity development. *The Counseling Psychologist*, *13*(4), 695–709.

Fromm, E. (1969). *Escape from freedom.* Holt.

Hardy, K. V. (2023). *Racial trauma.* W. W. Norton.

Jacobs, E. E., Schimmel, C. J., Masson, R. L., & Harvill, R. L. (2016). *Group counseling: Strategies and skills* (8th ed.). Cengage.

Rogers, C. R. (1942). *Counseling and psychotherapy.* The Riverside Press.

Rosa, E. M., & Tudge, J. (2013). Urie Bronfenbrenner's theory of human development: Its evolution from ecology to bioecology. *Journal of Family Theory & Review, 5*(4), 243–258.

Titelman, P. (Ed). *Differentiation of self: Bowen family systems perspectives.* Routledge.

Yalom, I. D. (1980). *Existential psychotherapy.* Basic Books.

Yalom, I. D. (1985). *The theory and practice of group psychotherapy* (3rd ed.). Basic Books.

Yalom, I. D., & Leszcz, M. (2020). *The theory and practice of group psychotherapy* (6th ed.). Basic Books.

# 7

# Feminist Intersectional Couple, Relationship, and Family Therapy

## *Nicole Jackson Walker, Candace N. Park, Kristina S. Brown, and Takeesha Hawkins*

*Couples, relationships, and families all have embedded patriarchal expectations of the rules, roles, dynamics, and concepts of love that are expected in these relationships.*

A feminist intersectional theory applied to couples and family therapy has many unique challenges related to dynamics and systems, considering the foundational assumption that oppressive, Eurocentric, heteronormative, Christian-dominant, patriarchal systems are the etiology of much psychological suffering (Brown, 2018; McGoldrick & Walsh, 2017). Feminist couples, relationships, and family therapists face particular challenges, given people with different intersectional identities and oppressions involved in these relational dynamics are raised with these messages and role expectations. The relational dynamics that develop from oppressive social, cultural, and political macrosystems impact each person differently based on their unique intersectional identity. Couples, relationships, and family systems are often built on the foundations of these passive embedded messages of privilege, oppression, and normalcy.

Feminist clinical foremothers of the second wave of feminist evolution explored the implications of family theory with gender and women's issues as the focus of treatment, recognizing specific oppressions such as domestic violence, sexual assault, and the like (McGoldrick & Walsh, 2017). More recently with the third wave of feminist theory, feminist family therapists have included intersectionality, first introduced by Crenshaw (1989), in honoring the importance of multiple oppressions (McGoldrick & Walsh, 2017).

## Feminist Family Therapy Emerges

Feminist family and couples therapy rises from a collective of feminist clinical thoughts. The need for a feminist approach to systemic therapy was born out of concern that traditional approaches reinforce gender roles, hierarchical structures, oppression of marginalized persons, societal values, systemic influences, and common definitions of couple and family (Hare-Mustin, 1978). Indeed, early approaches to family therapy paid little attention to gender dynamics within the home, often contributing to an imbalance in power (Bitter, 2021; Hare-Mustin, 1978). Working with couples and families requires understanding gender and cultural influences within the home. While the pioneers of family therapy (e.g., Ackerman,1966; Bateson, 1979; Bowen, 1978; Haley, 1976; Madanes, 1981; Minuchin, 1974) appear to have an evolving understanding of such issues in theory and practice, therapists must be aware of how these theories may reinforce the patriarchy and status quo (Bitter, 2021). Contratto and Rossier (2005) claimed that "[t]he feminist therapy movement emerged from some of the major questions that women, practitioners, and theorists struggled with" (p. 9).

The influence of the "theory and philosophy of consciousness-raising" applied to family therapy began to emerge to a broader audience in 1978 with the contributions of Rachel Hare-Mustin (p. 181). As the first person to openly address how traditional family therapy failed to examine the negative impact of socialization practices on women, Hare-Mustin (1978), formally offered an alternative approach to family therapy informed by feminist values and interventions. As feminist voices began to rise in the family therapy literature, the *Journal of Feminist Family Therapy* was launched in the mid-1980s (Kaslow, 2007). Feminist family practitioners also rose to meet the needs of the field.

In 1984, approximately 47 female leaders in marriage and family therapy met at the initial Stonehenge conference (McGoldrick & Walsh, 2017). Organized by Monica McGoldrick, Froma Walsh, and Carol Anderson, the conference's goal was to address ongoing gender-based needs for women and practice, theory, and research in family therapy. The conference provoked reactions not only from male therapists but also from female therapists. Some female therapists may not have thought that gender was an issue or may have been concerned about retribution from their male colleagues. Following the Stonehenge conference, the Women's Project in Family Therapy was formalized, which provided a space for open dialogue (Bitter, 2021; Silverstein, 2003; Walters et al., 1988).

Marrianne Walters, Betty Carter, Peggy Papp, and Olga Silverstein, the originators of the Women's Project, also wrote *The Invisible Web: Gender Patterns in Family Relationships* (Walters et al., 1988), a groundbreaking book analyzing traditional family therapeutic practice from a feminist perspective and providing feminist guidelines for family therapy. Thus, feminist family therapy, alongside other feminist therapists working in other models and populations, emerged. In the earlier waves of feminist family therapy, the focus was on issues of power and control inside the family but did not center on gender (Braverman, 1986). As pioneers persisted, a shift was evident as gender became a central focus (Hare-Mustin,1978; McGoldrick, 1998). Silverstein and Goodrich (2003) described feminist family, couples, or relationships therapy as focused on violence and injustice both within and upon the unit. The emergence of intersectionality (Crenshaw, 1991) in third-wave feminist theory also began to influence family therapists. (Comas-Díaz, 2010; Comas-Díaz & Byars-Winston, 2010).

The mantra of feminist therapy is "the personal is political," recognizing the psychological impact that the social, cultural, and political systems have on clients. Feminist therapists have a shared belief that sociopolitical systems impacting the individual will also impact the family or couple dynamics and systems in very personal ways. Additionally, feminist family therapists acknowledge that what has been upheld as the Eurocentric, heteronormative, Christian-dominant, patriarchal, "normal" family structure is often marginalizing, oppressive, and even rejecting for many families today (Hoffman, 1993; Kaschak, 1990, 2010; McGoldrick, 1998; Papp, 2000). Furthermore, social justice and advocacy are central features of feminist work with advocacy by clients being their choice.

# Contemporary Couples and Families

The concept of family has changed throughout recent decades, with increasing acceptance of "nontraditional" families. Historically, an acceptable family was seen as a heterosexual, same-race, cisgender couple, with children who were an extension of that dynamic. According to the Pew Research Center (2024), two-parent households are declining in the United States as divorce, remarriage, and cohabitation rise. Families, couples, and relationships are increasingly diverse in ethnicity, age, gender, and education. Additionally, traditional definitions of family, often limited to legal or blood relationships, often fail to account for social, cultural, and economic factors that shape family bonds.

Feminist couples, relationship, and family therapists must recognize the varied relational structures to provide ethical and unbiased therapy. In feminist family therapy, clients' narratives are honored, and they define their own family, often including those bound by mutual consent and shared responsibility for various activities of daily life, rather than the default of blood or legal ties. Feminist family therapists empower all family members to construct and deconstruct with autonomy and freedom.

Traditionally, couples are seen as two people in a committed relationship. In some cases, dyads may grow consensually to form a triad or quad, involving relationships of three or four individuals committed to one another in ethical, consensual non-monogamy (Rubel & Burleigh, 2020). These relationships, which may be polyamorous, can involve various genders, sexual orientations, living arrangements, and levels of commitment, whether monogamous or non-monogamous, married or unmarried, sexual or nonsexual.

# The Feminist Intersectional Couple, Relationship and Family Therapy Model

In feminist intersectional therapy with couples, relationships, and families, the feminist therapist is attending to multiple processes simultaneously, focusing on intersectional identities and the interplay of privilege, oppression, power, and empowerment within multiple systems. Unlike other theoretical orientations, feminist therapists prioritize understanding how historical, social, cultural, and political influences contribute to clients' concerns. The goals of a feminist therapist are to raise awareness about the role of culture, context, power, and social influences on the couple, relationship, or family and facilitate empowering each member to understand the context of their dynamics and take responsibility where appropriate. Lastly, understanding advocacy and what it means to advocate for oneself, a partner, or their family is prioritized. This model moves through five tasks:

## Task 0.5: Therapist Introspection

Feminist intersectional clinical practice with families, relationships, and couples begins before meeting with clients and continues throughout clinical practice. Feminist therapists, including those of families, relationships, and couples, must remain competent and congruent with their feminist thoughts and commitments to advocacy. This means remaining current on feminist literature and the social, cultural, and political norms as they evolve, which may have an oppressive impact on clients. It also may involve gaining supervision from other feminist couples, relationships, or family supervisors. Perhaps of most importance is the consistency of the feminist therapist's ongoing process of self-awareness and willingness to address one's privileges by examining one's biases and distortions. Brown (2018) suggests that feminist therapists ask themselves the following:

> What are the power dynamics in this situation? Where am I taking patriarchal assumptions for granted as true? What norms about power and powerlessness are so built into my assumptions, or those of my client, that I am taking them as unassailable? (p. 38)

As social, cultural, and political changes consistently occur, the feminist therapist must remember that all choices are made by clients and are entirely uninfluenced by the therapist's beliefs. The therapist may disagree with or even fear the client's choice, but as a feminist therapist, autonomy, and empowerment are the basic principles. The process of identifying ways in which one may inadvertently disempower one's clients is ongoing, as is the identification, development, and implementation of liberatory strategies that support empowerment (Brown, 2018).

## Task 1: Transparent Egalitarian Therapeutic Alliance

A core tenet of feminist theory is the emphasis on building and maintaining transparent egalitarian relationships that share equal power (Brown, 2018; McGoldrick & Walsh, 2017). Rapport building is challenging because the feminist therapist enters an existing power structure with many facets of dynamics. Feminist therapists must first understand this relational system to appropriately find ways to balance power. In couples, relationships, and family dynamics, power is often part of the presenting problem. Therefore, the feminist therapist must be transparent explaining that recognizing and addressing power is part of the therapeutic process. During this task, the feminist therapist validates the family's structure, strengths, values, and resilience. The therapist conceptualizes the family in an ecosystem of Eurocentric, heteronormative, Christian-dominant, patriarchal, oppression and privilege, prioritizing validation of personal narratives and experiences.

Some feminist therapists use self-disclosure as a means of transparency and balancing power. However, therapeutic self-disclosure is a skill that requires discernment. Self-disclosure can foster a sense of shared experience and be empowering, or it can have the unwanted outcome of taking power and voice from the clients by making the session about the therapist. According to Brown and Walker (1990), "This proactive embrace of self-disclosure is unique among theories of psychotherapy and reflects certain core tenets of feminist therapy theory regarding the relationship of client and therapist and the role of the therapist in the healing process" (p. 135).

### *Connecting with Couples and People in Relationships*

Couples (or other types of romantically tied relationships) therapy can be challenging because often relationships/couples enter therapy with expectations of the therapist taking sides. An unknowing therapist who is not focused on power might naturally side with the one who does not have the power. When building rapport, the feminist therapist must be careful not to align with anyone. Setting tones of balanced power can be achieved through collaborative agreements such as no secrets between the feminist therapist and individual members of the relationship, transparent communication, cancellation of sessions if one person cannot attend therapy, and so on.

## Connecting with Families

As with couples, a feminist family therapist enters a family that has existing structure and power differentials. A feminist therapist must first understand the family's power structure dynamic to understand how to navigate the egalitarian therapeutic position. When building rapport with families, it is important to consider the various developmental needs of members and each member's intersectional identities. Family members of oppressed groups may be more mistrusting and may require more time or varied approaches than other members to trust the therapist. The family must also be considered as a whole unit related to understanding privilege, resources, oppression, marginalization, and rejection from the larger community and systems. It is important to validate each family member's unique intersectional perspective and experience and question how much power they perceive themselves to have in the family and outside of the family.

# Task 2: Exploration of Patriarchal Influences

In this task, the feminist therapist will explore internal and external factors affecting the couple, relationship, or family. Collaboratively, everyone will explore members' identities and roles in the couple, relationship, or family and in the larger world. The feminist therapist will also examine how the hierarchal structure within the family and ecosystem has evolved into its current dynamics through an intersectional identity examination of the unit and each member's privilege and oppression.

## Feminist Intersectional Applications That Can Be Used in This Task

**Intersectional Power Analysis.** An intersectional power analysis consists of self-examining each person's identities (e.g., gender, sexuality, abilities, race, religious beliefs, socioeconomic status, etc.). After thoroughly examining their intersectional identities and the confluence of those identities, each considers ranking which ones are the most salient to them. Then, clients examine how their multiple identities are perceived socially, culturally, and politically and whether they carry privilege, oppression, or neither within the family and/or larger community. Clients may complete an analysis for each member of the system, as well as the whole system.

**Strengths Exploration.** After each member understands their intersecting identities, individual members of the couple, relationship, or family are asked to explore their strengths and present those to one another. Members are then asked to share what they see as the strengths of the other members. Then, each will share their perceived strengths as a family unit.

**Feminist Intersectional Genogram.** Tools feminist systems therapists may utilize are the critical genogram (Kosutic et al., 2009) and the cultural genogram (Shellenberger et al., 2007), both of which consider the multifaceted dynamics impacting an individual, such as race, class, and religion. Additionally, the feminist intersectional genogram is offered here. The purpose of using a feminist-compatible genogram is for the feminist intersectional therapist to gain a better understanding of what systemic influences are affecting the members of the couple, relationship, or family, also called critical consciousness. Critical consciousness can be considered an ability to recognize and understand systems of oppression and privilege that, in turn, allows for action that increases personal power and dismantles oppressive practices (Kosutic et al., 2009). The feminist therapist, by having a deeper conceptualization of the members and the many systemic and cultural influences upon its members, will be better positioned to work with them.

**The Feminist Intersectional Genogram Key Additions.** Remember, the feminist intersectional genogram differs from the McGoldrick and Gerson (1989) version in key ways. It is not linear, with each generation of people placed on the same plane. Varying horizontal positions of members will show slight to significant power differentials. Also, connections between members are directional, with power indicated by an arrow from who has more power to who has less power.

These feminist intersectional genogram symbol additions to the traditional genogram conceptualize the family in the context of society. Positioning does not represent the therapist's viewpoint at any time. Instead, it uses the total information provided by all members, combined with the therapist's understanding of intersectionality, the dominant culture, and the existing hierarchical structures. The goal is to have a diagram of the client's world and how it shapes them.

Relationships may be indicated as close, "broken," or "distressed" in a similar fashion to a traditional genogram (McGoldrick & Gerson,1989). However, rather than using the terms broken or distressed, a feminist therapist might consider that the end of a relationship may be a "fix" or "empowering." Therefore, words such as "chose to end" or "working toward a resolution" may be more appropriate.

*Power direction:* Use a power analysis and the questions provided as a guide to determine power dynamics, then consider how intersectionality impacts power dynamics within the genogram. Whenever possible, consider hierarchal structures and indicate those directionally. People with more power may be placed to the left or slightly above another with less power. This will immediately call the viewer or feminist therapist's attention to what power dynamics may be at play. This process can become challenging at times when a person may possess varied amounts of power based on different social locations (e.g., being male and bisexual). How has power played a role in the unit's dynamics? Have there been instances where someone challenged or broke away from these power dynamics? Power dynamics should be indicated directionally with the member in power pointing toward those who have traditionally held power in the unit.

*Gender roles:* Clients should not be limited to a binary representation with typical circles and squares. One should use an oval shape to depict those not identifying as one gender. They may also consider other shapes. How has gender played a role in the unit's dynamics? Have there been instances where someone challenged or broke away from these roles? For example, what symbol should be used to describe those who do not identify as male or female?

*Culture:* Have there been instances where someone challenged or broke away from these roles? There are many aspects of culture. At a minimum, use specific geometric symbols and colors to represent race, ethnicity, religion/spirituality, affectional orientation, socioeconomic status, immigration/acculturation status, and community membership(s) (see Figure 7.1 for details). In line with feminist theory, no standard set of symbols should be used so long as your key accurately identifies them for all. You may choose standard symbols or construct your own to indicate cultural aspects not identified here. You must, however, keep in mind where symbols represent binary structures. How has culture played a role in the unit's dynamics?

## KEY

| | | | |
|---|---|---|---|
| African American | ◯ Female | ▲ Heterosexual | ⬤ Community Connections |
| Native American | ▢ Male | ◆ Pansexual | ◯ Fictive Kin |
| Pacific Islander | ◯ Transgender male to female | ⬢ Bisexual | ⨝ Above Poverty Line |
| Hispanic/ Latino/Latinx | ⬭ Transgender female to male | ⬠ Homosexual | ◇ Below Poverty Line |
| White/Caucasian | ⬡ Non-Binary | ⬣ Asexual | ✚ Adequate Resources |
| Asian | ⋈ Two-spirit | ▆ Queer | ▬ Limited Resources |
| Middle Eastern /North Africa | | ▰ Ally | |

★ Religious
☆ Spiritual
⚡ Trauma
〜 Mental Health Condition
≈ Invisible Disability
≋ Visable Disability
⁄ Working Toward Resolution
↗ Power Line

▢ _____

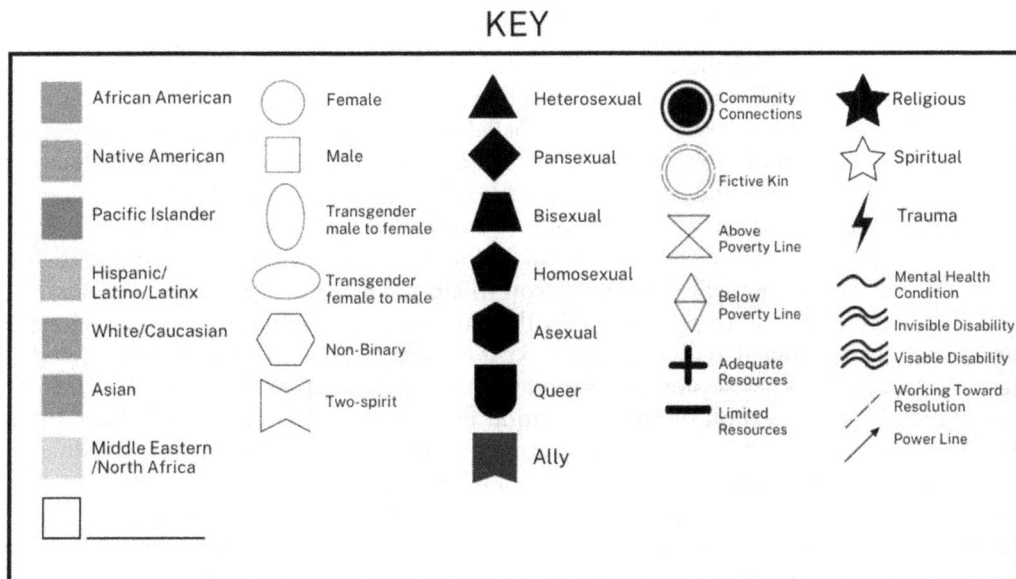

FIGURE 7.1 *Genogram Key.*

# Task 3: Higher Consciousness and Choices

Task 3 explores consciousness raising and the opportunity for change. Feminist intersectional clinical applications and interventions are only suggested to explore new thoughts with clients, emphasizing creativity, equal power, and collaboration. Traditional and new interventions can be adapted for feminist therapists working with systems modalities, just with a different focus on intersectional identities and association privileged marginalizations and oppressions. The goal here is to aid clients in gaining a new level of awareness, allowing them to make more conscious choices while embracing client autonomy. Once awareness is gained, all choices are free and equal.

## *Collective Consciousness Raising*

The goal of the feminist couple, relationship, and family therapist is to increase clients' awareness of how social, political, and cultural influences affect them, using that information to empower them toward a more robust human experience. There are many options for creative therapists to engage in the exploration of awareness. Understanding how beliefs, norms, and ideas of "right" came to be may help individuals increase awareness about their personal, relationship, and familial suffering. When working with couple, relationships, and families, giving context to their problems and the freedom to make new choices will allow members to no longer hold each other solely accountable for their suffering. Although much of the etiology of suffering may stem from oppressive systems, the relational units are still responsible for navigating and managing it through empowerment. Because the clients have a new examined awareness, they can choose to change or not and decide together what to do with this new consciousness.

## *Feminist Content and Process and the Here and Now*

The feminist intersectional therapist will use their understanding of content and process to illustrate to the members in real time the ways that they may be consciously or unconsciously expressing traditional patriarchal-embedded beliefs or enacting oppression upon each other. Content can be thought of as the "what," and feminist process is the "why and how." Members of couples, relationships, and/or families will bring to sessions the "what." For example, parents might complain that their child is misbehaving. They may recount an incident from the previous week where the child snuck out of the house and then later, when discovered, lied about it. The parents will likely want you to aid in changing the child's behavior. The child will likely want you to point out that the parents are too restrictive. While a feminist therapist might be tempted to dive into the story, it is far more productive to observe ways that the child "misbehaves" in session and the ways that the parents are "restrictive" in session. Through careful observation of communication patterns, the therapist might observe that the parents are talking down to the child or might notice ways the child is being dishonest. The feminist therapist might question what is causing the parents to "talk down" to the child in the moment or what is causing the child to be less than forthcoming. It is possible that in the answers to these questions, you might discover that the parent holds some patriarchal hierarchal notions about what it means to be a parent and a child, or are simply repeating how they were parented without a conscious examination. The feminist therapist may also discover that the child fears the parents and lies are attempts to control the situation and feel empowered. This is a challenging scenario for a feminist therapist because there is a fine line to walk between not disempowering parents while empowering the child. It is important to note that empowering and validating does not mean getting one's way. Being heard does not mean that people will agree. Empowerment is in the process, not the content.

**The Feminist Active Listening Experience.** Utilizing the active listening experience is psychoeducational and experiential. The feminist therapist first teaches and models active listening skills, then encourages the members to do so for one another. Each member listens for: empowerment, learned helplessness, embedded patriarchal messages, imposter syndrome, and any type of suffering caused within the Eurocentric, heteronormative, patriarchal ecosystem. As each member shares, the others may seek clarification when necessary and ensure they have understood the experience correctly in macrosystemic context. Each member then comments on what they have heard and confirms their understanding of the experience. In feminist couple, relationship, and family therapy, particular attention is given to the notion that under many circumstances, less empowered members will be accustomed to not having their voices heard. The therapy session may be the first and/or only time when other members are expected to listen to them.

**Feminist Evoking Empathy.** The evoking empathy experience involves using various techniques (e.g., role play, perspective taking, intersectional identity swap, etc.) to encourage a couple or family member to share a meaningful story from their life when they experienced victimization, oppression, powerlessness, helplessness (learned or otherwise), or were vulnerable to society's norms. For example, a member might share about a time when they felt victimized because of their ethnicity, gender, and so forth, but felt it was pointless to bring it up. The feminist therapist encourages affective expression while sharing and then asks the other member(s) to express an affective response. In couples/relationship therapy, this technique is used to deepen the emotional connection between partners through understanding their existence and experiences related to patriarchal injuries in the larger community. In family therapy, "evoking affective empathy" expands to include multiple family members. Each family member is invited to share an experience of vulnerability as described previously.

This exercise might contribute to a shared understanding of each family member's unique challenges, promoting empathy within the family unit for each other's experiences, different intersectional oppressions, and vulnerabilities. The hope is that this newfound construct of empathy creates a more compassionate and supportive family dynamic with an overall higher consciousness.

To take it a step further, a therapist might use the feminist intersectional role play in session. In couples or relationship therapy, feminist intersectional "role play" might focus on the power dynamics between the partners. A therapist might suggest an intersectional identity swap to take it even a step further. The swap is an in-vivo method whereby members are urged to experiment by taking on one another's intersectional identity positions as homework in real life.

**Power Understanding Skills.** The feminist therapist models and collaborates on effective communication skills related to power. For example, the therapist encourages the use of "power" statements. These statements are in the following format: When I (fill in the blank), I, standing in my power, feel (fill in the blank). Conversely, each member would also examine, "I feel no power when I (fill in the blank)." Ideally, this allows each member to understand how to empower and disempower each other. This can be used throughout down the therapeutic process as a note when a member feels either way.

**Assertiveness Experiencing.** Assertiveness is an underpinning of feminist therapy. It allows individuals to take personal power and responsibility over their lives. Identifying how people currently seek power (e.g., passive-aggression, internalizing, self-destruction, aggression, etc.) is the first part of each member's process toward assertiveness. A feminist therapist might also explore how each member came to their style of power through social construction and expectations based on intersectional identities. The feminist therapist must remember that assertiveness will have different norms, implications, and consequences for everyone. Exploring it as a system might allow each member to understand other assertiveness styles.

**Smash the Patriarchy Question.** The "smash the patriarchy" question allows people to explore their relational wants and needs that are limited by social, cultural, and political norms, constructs, and expectations. The feminist therapist might ask, "If there were no social, political, or cultural forces acting upon you, what would be different in this relationship/family?" Responses to this question might help partners align their visions for the future and find shared goals beyond societal expectations. They could also help a family determine members' aspirations that may lead to creating a shared vision for the family that transcends external patriarchal pressures. This question may need to be adjusted to match the developmental and cultural needs of members. For children, this question may sound like, "If you had superpowers and nothing could affect you, what would you tell your parents when (fill in the blank)?"

**Navigating Systemic Non-Negotiable Power Structures.** When equal power cannot be shared (e.g., parent-child, employer-employee, legal system-accused, etc.), clients may need aid in navigating non-negotiable power structures. Although the goals of feminist therapy are for empowerment, there will be situations where uneven power differentials are unavoidable. For example, children will not have the same power as their parents in the family system. Navigating power within a family would allow a child to realize process power (i.e., being understood) and have a voice even when overruled. Often, people equate "You didn't hear me" with "You do not agree with me." There must be a clear delineation between these two things when navigating power. When people find themselves in relationships or systems where they do not have full power over their lives, people have the choice to continue in the system as is or to make a change. The couple or family can then engage in open dialogue about the topic and how it applies to their current circumstances.

## Task 4: Advocacy and Ongoing Empowerment

When a feminist therapist and clients agree that it is time to end therapy, it is often because the clients have reached goals related to higher consciousness and reducing the impact of the embedded historical patriarchal influences. They have established a sense of personal, couple, relationship, and/or familial power. Within feminist therapy, there is an underlying sense of advocacy as part of the therapeutic process, and it can take many forms. Advocacy can be part of the healing process (Adler, 1956/1964). It can also be discussed at the end of therapy how the relational unit can continue to advocate for themselves once the therapy ends. Advocacy can range from being assertive within the family to protesting or running for legislative positions. The relational unit should feel no pressure from the therapist to advocate. However, clients may wish to discuss addressing any micro and macro problems they encountered during therapy.

## Feminist Intersectional Relationship Model Example: Meet Juanita, Kasey, and Wayne

Wayne, Juanita, and Kasey identify as having a polyamorous relationship. Juanita (25; she/her) and Kasey (25; they/them) have been together since the first year of college. They identified as being in an open relationship. Juanita and Kasey had previously utilized therapy to negotiate the boundaries of their relationship. Recently, they decided to shift from an open relationship to a closed polyamorous triad with Wayne (27; he/him), a cisgender African American man, who moved in with them a month ago.

Juanita is a first-generation Honduran American who identifies as bisexual. Her parents immigrated to the United States before her birth. The family is Catholic and operates from a patriarchal structure. Juanita's mother has always stayed at home to take care of everyone. Now that the youngest has moved out, and only her own mother is alive, she is pushing her children to get married and have babies. Though her brothers are included in this, the primary focus has been on Juanita as the only girl. She has not "come out" to her family of origin. who believe that she and Kasey are simply roommates.

Kasey, originally from Alabama, is a white transgender woman who identifies as pansexual. Kasey was raised by a single mother and has no knowledge of their father. Kasey's immediate family is close. Their extended family are self-proclaimed conservatives. They have a twin brother. Both the mother and brother are supportive of Kasey, yet do not discuss Kasey's identity with extended family. Their mom shared that she had recognized some gender and sexual struggles in high school and when Kasey went to college, their mom has been supportive. They have brought Juanita home for holidays, and Kasey's family is aware of their relationship status.

Wayne first met Kasey two years ago through a dating app. Kasey later introduced Wayne to Juanita. They are experiencing some issues of jealousy within their relationship. Kasey struggles with their weight and worries that Wayne has begun to prefer Juanita sexually.

### Working with This Relationship

*Task 0.5:* The feminist therapist first self-examines their idea of what constitutes a couple. If they discover that they hold a more traditional view, they work to expand their perception. The feminist therapist, in this case, is heterosexual and in a monogamous relationship with only one partner. Because this is the predominant structure of couples in America, this therapist acknowledges the privilege that they have when loving another just one other person. The feminist therapist engages in an ongoing exploration of any potential bias that exists concerning affectional relationships and makes all efforts to avoid proceeding in ways that might be harmful to the therapeutic alliance.

*Task 1:* The feminist therapist begins with informed consent that sets the ground rules for working with this "throuple"/triad relationship. They emphasize that they will communicate with all three clients via text using a group chat, rather than communicate with one member. They then address inherent power differentials in the relationship and ways to minimize them. For example, the therapist disavows any belief that they are the expert in the room and reminds the relationship that each member brings their expertise. In joining with the triad, the feminist therapist is mindful of taking on the role of a less empowered member of the structure not to disrupt any homeostasis. The feminist therapist uses transparency to discuss how their culture and social location may impact the relationship. They allow room for the clients to ask questions and construct a collaborative agreement for therapeutic goals and processes. Working together in this capacity continues throughout therapy to maintain an egalitarian relationship.

*Task 2:* The feminist therapist completes a power analysis with each of the three individuals and then collaborates to complete an intersectional power analysis for the relationship. The therapist also completes a feminist genogram in collaboration with all three clients, Figure 7.2, and the ensuant comments contain an analysis discerned by all of the relationship members based on the information shared. All of this information garnered fruitful discussions and raised consciousness about themselves and each other.

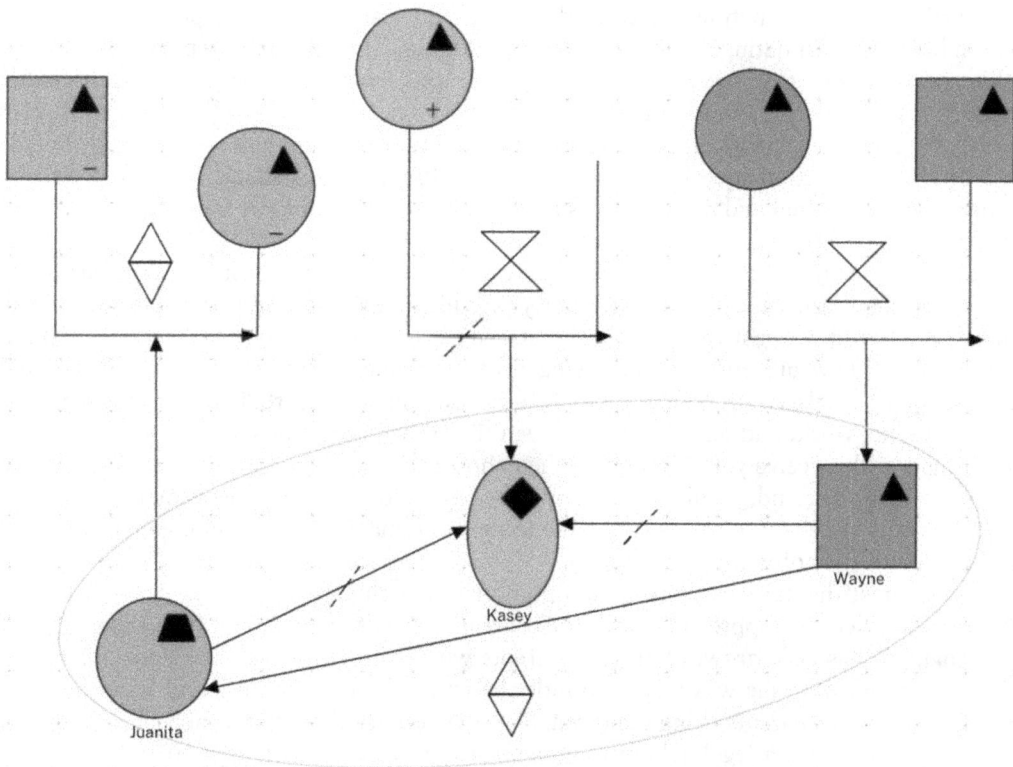

FIGURE 7.2 *Juanita, Kasey, and Wayne's Genogram.*

This feminist intersectional genogram denotes several critical factors related to intersectionality. Note that it may look slightly different depending on the various members' power analyses and individual contributions. These are some of the many considerations that may be reflected in a feminist intersectional genogram.

First, Juanita's parents are immigrants from Honduras; both their immigrant status and ethnicity are depicted in the hierarchy slightly below Kasey's parents, who are American-born and White. Since her parents' relationship is comprising a male-dominated hierarchy, an arrow points from the male to the female partner, with the male appearing on the left. Wayne's parents, who are of African American descent while not married, remain in a committed relationship. This female-dominated hierarchy denotes power from the female to the male; the mother is on the left. Kasey's mother is a single parent with no partner and, by virtue of that, has more power than an absent father. Despite being a single parent, her whiteness affords her power. For this reason, she is depicted slightly higher. If she were married to a white male, Kasey's parent might have been placed even higher. The father is left off the diagram to depict his absence and an arrow points in his direction.

Second, While Juanita is her parents' child, she reports that her American citizenship and her first language, English, have given her more power in navigating most environments over her parents. For this reason, you see an arrow pointing upward toward her parents. Third, in Juanita and Kasey's relationship, although you see an arrow pointing from Juanita to Kasey (because Juanita is cisgendered and Kasey is transgender), you will also notice that Kasey is situated slightly higher on the diagram than Juanita to indicate that being white has been reported by Kasey as providing them an element of power in the dominant culture, especially when others are unaware of their transgendered status.

Fourth, the power analysis indicates that Wayne as a male possesses power over Kasey whom he first began dating. He is cisgender and African American, and reports that Kasey's whiteness allows them to "generally be on equal footing" with him despite their transgender identity. For this reason, you see them on the same level in the diagram. The therapist also noted that he is depicted slightly higher in the diagram than Juanita who is both female and of Honduran ethnicity. According to Juanita, although he is Black, he is perceived by society as heterosexual and male and this affords him power, while her identity as a bisexual Honduran female often presents her with many challenges.

*Task 3:* From an intersectional power analysis, the feminist therapist begins to garner an understanding of their lived experience. They provide an empathic response and state, "You all live in a world where it would appear that you are not free to love who you love without judgment, and laws prevent you from living as others might, having the same rights. I would imagine that this places stress on each of you. Kasey, you are hurt that you are not seen as a woman by the world and fear that that is even true in your relationship. Wayne, you worry that others will perceive you differently when choosing a partner whom the world does not accept as a woman. And, Juanita, you want to be free to love your partners equally but know that laws will force you to choose only one to marry. I imagine this might create feelings for you at the injustice of it all."

The feminist therapist uses the technique of evoking empathy. They ask each partner to share an experience of oppression while the other members actively listen. Juanita shares how challenging it has been growing up with parents who did not always have legal citizenship. She talks about how she was forced to hide the truth about her family and how she often lived in fear of her parents being deported. She shares that this is why it hurts her so deeply that she cannot have a legal acknowledgment of both of her partners. Further, she knows that there are feelings of jealousy from Kasey about her relationship with Wayne, and she believes that if she has biological children with Wayne, that furthers any conflict, despite her awareness that from a legal standpoint, this is the easier option. In sharing her story, both Wayne and Kasey can appreciate the complicated situation that Juanita is in.

Wayne shares a story about a time when he was pulled over by the police and interrogated. He shares that he was informed that he fit the description of a suspect but that he believes he was pulled over for being a Black man. He describes how he was belittled by the police officer who called him "son." He then goes on to share about what life was like growing up. He describes his father as being emasculated by his mother because his father never seemed to have a job for very long or struggled to have one. He states that often his mother would exclaim to his father "you're no man" and then remind him of the importance of being nothing like his father. From his sharing, his partners gain an understanding of why he is often so bothered when others accuse him of not being manly for dating a transgender woman. They even begin to understand how on some level he may prefer Juanita over Kasey, as he too is a victim of a system that biases people, even if implicitly.

Kasey shares a story from their childhood before their transition about being the last to be chosen for sports. They talk about their feelings of rejection when others did not want them on their team. Kasey had been accused of not being a very good athlete, as they were overweight, could not run very fast, and played sports timidly. They go on to explain that they were always told that they "played like a girl." Kasey exclaims "I've never been picked, that's why it was so meaningful when I was picked by both Juanita, and later Wayne." From this story, their partners can have an understanding of Kasey's jealousy. Kasey has difficulty trusting that they will continue to pick them.

The feminist therapist encourages communication by offering a power statement to the triad. Kasey, feeling empowered, states, "When you, Wayne, and Juanita, spend time together that does not include me, I feel rejected, therefore I, standing in my power, would like to establish a rule that time alone with one partner must be agreed on by all." The other members utilize active listening to mirror what they heard before the therapist encourages a deeper exploration of Kasey's request. When the therapist notices Wayne monopolizing or talking over his partners, they utilize process commentary to highlight behavior that might impact the triad. In the here and now, the feminist therapist will process with Kasey and Juanita how they feel when Wayne talks over them. The goal of this is to raise consciousness about the power dynamics in the relationship. Wayne, as a male, may be inadvertently repeating patterns of communication that are seen in society. This may prevent his partners from speaking up as much as they want. Wayne begins to notice how society influences his "manliness" and begins to reject such. Conversely, Kasey begins to understand how they may not feel "womanly" enough. They, too, begin to reject such notions after Wayne shifts. In time, Juanita begins to shift her perspective on marriage and children. She offers to her partners that they should legally marry. She will carry children for the family that are both biologically Kasey's and Wayne's. In time, this triad will become a family.

*Task 4:* Closure is obtained when the triad begins to see how their sexuality, gender identity, ethnicity, and race have contributed to their challenges. They begin to understand that the patriarchal society has imposed expectations upon them about what it is to be male or female. They begin to shift their perspective and reject society's narrowed definitions. Having raised their collective consciousness, they begin to improve communication, express their power, and reject ways in which they might inadvertently have oppressed one another.

Although this case is framed with a triad, this model can also be used with families and with couples. All the feminist intersectional applications can be adapted to a larger or smaller system.

# Special Considerations with Couples, Relationships, and Families

## Divorce

Divorce is a legal process that is wrought with unequal Eurocentric, heteronormative, Christian-dominant, hierarchical, patriarchal systemic challenges. Systemically, one can acknowledge the intersectional patriarchal influences of the legal system in disproportioned rulings, child custody assignments, and so on. Divorce can be a disempowering process for all involved, from the marital partners to the children to people with no legal rights in their states, as well as future new family members (i.e., stepparents). In heterosexual marriages, divorce is not just about interpersonal difficulties but instead a process affected by gender, cultural socialization, and society (Lund, 1990). By and large, inequity is easily witnessed and not easily rectified; one should be mindful of power dynamics and accusations (i.e., parental alienation) that might emerge (Paquelet & Brown, 2022).

## Working with Feminist-Resistant Clients

Feminist couple, relationship, and family therapists will engage with clients who do not share feminist ideology. This requires a nuanced and respectful approach to ensure an inclusive therapeutic space that acknowledges diverse perspectives. Therapists maintain an open dialogue about feminist therapy concepts while avoiding language that may be perceived as narrow. For example, a therapist will accept other ways of knowing during consciousness raising. Understanding that social, cultural, and political messages often serve as defense mechanisms, the feminist therapist must not force ideas onto clients.

It is vital to share feminist intersectional values without imposing them upon clients, framing this viewpoint as one of several perspectives. This approach highlights the intersectional diversity within feminism and adapts to different worldviews. Empowerment, a central goal for feminist therapy, is demonstrated through choice in the therapeutic process, allowing clients to decide the extent to which feminist principles are integrated into their therapeutic journey. By adopting a client-centered (Rogers, 1995) and inclusive approach, feminist couple, relationship, and family therapists can engage effectively with clients who may not identify with feminist principles, creating a safe and respectful space where diverse perspectives are acknowledged and valued.

# What If?

What if there were no social hierarchies and every family member was really seen as equal?

What if there were no gendered social constructs for life tasks (career, relationships, etc.)? How would that impact relationship systems?

What if gender roles were reversed and tasks traditionally assigned to one gender were given to another? What would relational roles look like?

What if children were empowered to make more decisions in families earlier on? Would childred become decision-makers?

What if marriage and divorce were no longer legal constructs, but choices instead? Would anyone get married?

# References

Ackerman, N. W. (1966). *Treating the troubled family*. Basic Books.
Adler, A. (1964). *The individual psychology of Alfred Adler*. Harper Perennial. (Original work published 1956)
Bateson, G. (1979). *Mind and nature: A necessary unity*. Hampton Press.
Bitter, J. R. (2021). *Theory and practice of couples and family therapy*. American Therapy Association.
Bowen, M. (1978). *Family therapy in clinical practice*. Jason Aronson.
Braverman, L. (1986). Beyond families: Strategic family therapy and the female client. *Family Therapy, 13*(2), 143.
Brown, L. (2018). *Feminist therapy* (2nd ed.). American Psychological Association.
Brown, L. S., & Walker, L. E. A. (1990). Feminist therapy perspectives on self-disclosure. In G. Stricker & M. Fisher (Eds.), *Self-disclosure in the therapeutic relationship* (pp. 135–154). Springer. https://doi.org/10.1007/978-1-4899-3582-3_10
Butler, J. (1992). Contingent foundations: Feminism and the question of "postmodernism." In J. Butler & J. Scott (Eds.), *Feminists theorize the political* (pp. 3–21). Routledge.
Comas-Díaz, L. (2010). *Multicultural care: A clinician's guide to cultural competence*. American Psychological Association.
Comas-Díaz, L., & Byars-Winston, A. (2010). *Race, ethnicity, and culture in career counseling*. In D. R. Brown & R. W. Lent (Eds.), *Handbook of counseling psychology* (4th ed., pp. 105–120). Wiley.
Contratto, S., & Rossier, J. (2005). Early trends in feminist therapy theory and practice. *Women & Therapy, 28*(3–4), 7–26. https://doi.org/10.1300/J015v28n03_02
Crenshaw, K. W. (1989). Demarginalizing the intersection of race and sex: A Black feminist critique of antidiscrimination doctrine, feminist theory and antiracist politics. *University of Chicago Leagan Forum, 1*(8), 139–167. https://chicagounbound.uchicago.edu/uclf/vol1989/iss1/8
Crenshaw, K. W. (1991). Mapping the margins: Intersectionality, identity politics, and violence against women of color. *Stanford Law Review, 43* (6), 1241–1299. https://doi.org/10.2307/1229039
Haley, J. (1976). *Problem-solving therapy: New strategies for effective family therapy*. Jossey-Bass.
Hare-Mustin, R. T. (1978). A feminist approach to family therapy. *Family Process, 17*(2), 181–194. https://doi.org/10.1111/j.1545-5300.1978.00181.x
Hoffman, L. (1993). *Exchanging voices: A collaborative approach to family therapy* (p. 93). Karnac.
Kaschak, E., (1990). How to be a failure as a family therapist. In H. Lerman and N. Porter (Eds.), *Handbook of feminist ethics in psychotherapy*. Springer.
Kaschak, E. (2010). The mattering map: Morphing and multiplicity. In C. Bruns & E. Kaschak (Eds.), *Feminist therapy in the 21st century*. Taylor & Francis.
Kaslow, F. W. (2007). A brief history of the field of family psychology and therapy. In F. Shapiro, F. Kaslow, & L. Maxfield (Eds.), *Handbook of EMDR and family therapy processes* (pp. 438–454). John Wiley & Sons.
Kosutic, I., Garcia, M., et al. (2009). The critical genogram: A tool for promoting critical consciousness. *Journal of Feminist Family Therapy, 21*(3), 151–176.
Lund, K. (1990). A feminist perspective on divorce therapy for women. *Journal of Divorce, 13*(3), 57–68. https://doi.org/10.1300/J279v13n03_05
Madanes, C. (1981). *Strategic family therapy*. Jossey-Bass.
McGoldrick, M. (1998). *Re-visioning family therapy: Race, culture and gender in clinical practice*. Guilford Press.
McGoldrick, M., & Gerson, R. (1989). Genograms and the family life cycle. In E. A. Carter & M. McGoldrick (Eds.), *Changing family life cycle* (pp. 164–189). Allyn & Bacon.
McGoldrick, M., & Walsh, F. (2017). Stonehenge conference on women in families family therapy. In J. Lebow, A. Chambers, & D. Breunlin (Eds.), *Encyclopedia of couple and family therapy*. Springer. https://doi.org/10.1007/978-3-319-15877-8_624-1

Minuchin, S. (1974). *Families and family therapy*. Harvard University Press.

Papp, P. (2000). *Couples on the fault line: New directions for therapists*. Guilford Press.

Paquelet, D. R., & Brown, K. S. (2022). Parental alienating behaviors in Noah Baumbach's high-conflict divorce films, the *Squid and the whale* and *Marriage story*: A cinematherapy tool for (training) mental health providers. *Contemporary Family Therapy 45*, 450–462. https://doi.org/10.1007/s10591-022-09656-3

Pew Research Center (2024). *Family and relationships*. Washington, DC Family & Relationships. Research and data from Pew Research Center.

Rubel, A. N., & Burleigh, T. J. (2020). Counting polyamorists who count: Prevalence and definitions of an under-researched form of consensual nonmonogamy. *Sexualities*, *23*(1-2), 3–27. https://doi:10.1177/1363460718779781

Rogers, C. R. (1995). *On becoming a person* (2nd ed.). Houghton Mifflin.

Rossiter, A. (2000). The postmodern feminist condition. In B. Fawcett, B. Featherstone, J. Fook, & A. Rossiter, *Practice and research in social work*, 24–38.  4th Wave Feminist Theory.

Salih, S., & Butler, J. (2004). *The Judith Butler reader*.

Shellenberger, S., Dent, M. M., Davis-Smith, M., Seale, J. P., Weintraut, R., & Wright, T. (2007). Cultural genogram: A tool for teaching and practice. *Families, Systems, & Health*, *25*(4), 367–381. https://doi.org/10.1037/1091-7527.25.4.367

Silverstein, L. B. (2003). Classic texts and early critiques. In L. B. Silverstein & T. J. Goodrich (Eds.), *Feminist family therapy: Empowerment in social context* (pp. 17–35). American Psychological Association.

Silverstein, L. B., & Goodrich, T. J. (Eds.). (2003). *Feminist family therapy: Empowerment in social context*. American Psychological Association. https://doi.org/10.1037/10615-000

Walters, M., Carter, B., Papp, P., & Silverstein, O. (1988). *The invisible web: Gender patterns in family relationships*. Guilford Press.

# 8

# Feminist Intersectional Therapy and Substance Use

## Kathleen McCleskey, Justin Jordan, Liz Curtis, and Joanne Jodry

*People coping with addiction are often oppressed by a social stigma based on limited patriarchal constructs of success. The oppressive patriarchal views around addiction can also be reinforced socially, culturally, and politically both in treatment and outside of it.*

Feminist intersectional therapy calls on feminist therapists to provide egalitarian collaborative care that is transparent and empowering to the individual(s) affected by substance use. Addiction and substance use treatment represent challenges as many clients are mandated to receive care and face legal or other consequences if they avoid treatment. Additionally, a "person who uses substances" (PWUS) is a marginalized identity in society, with stigmas related to substance use still being perceived as a wrong moral choice that can be easily fixed by instead making the right decision. Despite new evidence-based scientific and therapeutic conceptions to better understand and treat substance use, the negative associations still prevail in a society that continues to marginalize and oppress the PWUS. The social stigma, employment concerns, and internalized and externalized judgments often leave PWUS fearful, depressed, isolated, and lonely as they try to make meaningful changes. Feminist therapists must examine and acknowledge any oppressed intersectional identities that serve to complicate the stigma associated with addiction and the unique experiences that PWUS clients suffer while trying to cope with their substance use.

Another challenge for feminist therapists is how to help empower individuals struggling with substance use to recognize systems of oppression while supporting individual responsibility in pursuing sustained recovery. This may include acknowledging that White heteronormative males designed the addictions treatment system. Therefore, the current traditional recovery models may not match all diverse clients' needs due to societal systemic biases that can permeate the process. Marginalized populations are always more impacted by majority power and views. For example, women face multiple barriers in seeking treatment for substance use disorders, including stigma, cost, and family responsibilities, with only approximately 11% of those diagnosed receiving treatment (Apsley et al., 2023). A 2020 study from the National Institute on Drug Abuse (NIDA), showed that more than 20% of sexual minority (LGB+) individuals in the United States have an alcohol use disorder. There is also evidence that Black and Brown Americans may be more likely to seek support through mutual self-help and clergy than professional services (Perron et al., 2009). Older adults and teenagers face unique hurdles in accessing providers knowledgeable about substance use in their age group. Additionally, an ongoing drug war in the United States has disproportionately targeted Black and Brown Americans, leading them to face more severe consequences for illegal drug use and often sowing distrust in professional helpers due to mandated care referrals in the process (Alexander, 2020). All of this points to unique needs and barriers that individuals face in engaging in therapy for addictions based on multiple, intersecting identities.

## History of SUD Treatment and Addiction Systems

Substance use treatment in the United States over the last century has been influenced by the Temperance Movement and the subsequent development of Alcoholics Anonymous (AA) in the 1930s (Lassiter & Spivey, 2017). This led to an approach to treatment focused on abstinence and based on the Twelve Steps of AA. This is also where the moral model of addiction began with its subsequent harsh stigma related to substance use. Interestingly enough, Lassiter & Spivey (2017) state that "excessive drunkenness led to domestic violence and the abuse of women and children, which resulted in a call for moderation" (p. 28), suggesting that the original intention of the Temperance Movement may have had feminist underpinnings. Religious clergy became the figureheads of the movement, and religious-based shame became the overwhelming message associated with PWUS that continues to perpetuate a "moral deficiency" stigma today.

Although substance use affected all social classes, races, and genders around the turn of the century, racial minorities suffered the most. Lassiter and Spivey (2017) reported, "There was a fear among some in White society that cocaine would empower African Americans to fight against the oppression and discrimination they were experiencing at the hands of the dominant white leaders" (pp. 30–31). The creation and enforcement of the U.S. Drug Enforcement Administration in 1973 (USDEA, n.d.) has disproportionately targeted Americans who are Black, Indigenous, and People of Color (BIPOC) (Earp et al., 2021). Institutional racism in the criminal justice system has led to a treatment system in which privileged individuals may be shielded from serious social consequences of addiction, while minoritized individuals face severe outcomes if they do not achieve and sustain abstinence from certain substances or behaviors (Alexander, 2020). Minorities are still jailed at alarmingly disparate rates for drug-related crimes compared to their White counterparts (Earp et al., 2021). For example, in 2019, Black people made up 12% of the U.S. population but made up 27% of U.S. drug arrests (Pew, 2022).

All this social, cultural, and political systemic history continues to permeate current attitudes about substance use. A currently accepted model of addiction is the disease model, which posits that addiction progresses in stages and is influenced by genetics and environment; it includes phases such as relapse and remission, and brain circuitry is modified (National Institute on Drug Abuse [NIDA], 2018a). This disease model puts addiction in the same category as diabetes or cancer and is biologically focused as opposed to morally focused while still recognizing the influence of the environment and access to care as complicating factors. Although the disease model is more compassionate and forgiving, it still has not served to eliminate the moral failure perception and social stigma that a PWUS experiences.

# Mandated Clients and Feminist Intersectional Therapy

Many addiction treatment clients are mandated to receive services by a legal or governmental authority, with painful consequences if they do not comply with that mandate (Hart, 2022). With legal or agency mandates often comes threats (jail, loss of children, etc.); urine drug screenings, mandatory number of meetings at specific times (convenient or not for the client's employment); and/or other severe consequences for noncompliance to authority. Additionally, there are agencies and systems (drug court, child protective services, probation/parole, divorce lawyers, etc.) that the client (and often feminist therapist) must engage with to avoid harsh consequences.

These institutional barriers and stigmas may impede the sense of autonomy and empowerment of a PWUS. How can the feminist therapist not be seen as just another gear of this oppressive system? Feminist therapists can support PWUS entering treatment by openly acknowledging the power dynamics and oppressive systemic issues contributing to mandated treatment protocols. Transparent discussions of systemic injustice and the conceptualization of addiction as "criminal" and "immoral" alongside the public health responses may help reduce natural defensiveness and improve the alliance between client and therapist. The feminist therapist can then genuinely support clients in their chosen goals while helping them navigate oppressive systems.

# Health Systems and Feminist Intersectional Therapy

Mental health struggles are correlated with substance use (NIDA, 2018b). Some clients may feel their concerns about depression, anxiety, psychosis, trauma, or mood instability are dismissed by medical providers who often focus on substance use first. It has been common for some medications or other services to be contingent on abstinence or changes with substance use, sometimes for justifiable reasons (such as drug interactions or evaluating if symptoms are caused by the substances).

It is noteworthy that a large number of Americans receiving medical care without these barriers are regular users of addictive substances, such as alcohol, tobacco, or caffeine. Still, the social constructs around addiction, stigma, assumption of drug seeking, and power dynamics may place the PWUS at a disadvantage in their recovery. Intersectional identities with additional marginalizations only serve to increase the barriers to recovery. Feminist therapists help PWUS clients navigate biased health systems and empower them to advocate for themselves for the best advantages possible in their recovery. The feminist therapist might also collaboratively advocate for individuals and systems.

# Holistic Lifestyle Barriers for People with SUD

In addition to social stigmas, public and private policies can create additional barriers for PWUS in their recovery process. For example, PWUS often experiences discrimination when trying to move forward in their wellness. Clients with histories of substance use disorder (SUD) can face barriers to employment in a variety of fields where having a drug-related conviction may represent the cause of termination of employment or not being considered for hiring (Hart, 2022). Substance use convictions also might result in barriers to enrollment in higher education or lead to suspension or removal from public K–12 schools or colleges. While not all individuals who use substances meet the criteria for a substance use disorder, a positive drug screen or test is often seen as a "red flag" for employers, indicative of moral deficiency, illegal behavior, instability, or unreliability. These situations represent lifestyle barriers that must be addressed in a holistic approach to recovery. The feminist therapist helps the clients examine and navigate the biased, oppressive systems that prevent their recovery and path to wellness.

## Systemic Advocacy

Feminist intersectional therapists embrace an advocacy and social justice mindset in their work with clients and society. While this work includes helping individuals advocate for themselves and taking direct action on their behalf within systems of immediate influence (e.g., the treatment agency, the criminal justice system, and their medical providers), it also often involves large-scale systemic advocacy. Working to dismantle systemic discrimination and oppression within a society and its government calls on feminist therapists to take action beyond the direct therapy relationship. Therapists embracing this feminist intersectional approach to healing have the opportunity to champion causes that lead to an equitable and just society. This can range from acknowledging the disproportionate targeting of BIPOC individuals in the enforcement of drug laws to encouraging governments, from local to state to federal, to spend less effort "catching" nonviolent PWUS.

Additionally, the feminist counselor may engage in dialogues with referral sources, such as drug court personnel, child protective services staff, and probation officers, about multiple pathways to recovery. Finally, a feminist therapist seeing little change through legislative policy or direct advocacy with local authorities may take the additional step of using their expertise and position of power to voice a need for change in protests, rallies, local town halls, interpersonal relationships, and via social media.

There are multiple levels and avenues of systemic advocacy for therapists treating PWUS, as these are just a few brief examples. While questioning a problematic status quo may lead to tensions and frustrations, it can also be appreciated as evidence of authenticity in the therapist's mission to cultivate positive change for individuals and communities. Just like with client autonomy, it is up to individual feminist therapists where and how they want to use their efforts; and to what level they are willing to go to be congruent with their personality traits, beliefs, and feminist principles.

# Feminist Intersectional Therapeutic Relationship

## Egalitarian Power Sharing

Fundamental underpinnings of a feminist therapeutic relationship are built on an egalitarian relationship. Brown (2018) defines this as "[a] relationship model for psychotherapy that simultaneously recognizes inequities of power inherent in the psychotherapy relationship and builds into that relationship systemic strategies for making power more equal" (p. 151). Examining and acknowledging the therapeutic power dynamics are essential to the feminist therapeutic process. Attempts to share power in this relationship value that both client and therapist bring expertise to the work—the client is the expert in their life, and the therapist brings training and experience to the relationship. All parties equally value both forms of knowledge.

## Collaboration and Transparency

In congruence with the feminist principle of demystifying the therapeutic experience for transparency, clients must understand and collaborate in all facets of the therapeutic process. No client is left wondering why a treatment choice was made for them instead of with them or why a document was signed because they had no choice. These feminist values become especially pertinent for mandated clients. For example, when a client is mandated to attend therapy for a substance-related charge, they are often thrust into a criminal justice system, which may immediately strip them of all power and autonomy that, in turn, forces therapists to become a part of that system by proxy. This is completely antithetical to feminist ethos. It is imperative that a feminist clinician working with a mandated client seeks out every opportunity for the client to make individual choices.

## Self-Disclosure

In attempts to flatten hierarchies, the feminist intersectional therapeutic relationship may be more accepting of self-disclosure than other therapeutic models. Self-disclosure of recovery status for feminists in clinicians needs to be considered with discernment and is encouraged when it may be appropriate and helpful. Because of its heavy emphasis on egalitarianism and client-as-expert credo, the feminist therapist is careful not to posit themselves as the omniscient being with the key to recovery. Forrest (2010) writes, "Healthy self-disclosure is a core ingredient in all effective psychotherapy relationships. Self-disclosure, transparency, and authenticity are essential to optimal human adjustment" (p. 106). In our model of working with addiction, we believe in being radically transparent with clients about how the system works. This radical transparency includes therapist self-disclosure of recovery status if that information is beneficial, relevant, or requested.

## Ongoing Self-Examination

A feminist clinician is encouraged to chronically examine their thoughts, values, and beliefs about substances and the people who use them. Thoughts and beliefs may be altered by personal life events, previous clients, mental health systems of employment, burnout, or compassion fatigue, and so on. Feminists or other therapists are not immune to embedded Eurocentric, heteronormative, Christian-dominant, patriarchal legacies of social norms and stigma messages, disempowering labels, and assimilated values. Since this client population has been so devalued, marginalized, and often rejected, an ongoing self-examination is critical to ensure that the feminist therapist does not replicate these oppressions in the therapeutic relationship.

# Feminist Intersectional Healing Factors

## Acknowledgments and Validation of Oppression

Feminist clinicians recognize and respect current and past coping skills that have helped clients navigate patriarchal influences thus far (Brown, 2018) and include and build on those skills as appropriate in current clinical work. Examining past and present intersectional injuries and the subsequent reactions (sometimes including the substance use itself) to them is acknowledged and validated. Understanding the systems of oppression does not remove personal responsibility but raises consciousness to prepare better tools for future success in recovery and life.

## Empowerment

When considering healing factors from a feminist perspective, empowerment is critical. It is, therefore, essential to consider how any client has experienced and is experiencing disempowerment, to examine that through an intersectional lens, and to explore how those experiences may connect to the use of substances. Oppression can be experienced in relation to any identity—gender, age, race, religion, affectional orientation, accused or convicted criminal, economic location, abilities, and so forth, as well as any other potentially marginalized area including being a PWUS. The feminist therapist realizes and works toward helping clients find personal power to assert themselves in these oppressive systems.

## Responsibility and Navigation

Validating and empowering PWUS around systemic bias and often counterproductive social and cultural pressures allows them to take fully conscious responsibility for navigating through these patriarchal systems with more power. A client could become stuck in an overwhelming amount of oppression, and experience learned helplessness (Peterson et al., 1993). Responsibility is only a healing factor if the client can hope to navigate the oppression.

## Advocacy

The feminist clinician advocates, with clients' permission, on their behalf, often with probation officers, lawyers, judges, and others, maintaining the feminist value of social justice advocacy. Intersectionality and multiple oppressions must be acknowledged with all clients; the systems (legal, educational, criminal justice, etc.) have often been the most punitive with those who are the most marginalized. For example, the feminist clinician remembers that clients coming to mandated therapy on the same legal charge may not have ultimately received the same sentencing or probation requirements due to their privileged or oppressed status. Part of the strength of modeling advocacy for clients is helping them understand that advocacy does not always give the desired result but that it is nevertheless vital to have our voices heard and to consider long-term objectives as well as short-term ones.

# A Feminist Intersectional Model of Working with Substance Use and Addictions

# (McCleskey & Jodry, 2016)

*This is an updated version of McCleskey & Jodry's (2016) feminist model working with addictions.*

## Welcoming and Honoring the Client

This initial stage involves the feminist intersectional therapist creating a connection with the client by introducing and implementing an egalitarian therapeutic relationship. This includes the therapist being genuine, congruent, accepting, inclusive, affirming, and introducing transparency about the therapeutic process. Role induction is especially important to clarify expectations that the client and feminist therapist will work collaboratively and that the process will be transparent for the client. This initial stage aims to begin the authentic, power-sharing partnership with the client through flattening the hierarchical relationship that often occurs with treatment providers.

## Understanding the Client's Intersectional Experience with Substances

In this early stage, feminist intersectional therapists transparently invite and accept and honor the client's narrative, acknowledging strengths in the client's story. This includes accepting and acknowledging the client's fear, defensiveness, and/or any desire to withhold some information. Feminist therapists understand that people develop strategies to survive when living in disempowering circumstances and these can be seen as strengths (Brown, 2018); resisting systemic requirements can be useful ways to retain personal power, including in therapy. Feminist clinicians can accept natural resistances and honor them as survival skills and empowerment strategies.

Collaboratively, the feminist therapist seeks to understand the client's addiction journey, their intersectional identities, and how those impacted their addiction story, their motivation for the amount of change or no change they desire, their fears and expectations of the therapist, and how they view the therapist being part of the oppressive system or not. In addition to learning about the client's history and experiences of substance use, the feminist therapist can begin to gather data about any developmental oppressions that may have an impact on their current substance use issues. This might include and exploration of any intersectional oppressive or limiting micro or macro systemic factors—abuse, neglect, family unemployment, and poverty, as well as personal and family experiences of racism, sexism, and other marginalization (Slaughter-Acey et al., 2023). This might also be the time that the client examines their intersectional social and cultural identities and identify salient intersections of identities. In all discussions, the feminist therapist endorses that the client can choose to not answer any questions that create fear or discomfort, with no therapeutic consequences for a client "passing" on a question or request.

## Feminist Intersectional Work: Raising Consciousness

In this phase of the therapy, the feminist clinician can collaborate with the client to examine the client's addiction journey within all the intersecting oppressive patriarchal contexts. Based on the client's perspective and reactions, this can be done using feminist terms (such as patriarchal messages and impacts) or less "feminist" explanations about how systems can impact everyone. How have systems injured them? Have any systems been helpful? How do/ have social and cultural systems encouraged or supported substance use? How have they supported the client's recovery goals (if that is the goal) or undermined recovery? Where does the client experience personal intersectional oppression and privilege unrelated to substance use? What systemic (Eurocentric, heteronormative, Christian-dominant, patriarchal) messages have they received about their intersectional identities? How do social intersectional identities connect to substance use? What identity labels related to substance use does the client use to describe themselves (addict, PWUS, person in recovery, etc.) and how do these identities help or hinder being empowered? See all feminist counseling techniques offered as tools to examine these questions.

## Feminist Intersectional Holistic Healing Process

Feminist intersectional therapists use a collaborative perspective to co-create holistic, meaningful goals. Plans for addressing substance use go beyond focusing only on a specific pattern of use, limiting use, or abstinence to include empowering the client in connection to the self and systems. Feminist clinical applications explore with the client many areas of holistic growth and empowerment while addressing their substance use treatment options. In this stage, there is a synthesized focus on the client's whole life, contextualizing substance use, understanding the privileges and oppressions of their social positioning, and promoting healing in all areas identified as harmful or limiting.

## Transforming Identities toward Wellness

Clients take the lead in defining who they are now related to substances and as a whole person. All identities and any connected internal or external labels may impact their recovery toward wellness. Some clients may have developed different language or self-concepts around their substance use that empower or limit their hope for the future. Some may be evolving or developing different identities. For example, some may be rejecting the identity of "addict" and replacing it with the identity of a PWUS. Feminist clinicians regularly help clients self-assess how the collaborative healing plan is working and what adjustments may be needed. Future challenges and barriers are anticipated, with potential plans to address those. Choices and decisions are not made reactively but proactively with freedom born from higher consciousness, forethought and intentionality, while also incorporating assertive empowerment skills gained in therapy. Clients leave the feminist intersectional therapeutic work with empowerment and with greater congruency in their intersectional identities.

# Feminist Intersectional 12-Steps

# (McCleskey & Jodry, 2016)

*This is an updated version of McCleskey & Jodry's (2016) feminist 12- steps with addictions.*

The Twelve Steps of Alcoholics Anonymous have been extremely helpful for countless people. At the same time, they are not universally endorsed by all clinicians or clients. PWUS may be mandated by the criminal justice system and by treatment programs to attend 12-step meetings and to "work the steps" in various ways. When this model works for clients and is consistent with their values and beliefs, it can provide a foundation for change. When this model does not fit a client's values and beliefs, being forced to work within it can recreate oppressive dynamics contraindicated to recovery.

This feminist intersectional 12-step model offers an additional perspective on the Twelve Steps that has been reimagined through a lens of feminist empowerment. Such a perspective may be useful for clients who have difficulty with the religious language of the Twelve Steps or with the emphasis on powerlessness and moral failure within them. If this model is also challenging for a client, it might be useful to work with the client to edit and adapt any model of the Twelve Steps, including this one, to create a version that is more consistent with the client's worldview.

12 Steps for Empowerment McCleskey & Jodry (2016):

1.  I recognize and believe that I have a choice to change my life, and with that recognition, I assert my power to help myself.

2.  I recognize that I need healthy, holistic support (physical, emotional, relational, psychological, spiritual) to help to change my life, and that asking for affirming help is a strength, not a weakness as framed by society.

3.  I make a decision to trust that I, and my supportive community of help, can work together to share in my holistic healing process.

4.  I will reflect on how I came to this point in my life, including both the internal and external forces that influenced my intersectional identities, my available choices, my levels of power, and any oppressive societal and cultural norms.

5.  I will examine and take responsibility for the complex choices I have made, contextualizing them in terms of my intersectional identities, my available choices, my levels of power, and any oppressive societal and cultural norms. I will move toward living more consciously and intentionally.

6.  I am ready to actively work to change my life, to focus on wellness and meaning, and to recognize my personal power while holistically living consciously and intentionally.

7.  I ask my supportive community for honest feedback and empathy, and to help me see my strengths and areas of growth, which I will openly reflect upon. I will decide what feedback is helpful in my future movement toward wellness and meaning.

8.  I recognize that as a human being, I may have both hurt others and may have been hurt by others. I may have also hurt or dishonored myself. I also recognize that oppressive societal and cultural norms contribute to all hurts.

9.  I will seek forgiveness with those I may have hurt, as long as doing so will not harm anyone. I will also seek to forgive myself, practicing self-compassion while taking responsibility for future behaviors in a conscious intentional manner.

10. I will continue to reflect on my holistic wellness and self-growth and strive to assert my choices and power in affirming ways. I will adjust as needed to stay on a healthy path of growth.

11. I will continue to seek a higher consciousness and understanding of holistic wellness to create and maintain a meaningful life path.

12. I can choose to be a part of other people's healing journeys toward holistic wellness and self-compassion, and to help others recognize their own strengths with raised consciousness and empowerment.

# Feminist Intersectional Clinical Applications

## Feminist Relational Transparency

Like existential psychotherapy (Yalom, 1980), the therapeutic relationship itself is a primary curative factor in feminist intersectional therapy. As stated before, one of the foundations of a feminist, egalitarian therapeutic relationship is transparency. What does it mean to be radically transparent with clients? It can be helpful to reflect on the kind of "behind the curtain information" therapists are currently comfortable sharing in a session. They were likely trained to keep staying focused on the client's problems and not share much information. However, withholding valuable information from clients about the sometimes-oppressive inner workings of the mental health system and our roles in it can disempower them. Feminist intersectional therapy always seeks to empower the client by flattening the hierarchy. Power can lie in knowledge. Any question a client has about how treatment systems works is valid, and feminist therapists seek to completely demystify the therapeutic experience. They will provide all information needed about the treatment protocols and their relationship to other authorities and referral sources, allowing the client to make informed choices about their consent and service engagement. This underpinning of feminist clinical application further empowers the client to ask questions of other people they may view as authority figures.

As discussed, self-disclosure might be one area of feminist transparency. Please note that maintaining professional boundaries is an ethical requirement for feminist therapists, so this does not mean the dissolution of boundaries for the sake of self-disclosure or that the focus should be on the therapist rather than the client. The power-sharing dynamic in feminist therapy is not enhanced if the therapist takes a remote, standoffish stance; instead, therapists fully engage in the process with clients as whole human beings. Brown (2018) points out that the therapist who is not "known or knowable" (p. 87) risks retaining even more power over the client than is already structurally in place. At the same time, self-disclosure must not hinder the purpose of therapy, which is to benefit clients (Evans et al., 2011). From this perspective, as part of how therapists weigh how each self-disclosure could benefit the client, they can consider how sharing or withholding parts of themselves could impact the egalitarian relationship, and their use of power in that relationship.

## Patriarchal Intersectional Injury Analysis

Clients show up to sessions with their ways of viewing the world and their lives. Feminist therapists collaboratively help clients examine and reflect on their views in a social, cultural, and political context to increase awareness, self-efficacy, and empowerment. In the world of addiction, oppressed perspectives often filled with learned helplessness keep clients stuck in destructive patterns. Feminist intersectional therapy encourages clients to challenge the development of these perspectives at their original social source. This application asks the client to intersectionally examine Eurocentric, heteronormative, Christian-dominant patriarchal injuries that have individually impacted their substance use.

For example, a transgender male client may have increased his alcohol intake after medically transitioning in an effort to "pass" at work and fit in at happy hour with his cisgender male colleagues who are engaging in similar use patterns. This client may have embedded social messages that men drink to bond with one another, men consume higher volumes of alcohol to keep up with and compete with one another, and he believes this is an inherently masculine activity. The feminist therapist might explore with this client what person or system first illustrated this message about masculinity to him. Does he trust the sources of these messages? Did other men in his life model this behavior? Did others of any gender identity encourage these behaviors or beliefs? Does that idea of masculinity or substance use fit his current value system, or does it just fit the patriarchy's?

The goal is to help the client think and behave congruently with their personal value system, to return autonomy from embedded messages, and to empower the client to make choices from a higher consciousness perspective. The goal is never to move the client toward the feminist clinician's value system. The goal is to examine patriarchal injuries that they may have been previously unaware of and to let the client decide how that is going to help in their recovery.

## Feminist Intersectional Twelve Steps for Empowerment: Personalized

Feminist therapists can introduce clients to the Feminist Intersectional Twelve Steps for Empowerment (MCleskey & Jodry, 2016). These Twelve Steps could be compared and contrasted with the traditional Twelve Steps of Alcoholics Anonymous and/or with other versions of the Twelve Steps. Collaboratively, the feminist therapist and client could identify which version they are drawn to and what resonates with them. The client and the therapist then might edit/modify any version of the Twelve Steps to more closely align with the client's perspective on recovery. Once the client has decided what their personal 12 steps of recovery will entail, copies can be made for a future roadmap as a tool for recovery.

## People, Places, Things, Power

In traditional substance use counseling, a helpful technique is to ask clients to identify people, places, and things that they associate with substance use (Giordano, 2021). This can include examples such as people they have often used substances with, places where they bought or used substances or where substances are readily available, items that they used in consuming substances, or sensory experiences associated with them. Because of these associations, proximity to these can trigger conscious or unconscious thoughts and feelings about substance use, and it is recommended to avoid these, at least for a period of time. A feminist therapist can include power as part of this list. Clients can identify which experiences of having power, being disempowered, giving power away, having power taken away, and so on, are associated with their past substance use. Adding the dimension of power to this list can help clients raise their consciousness about when they do or do not have power. It can also help them plan for future experiences with power and any associated thoughts or feelings accompanying them.

## Feminist Intersectional Label Analysis

Feminist therapists inherently reject labels that might limit a client's future in tandem with pathology but must consider the idea that some clients find comfort in labels as it can contribute to a sense of community, belonging, and understanding. Herein lies the value of an Intersectional Label Analysis. Clients must grapple with the differences between how the world sees them versus how they see themselves (the personal is political, after all). Clients may need guidance in understanding how their intersecting identities make up their holistic identity.

Gender, race, ethnicity, ability, affectional and/or sexual orientation, religion, spirituality, and socioeconomic status are great places to start. Connecting these identities with addiction is the next step. Culturally, spiritually, or patriarchally, how do these identities interact with beliefs or patterns of substance use? Were there any ways in which using substances benefited the client in terms of their identity (e.g., a disabled person managing chronic pain, but their use ultimately became unmanageable)? Can the therapist find ways to help clients recover power through examining intersectionality and discovering how their inextricably intertwined identities make them better manage recovery? Finding strength and insight through Intersectional Label Analysis will be the goal here.

## Support and Resource Analysis

Feminist therapists promote collective support, thought, and action. Individual support can be contextualized through relationships. Recovery from addiction is an inherently supportive endeavor, with a heavy emphasis on group support. Some clients may reject the concepts of group support, and the support resources need to be tailored to the client's unique desires, which may be connected to their intersectional identities. Support and Resource Analysis asks the client to examine who is available to aid them through their journey through recovery and who will support their empowerment. Ideally, this will go beyond simply writing down three phone numbers. What if clients considered five people who have positively influenced them throughout their lives or served as models of encouragement and empowerment? Collaboratively, feminist therapists and clients could analyze the difference between who can get together for coffee or lunch and who can be called at 3 a.m. when they are urged to relapse.

On the other hand, the client can explore whom they need distance from, who disempowers them, who supports their use instead of their recovery, and who no longer aligns with their values. Clients can benefit from processing those who deserve a place in their journey. Support and Resource Analysis should also include a discussion of whether or not the client wants to participate in recovery-oriented support groups, what the benefits and risks might look like, and whether those options will be empowering and how. Therapists discuss the choices of a feminist sponsor or feminist peer recovery coach relationship. Ideally, these supportive coaching relationships will be egalitarian in nature, because repeating oppressive dynamics is antithetical to recovery work. It might prove beneficial if the feminist therapist seeks feminist coaches for referrals when necessary.

## Recovery-Cultural Analysis

A Recovery-Cultural Analysis asks clients to consider their cultural relationship to recovery. From a sociological perspective, how have they been treated as "addicts" and/or PWUS? Additionally, some cultures embed substances and drinking alcohol into their daily way of life, and it is a familial lifestyle. Have they internalized any of these messages and, in turn, behaved accordingly? Perhaps they feel that they lack familial, social, and cultural connection by no longer participating in any substance-based rituals and traditions. Significant to consider as well is a client's potential reluctance to connect to support or recovery at all, as the United States' bootstrap mentality typically discourages the help-seeking inherent to recovery. It is helpful to collaboratively explore the societal and cultural beliefs that might be holding the client back from furthering their recovery and possible isolations associated with that recovery. A goal here is to help the client sift through cultural norms and views of substance use and discover their personal value system free from social and cultural messages.

## Group Work

Group therapy is an empowering atmosphere for a consciousness-raising activity, which is foundational to the roots of feminist therapy. There are many ways to help raise members' consciousness; they need not be overly complicated. A question posed to the group can be as simple as "In what ways has using substances made your experience as a person with/who is (a social identity/location) easier? Harder?" The idea is to let the collective speak for itself, to identify and normalize patriarchal injuries, and to illuminate addiction experiences that may be making group members feel isolated. Also, each feminist technique described here can be adapted for group work. Unique to recovery work is the prevalence and evidence-based support of peer-led support groups such as Alcoholics/Narcotics Anonymous, SMART Recovery, Women for Sobriety, and many others. These groups are inherently voluntary, and though clients may be encouraged to attend, autonomy should be respected if a client chooses not to engage in group work. If clients are forced to go by a treatment program, this could be an opportunity for advocacy by the clinician and/or by the client. A goal would be to explore the client's desire or hesitation to create a recovery community and any potential barriers.

## Advocacy

Feminist theory is historically and inherently tied to intersectional social justice work. "The personal is political" is not feminism's battle cry by accident. Feminists believe in power through collective action. As Walker (2014) said, "the most common way people give up their power is by thinking they don't have any." Feminist therapy always seeks to empower the client. Healing and empowerment can lie in advocacy, social justice, and intentional activism. However, it is solely up to the client to choose the type of advocacy they might want to engage with while using their power. Advocacy ranges from deciding to have self-compassion and advocate to yourself for yourself, to self-advocating by speaking up with your assertiveness, to marching in protest. It is very important that the feminist clinician does not pressure clients to advocate beyond their desire. Additionally, feminist clinicians may advocate on their clients' behalf with the permission of the client and when applicable, whether this be on an individual scale like with their probation officer, or on a collective scale, like with their local representative.

# Feminist Intersectional Application Example

In this example, we are applying the feminist intersectional model with an individual client for clarity. We recognize that many services for PWUS occur in group settings, and this model can be adapted for group work, as can the interventions discussed previously.

Dedra is a 28-year-old, cisgender, Latina referred to Derron's community mental health agency for substance use assessment and services. Derron is a 30-year-old, cisgender, Black male with a master's degree and state licensure. Dedra was referred by her probation officer,

Gia, due to testing positive for cannabis on her initial drug screen. Dedra's probation stems from larceny charges. Derron has several years of experience providing counseling for clients who use substances. During the intake assessment, Dedra reports a history of cannabis, alcohol, and methamphetamine use. She is referred to meet with Derron for weekly individual therapy. Members of this mandated program are regularly drug screened by agency staff and are required to pursue abstinence. Additionally, Gia will receive monthly reports about Dedra's participation in the program.

## Welcoming and Honoring the Client

In her first session with Derron, Dedra shares that she has never been to treatment before this incident. Derron uses transparency to have a conversation with Dedra about informed consent, confidentiality, what he will record in his notes during sessions and that she is free to see those notes, required drug screening, and what he is required to share with Gia. Dedra had already signed a release of information form for communications with Gia, as well as a confidentiality form outlining 42CFR-Part 2 in addition to the program intake paperwork. As they began talking in session, Dedra appears angry and says she should not be punished for using cannabis, which is legal in many states and should not have to do drug testing (she happens to be in a state that prohibits recreational use but does allow medicinal use; Dedra does not have a prescription currently). Derron normalizes Dedra's frustrations and self-discloses that he is also frustrated by some of the systemic requirements of the treatment, particularly when probation mandates are added.

He describes his approach to Dedra and explains that she is the expert on her own life, her experiences, and her desires for the future. He has training and experience that has been helpful with others. He hopes they can partner together to discover what will be helpful for her growth, including becoming more empowered by getting off probation. Dedra is quiet at times and does not offer much information beyond what is on the initial paperwork. Derron assures Dedra that he wants her to set the pace for sharing information with him.

## Understanding Client's Intersectional Experiences with Substances

In the next individual sessions, Derron continued to use transparency and some self-disclosure with Dedra. Dedra asked Derron if he was in recovery or not. He decided to share with her that he does not identify as a person in recovery. His self-disclosure felt important to him so that Dedra would feel his openness to "being real" about recovery and sharing that he had not had a substance use recovery journey of his own. Dedra seemed receptive to that. He also invited her to share her story of substance use to the extent that she was comfortable doing so. He suggested that she consider doing an Intersectional Label Analysis with him. She agreed to do this and together, they identified that ethnicity, gender, SES, and age were important intersections for her. Derron noticed that Dedra was more energized to share about her intersecting identities than discussing substance use directly at this stage of the therapeutic process. Derron began exploring how her identities may have impacted her initial use and progression of substances use, especially cannabis, as well as how she perceives her drug use currently. She admitted it was currently hard not to use cannabis, the only substance she had been using recently.

Derron introduced a Patriarchal Injury Analysis to invite Dedra to name the systems that have or that continue to oppress her. This leads to a discussion about systemic issues with probation and the criminal justice system and how Dedra intersectionally experienced oppression in terms of her ethnicity and gender. Dedra shares that she thinks her family is targeted by law enforcement in the area due to their ethnicity, and that being Latina, she feels stereotyped often. Dedra also identified the educational system as one that was not supportive. She felt frustrated by the lack of encouragement she felt in high school from teachers and staff; she started college at a predominantly White institution but left after a year because she did not feel valued or seen there. Dedra told Derron that she appreciated being able to be honest about her experiences, especially him affirming racial biases in the criminal justice system and in education systems.

## Feminist Intersectional Work: Raising Consciousness

Derron and Dedra use many of the techniques listed previously to uncover systemic context for Dedra's experiences. In the Recovery-Cultural Analysis, Dedra shares that she has felt pressure to be a positive role model for her younger siblings but also felt pressure to go along with friends' and boyfriends' substance use. Using the People, Places, Things, and Power exercise, Dedra shared that she felt powerful setting boundaries with some friends by saying no to using methamphetamine regularly but had a harder time holding that boundary with one boyfriend. She identified places where it was hard to avoid people who were using and pointed out people who still used cannabis with whom she did not want to sever ties. She and Derron processed what she wanted from those relationships, what she got from them, and how to navigate the risks of sustaining these relationships. She identified her culture and identity as a Latina as being a source of strength and pride for her. She is proud to be close with her family and regularly celebrates holidays and significant events with them.

## Holistic Healing Process

Derron and Dedra worked collaboratively to set goals. Dedra decided that she wanted to be off probation and so needed to follow the requirements even though they felt it was unfair. She also wanted to get a better job; doing some career counseling was another goal. Dedra was not convinced that she was an addict and did not like that label. She admitted that her use had been part of what got her in trouble. Dedra is committed to abstaining from cannabis while on probation, but she was not sure if she would go back to using it once she completes probation. Derron collaborated with Dedra to create a treatment plan that would fulfill the requirements for probation and help her work on her career goals. They also did a Support and Resource Analysis to identify five people who Dedra thought would help her grow her sense of power. This included a heavy emphasis on family relationships.

## Transforming Identities to Wellness

Derron shared the Feminist 12 Steps for Empowerment and the Twelve Steps of AA and asked Dedra her thoughts. Together, they compared and contrasted them. Dedra liked the empowerment focus of the feminist version as that was more consistent with her identity and goals. She did not identify as addicted and instead viewed herself as a person growing into herself who made some poor choices but for understandable reasons. Importantly, Dedra felt a sense of control over the focus of individual sessions, despite feeling disempowered by the justice system. Dedra's collaborative work with Derron in individual therapy allowed her to increase self-awareness, embrace what was within her control, and feel empowered to make conscious choices about substance use and relationships.

# Potential Challenges of a Feminist Intersectional Approach in Substance Use Work

One potential challenge of using a feminist approach is that people can have misunderstandings about feminism and can also have negative attitudes about it. Many people still associate feminism with second-wave feminism, which centered gender as the only critical social location and which centered on the needs of White, middle-class women and White women's rights. Contemporary feminism still has an emphasis on gender, but on the full range of genders, and recognizes all social locations that are oppressed or privileged, not just gender. In addition, the intersectionality of social identities is a crucial emphasis of fourth-wave feminism today. Clients may have negative attitudes about feminist therapy without truly understanding what it is in its current evolution.

Similarly, mental health colleagues may misunderstand this approach, have negative attitudes about it, and/or not feel comfortable with the way feminist therapy seeks to disrupt systems of oppression, which can include the systems within which they work. A feminist therapist is more likely to "make waves" by questioning policies and procedures and advocating for organizational change. As an example of this, feminist therapists may be more likely to react differently to things like diagnoses, treatment planning, requirements that clients attend 12-step meetings, and punitive responses from programs and other systems than are therapists rooted in other theories. Feminist therapists will generally see clients' problems as being caused by or exacerbated by systemic oppressions and limitations; this is a different perspective than many therapeutic theories. Feminist therapists may need to educate colleagues, as well as clients, in this approach.

Feminist therapists also tend to question the status quo of traditional treatments. Much of SUD therapy was formed from a middle-class male perspective, much of the addictions research has focused on males, and the dominant underpinnings of substance use treatment are drawn from the medical model (Peralta & Jauk, 2011). All of these traditional aspects of substance use conceptualizations and treatments are, therefore, rooted in patriarchal systemic thought. Feminist therapists are likely to questions these assumptions and models and any vestiges of these that remain in treatment programs. This questioning may feel threatening or invalidating to people who are invested in traditional systems of thought and treatment.

# Additional Considerations

## Feminist Motivational Interviewing

Patriarchal models of addiction treatment exploit the power dynamic between therapist and client, a dynamic that may have already begun in the courtroom for mandated clients. Even the well-accepted disease model is a medical model that puts the feminist clinician in a position to say, "You have a disease that only I know how to treat, and furthermore, there is only one way to treat that disease." This one-size-fits-all perspective does not respect client autonomy, which is central to the feminist model. Motivational interviewing is perhaps the closest match in terms of feminist ethos when it comes to currently accepted addiction treatment models. Motivational interviewing (MI) is defined as being rooted in a spirit of how to be with people (Miller & Rollnick, 2023) as opposed to a rigid list of protocols. MI includes critical concepts such as honoring client autonomy, remaining curious and open, collaborative goal-setting, and allowing the client to create their meaning; this is congruent with feminist principles. A feminist clinician practicing MI might be keen to relinquish power and collaboratively examine the client's readiness to change at their pace. Client strengths will be highlighted and used as anchors to facilitate recovery. It could be argued that motivational interviewing is a feminist model of dialogue.

## Harm Reduction: Individual Impact

Patriarchal models of addiction require total abstinence for entry and participation in treatment, foregoing the notion that clients are capable of making alternative choices for themselves. By contrast, a feminist model of harm reduction might aim to accept the client's unique voice and meet them where they are in terms of readiness for change (Collins & Clifasefi, 2023). Patriarchal models often seek to move the client into the action stage immediately, and anything less is seen as a personal failing of the client's motivation and drive. Feminist theory and harm reduction promote the idea that clients move at a pace that aligns with the client's experience and available resources.

In keeping with the core feminist tenet of an egalitarian therapeutic relationship, harm reduction directly promotes this by allowing the client to create their meaning out of sobriety. In other words, "It is accepted that the therapist does not have a greater grasp on truth than the patient, and there is an emphasis on the co-construction of meaning by patient and therapist" (Tatarsky & Kellogg, 2011, p. 40). Harm reduction coloration might mean co-creating goals, which can include targets like using alone or in a group setting, joining a needle-sharing program, or modifying the amount of substances they used. At the individual level, harm reduction means accepting small incremental changes as progress, promoting and highlighting client strengths, empowering client use of choice and autonomy, destigmatizing use, utilizing psychoeducation when necessary, and checking for safety.

## Working with Paraprofessionals

Peer recovery specialists who use their lived experiences to guide individuals pursuing addiction recovery are now a large portion of the addiction treatment workforce (Fortuna et al., 2022), in addition to bachelor's level case managers and paraprofessionals. Feminist therapists can offer valuable knowledge and treatment skills to treatment teams and may be called on to supervise and/or mentor these paraprofessionals. Working from a feminist lens can enhance these collaborations, including providing education about systemic issues facing clients and emphasizing multicultural and social justice conceptualizations of client needs in treatment. While the roles of these helpers will vary, therapists should strive to understand their strengths in meeting clients' needs and seek to utilize their roles and skills to enhance client success. For instance, a peer recovery specialist may be able to help clients navigate fears and possible disaffirming experiences with mutual self-help groups in ways a feminist therapist cannot due to ethics and boundary issues.

# What If?

What if there were no stigmas associated with addiction? How would life be different for those in recovery?

What if all treatment facilities for addictions were free of financial charges? Everyone was treated equally?

What if the insurance companies offered up to a year of residential treatment for those who needed it on the first inpatient experience?

What if addiction was truly seen as a medical disease and was treated as such, with compassion and understanding?

What if we could go back in time and erase the perspective of moral failure in addiction? What alternative explanations of addition might we have today?

# References

Alexander, M. (2020). *The new Jim Crow: Mass incarceration in the age of colorblindness*. The New Press.

Apsley, H. B., Vest, N., Knapp, K. S., Santos-Lozada, A., Gray, J., Hard, G., & Jones, A. A. (2023). Non-engagement in substance use treatment among women with an unmet need for treatment: A latent class analysis on multidimensional barriers. *Drug and Alcohol Dependence, 242*.

Brown, L. S. (2018). *Feminist therapy*. American Psychological Association.

Collins, S. E., & Clifasefi, S. L. (2023). *Harm reduction treatment for substance use*. Hogrefe Publishing.

Earp, B. D., Lewis, J., Hart, C. L., & with Bioethicists and Allied Professionals for Drug Policy Reform. (2021). Racial justice requires ending the war on drugs. *The American Journal of Bioethics, 21*(4), 4–19.

Evans, K. M., Kincade, E. A., & Seem, S. R. (2011). *Introduction to feminist therapy: Strategies for social and individual change*. SAGE.

Forrest, G. G. (2010). *Self-disclosure in psychotherapy and recovery*. Rowman & Littlefield.

Fortuna, K. L., Solomon, P., & Rivera, J. (2022). An update of peer support/peer provided services underlying processes, benefits, and critical ingredients. *The Psychiatric Quarterly, 93*(2), 571–586. https://doi.org/10.1007/s11126-022-09971-w

Giordano, A. L. (2021). *Why change people, places, and things in early recovery? It's all about conditioning*. https://www.psychologytoday.com/us/blog/understanding-addiction/202106/why-change-people-places-and-things-in-early-recovery

Hart, C. L. (2022). *Drug use for grown-ups: Chasing liberty in the land of fear*. Penguin.

Lassiter, P. S., & Spivey, M. S. (2017). Historical perspectives and the moral model. In P. S. Lassiter & J. R. Culbreth (Eds.), *Theory and practice of addiction counseling* (pp. 27–46). SAGE Publications.

McCleskey, K., & Jodry, J. (2016, July). *The personal is political in addictions: Feminist applications with the 12 steps*. Workshop presented at the meeting of the American Mental Health Counselor's Association, New Orleans, LA.

Miller, W. R., & Rollnick, S. (2023). *Motivational interviewing: Helping people grow and change*. Guilford Press.

National Institute on Drug Abuse (2020). *2020 National survey on drug use and health*. retrieved from https://www.samhsa.gov/data/sites/default/files/2021-10/2020_NSDUH_Highlights.pdf

National Institute on Drug Abuse (2018a, January 17). *Principles of drug addiction treatment: A research-based guide* (3rd ed.). Retrieved from https://archives.nida.nih.gov/publications/principles-drug-addiction-treatment-research-based-guide-third-edition

National Institute on Drug Abuse (2018b, August 15). *Comorbidity: Substance use and other mental disorders*. https://nida.nih.gov/research-topics/comorbidity/comorbidity-substance-use-other-mental-disorders-infographic

Peralta, R. L., & Jauk, D. (2011). A brief feminist review and critique of the sociology of alcohol-use and substance-abuse treatment approaches. *Sociology Compass, 5*(10), 882–897. https://doi.org/10.1111/j.1751-9020.2011.00414.x

Perron, B. E., Mowbray, O. P., Glass, J. E., Delva, J., Vaughn, M. G., & Howard, M. O. (2009). Differences in service utilization and barriers among Blacks, Hispanics, and Whites with drug use disorders. *Substance Abuse Treatment, Prevention, and Policy, 4*, 1–10.

Peterson, C., Maier, S. F., & Seligman, M. E. P. (1993). *Learned helplessness*. Oxford University Press.

Pew Research Center. (2022). *Drug arrests stayed high even as imprisonment fell from 2009 to 2019. https://www.pewtrusts*.org/en/research-and-analysis/issue-briefs/2022/02/drug-arrests-stayed-high-even-as-imprisonment-fell-from-2009-to-2019

Slaughter-Acey, J., Simone, M., Hazzard, V. M., Arlinghaus, K. R., & Neumark-Sztainer, D. (2023). More than identity: An intersectional approach to understanding mental-emotional well-being of emerging adults by centering lived experiences of marginalization. *American Journal of Epidemiology, 192*(10), 1624–1636. https://doi.org/10.1093/aje/kwad152

Tatarsky, A., & Kellogg, S. (2011). Harm reduction psychotherapy. In G. Alan Marlatt, Mary E. Larimer, & Katie Witkiewitz (Eds.), *Harm reduction: Pragmatic strategies for managing high-risk behaviors* (2nd ed., pp. 36–60). Guilford Press.

Understanding Motivational Interviewing. (2021). *Motivational Interviewing Network of Trainers*. Retrieved August 25, 2023, from https://motivationalinterviewing.org/understanding-motivational-interviewing

U.S. Drug Enforcement Agency. (n.d.) *Drug enforcement administration: The early years*. https://www.dea.gov/sites/default/files/2018-05/Early%20Years%20p%2012-29.pdf

Walker, A. (2014, October). Alice Walker: "People give up their power by thinking they don't have any." *Big Think*. https://bigthink.com/words-of-wisdom/alice-walker-people-give-up-their-power-by-thinking-they-dont-have-any-2

Yalom, I. D. (1980) *Existential psychotherapy*. Basic Books.

# 9

# Feminist Intersectional Theory with Crisis Intervention and Trauma

## *Dominique Maywald, Michelle Sunkel, Laura Dawson-Fend, Eunae Han, and Madalyn Stott*

*Crisis and trauma cannot be separated from existing embedded patriarchal privileged and oppressive beliefs, intersectional social positioning, and an existing sense of power or powerlessness that is impacted by these.*

Feminist intersectional theory has much to contribute to crisis and trauma conceptualizations and interventions. Crisis counseling and trauma work are intimately connected clinically and share therapeutic interventions. Although diverse definitions of "crisis" exist, a practical conceptualization views a crisis as a response to an event or situation that overwhelms an individual, challenging their coping mechanisms (James & Gilliland, 2017). Crisis reactions often manifest as short-term periods of disequilibrium, where therapeutic goals are focused on restoring the client's pre-crisis level of functioning. The subjective nature of crises is widely acknowledged (James & Gilliland, 2017; Sokoloff & Dupont, 2005; WHO, 2012), as personal and societal factors can influence whether an event is perceived as a crisis or an opportunity (Greenstone & Leviton, 2011). The broader societal perception of a crisis, including explicit and implicit biases, exploitation, and the suppression of narratives, significantly influences individual crisis reactions (Collins & Bilge, 2020; Crenshaw, 2017; Sokoloff & Dupont, 2005). Within third and fourth wave feminist paradigms, defining "crisis" becomes nuanced because feminist frameworks emphasize the intersectional nature of lived individual experiences (Sokoloff & Dupont, 2005). Accepting this perspective, a crisis is framed as an individual's reaction to a stressful event and a possible reflection of systemic inequality and power imbalances (Brown, 2018) within societies. This notion aligns with the World Health Organization's (WHO, 2012) characterization of crises as unforeseeable events with potential for harm, particularly in communities ill-prepared to respond to crises.

Feminist intersectional clinical theory contributes to understanding crises by adding social, cultural, and political lenses to both the crisis reaction and intervention strategies. Feminist scholars argue that crises disproportionately affect vulnerable communities and are not sudden events but represent the manifestations of harmful policies, oppressive structural inequities, and systemic discrimination (Brown, 2018; Collins & Bilge, 2020; Crenshaw, 2017). A crisis, as defined through a feminist lens, may be conceptualized as any event or situation that necessitates immediate support and intervention, wherein individuals or communities are confronted with circumstances that exacerbate existing inequalities and systemic challenges. This definition acknowledges the deep interplay of intersectionality, recognizing the diverse identities and social locations—shaped by factors such as gender, race, class, sexuality, and ability—interact with oppressive, unjust, or patriarchal systems and structures. This definition underscores that crises might also be represented as ongoing states of power imbalances generated and perpetuated by oppressive structures and systems.

There are many risks associated with crisis intervention. A significant risk in crisis intervention is the potential reinforcement of systemic inequalities. Everyone's experience of a crisis is uniquely shaped by their personal intersectional identities and societal contexts, leading to a wide range of interpretations and reactions. This subjectivity poses the danger of misaligned therapeutic interventions that do not fully acknowledge or address the important factors influencing the crisis reaction. This oversight can lead to ineffective and harmful therapeutic outcomes. The traditional focus on returning individuals to their pre-crisis level of functioning risks overlooking the transformative potential inherent in crisis situations. This approach can inadvertently contribute to a narrative that views individuals merely as victims of their circumstances, rather than as agents capable of resilience and change. Lastly, crisis situations from a feminist clinical perspective shine a light on the limitations and biases of systems, increasing the risk of pathologizing normal reactions to abnormal situations.

However, it is also crucial for feminist clinicians to recognize that within each crisis lies both danger and opportunity (Sue, 2016). A holistic understanding of an individual's unique intersectional crisis experience is fundamental to exploring clinical practice (Crenshaw, 2017; Brown, 2018). The person-in-environment perspective enables clinicians to identify client-specific rights, support needs, and advocacy strategies. With feminist principles, a crisis can be the catalyst for consciousness-raising (hooks, 2015), representing opportunities for both personal empowerment and societal transformation. Feminist clinicians must navigate crises with humility, empathy, and curiosity. Feminist intersectional crisis intervention requires a deep understanding of intersectionality and a commitment to advocating for change across practice levels.

# A Feminist Intersectional Model for Creating Brave Spaces during Crisis

This non-directive model takes a different approach to intervention within a crisis and will require more time spent with the client to attend to the principles of feminist intersectional theory.

## Creating a Brave Space and Building Connection-Dual Process

Feminist clinicians prioritize client safety by establishing brave spaces imbued with feminist ideals. This requires gaining informed consent and assent. This process begins with emphasizing client autonomy and control. Feminist clinicians engage in sensitive discussions such as potential harms affecting clients and their communities, navigating complex conversations surrounding the topics of suicide and homicide, with a focus on protecting the well-being and safety of all. It is crucial that clients understand the practitioner's role. Feminist clinicians are transparent, seek consent, clarify each step, respect the client's choice, and affirm that power resides with the client and not only in the clinician.

## Client Intersectional Narrative and Their Relationship to the World around Them

Feminist practitioners situate clients as credible sources of information. Understanding the client's narrative and their connection to the world around them is essential throughout the intervention process. Feminist clinicians listen attentively to the client's perception of the crisis, paying close attention to their language. Language choices can reveal the client's view of the crisis. Recognizing the client's intersectional identities and potential areas of privilege and oppression might inform the client's perceptions of capabilities and power. Do clients articulate a sense of empowerment or feelings of being trapped in narratives of colonization or victimization? Clinicians also consider the client's cultural norms, which may conflict with the individualistic, ableist, self-centered, nationalistic, patriarchal, and Christian-dominant values prevalent in Eurocentric heteronormative societies.

## Empowering Clients to Trust Themselves while Providing Support and Resources

Feminist clinicians encourage clients to discuss their coping strategies, connecting these skills back to their inherent strengths and resiliencies. The practice emphasis is on encouraging clients to trust in themselves and their choices as much as possible; in crises where there are dangers to the client or others, clinicians can honor the client by being receptive to their perspectives and desires. Feminist practitioners assist clients in exploring their position in and within the crisis. Feminist clinicians take on an advocacy role, challenging the patriarchal structures and oppressive systems that may contribute to the crisis reaction, striving to create more equitable systems. By providing support and culturally affirming resources, feminist clinicians aim to see clients emerge from the crisis empowered.

## Critical Reflection on Positionality

Critical reflection on positionality is an ongoing process throughout the intervention model. Clinicians engage in introspection, ensuring that their approach aligns with the feminist ideals of equality, empowerment, and dismantling oppressive structures. This self-reflection is crucial in maintaining adherence to feminist principles within clinical work, fostering continual growth and practice integrity. At times, egalitarian power may need to shift if danger is present.

| Brave Space | Understand | Encourage | Reflection |
|---|---|---|---|
| **BUILDING CONNECTION** | **CLIENT NARRATIVE** | **CLIENT EMPOWERMENT** | **POSITIONALITY** |
| • Prioritize Safety (Suicide, Homicide, etc.)<br>• Emphasize Client Control and Autonomy<br>• Egalitarian Relationship | • Respect Client as a credible source of information<br>• Active Listening<br>• Explore client cultural norms and perceptions of the crisis | • Identify client coping skills<br>• Connect the coping skills to client strengths<br>• Provide support and culturally affirming resources<br>• Clinician Advocates | • Clinician critically analyzes their role within the crisis through a feminist lens |

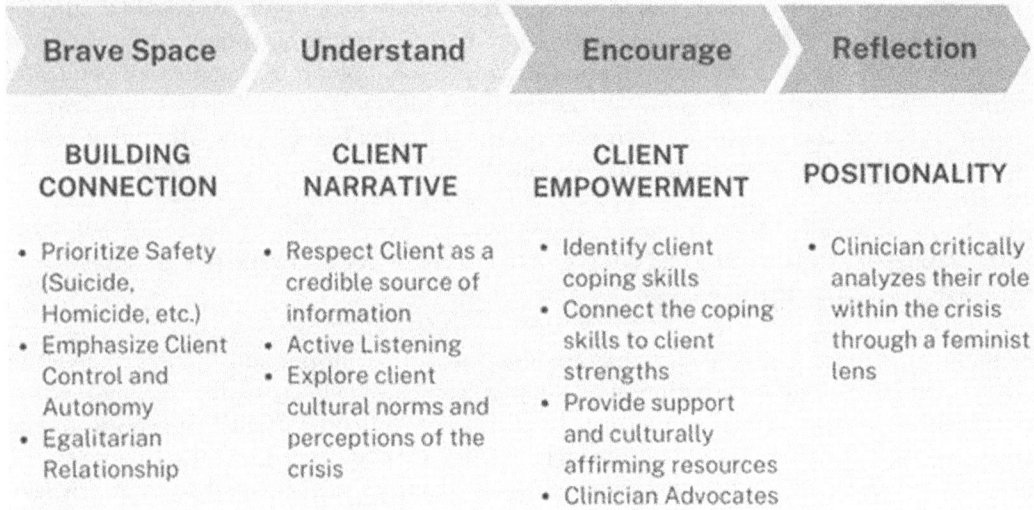

FIGURE 9.1 *Feminist Intersectional Model for Creating Brave Spaces during Crisis.*

# Feminist Intersectional Crisis Example: Roberta in Crisis

Roberta was referred to the crisis center when the police arrived at her residence to arrest her oldest son, Juan, on drug charges. Roberta is visibly upset and confused about her son's situation. Her primary concern is that her family will be deported as a result of her son's involvement with the legal system. Roberta is a 26-year-old undocumented female from Guatemala. She is married and has four children ranging in age from 1 year old to 10 years old. Roberta does not speak much English, but she is able to understand a little English. The family system is experiencing poverty and lives in a three-bedroom trailer. Roberta's husband, Jose, is the family patriarch; his primary role in the family system is to provide financial resources. Jose is a day laborer who is rarely at home, which means his interactions with his children are limited. Roberta discloses that she and Jose sometimes have loud arguments, and he physically "punishes" her in front of the children. The friction in the marriage has created difficulty in Roberta's parenting of Juan. Roberta reports that she has no control over her son and that he does not respect her. She is fearful, anxious, and uncertain of the next steps to take.

## Roberta Crisis Conceptualization

Roberta's crisis, underscored by her son Juan's detention over substance use charges, necessitates a nuanced approach that respects her fears and provides tailored support considering her family's undocumented status. In applying the Feminist Intersectional Model for Creating Brave Spaces during crisis to Roberta's case, it is good to remember that a crisis is immediate and time-limited, so time is of the essence. To create a brave space for Roberta, it is crucial for the counselor to address her multifaceted needs. It is not enough to only assess for suicidal and homicidal ideation and make sure the physical environment is safe; it is also important to address intersectional issues. How might a clinician accommodate Roberta's language barriers? Is there a certified translator who speaks Spanish and understands

Guatemalan society's cultural nuances? Working with the translator, the therapist explains the rules and limits to confidentiality, emphasizing that Roberta's documented status is not a reason to contact the authorities.

To build an understanding of Roberta and her relationship to the world around her, the clinician must remember to engage in open dialogue, ensuring Roberta is esteemed as the expert in her lived and living experience(s). Practitioners can ask clients if there is anything else that is important for them to know within their professional role. Questions to consider when supporting Roberta's family during the crisis reaction and to engage in bravery include the following: Does the family have safe housing, food, water, and electricity? Is the home physically safe? Does everyone have clothing that is seasonally appropriate? Is there formula and diapers for the baby? Does the family have access to societal benefits? As the family is undocumented, they may not be able to use any of the social safety nets that documented clients may access; this would require the clinician to be creative when navigating resources. What supports and healthy coping skills are available to the family? What are the ongoing concerns that Roberta has and how can the practitioner assist in de-escalating those concerns? This includes discussing substance use within the family, the impact of Juan's detention, and fears of deportation, ensuring a feminist approach that validates her emotions and stresses the importance of understanding her legal rights in the United States. These efforts reshape the crisis evaluation putting the client at the center of the intervention and ensuring that all information the client feels is relevant and important is shared. A brave space is about creating a safe egalitarian alliance between the client and the clinician. Practitioners acknowledge that they are working with people experiencing a crisis. Clients experiencing a crisis may be exhausted, exploited, distressed, and highly vulnerable to increased oppression. Practitioners work to reinforce autonomy, understanding, and clarity, while providing intervention services with compassion and empathy.

Roberta is empowered to trust in herself and her choices. As the clinician walks beside Roberta through her crisis reaction, they strive toward equity and advocacy. This approach is rooted in mutual respect and trust, affirming Roberta's courage in seeking help. The clinician must be well versed in the concepts of poverty, racism, xenophobia, and scapegoating that impact marginalized clients. Addressing domestic dynamics within the family, the clinician explores intimate partner violence (IPV) without judgment, recognizing Roberta's experiences with oppression and financial dependency. The goal is empowerment, respecting Roberta's autonomy in decision-making, and fostering situational resilience. Is Roberta open to a protective shelter? Are there shelters prepared to respond to the needs of Roberta and her children? Will Roberta be free from deportation if she accesses IPV services? Does Roberta believe the couple should stay together? Roberta may choose for any number of reasons not to address the issue of IPV. If that happens, the clinician might ask questions related to how they could best support the family right now. The practitioner knows to be cautious when working within systems and connects Roberta to culturally affirming legal and community resources. The practitioner verifies that all resources are aligned with intervention goals, facilitating a warm handoff to agencies equipped to support undocumented families. As practitioners connect clients to resources, they continue to build and reinforce healthy referral mechanisms. This case, while complex, has the potential to connect this family to resources to improve their current circumstance, perhaps creating a pathway to citizenship and increased community support.

Once the immediate stress of the crisis has passed and Roberta has been referred to agencies that will help her navigate the longer-term impacts of the crisis, the practitioner must examine their position to and within the crisis. Post-crisis, the practitioner reflects on their practice of the feminist model for creating brave spaces during crisis. Was the clinician able to manage their biases and expectations? Was Roberta allowed to lead her treatment experience? In light of Roberta's case, what new insights were gained? How does this case enhance feminist practice moving forward? If the clinician finds that they are unable to locate their position to or within the case, feminist principles and assumptions were not followed, or the practitioner lacked cultural humility, supervision and consultation must be sought.

As a feminist practitioner, it is essential to understand how systemic inequalities intersect with individual experiences of crisis and trauma. A crisis represents a significant disruption in a person's life that demands immediate attention. While it can be distressing, not all crises lead to trauma. A key differentiator is that a crisis is often acute and temporary, requiring prompt intervention often dictated by agency protocols and available resources. Trauma can have a deeper, long-lasting impact on an individual's psyche, perhaps resulting from prolonged exposure to distressing events or repeated violations of personal boundaries and capacities. Trauma is not just the event itself but the lingering effect on the person's mental, emotional, and physical well-being. It is critical to acknowledge how societal dynamics, such as oppression, marginalization, bias, and othering can exacerbate both crisis and trauma, necessitating a tailored, empathetic response that recognizes these broader contexts.

# Feminist Intersectional Therapy and Trauma: Inclusive Understanding

## Overview of Trauma

There are many definitions of trauma. The Substance Abuse and Mental Health Services Administration (SAMHSA, 2024) defines individual trauma as "an event or circumstance resulting in: physical harm, emotional harm and/or life-threatening harm. . . . [The event or circumstance] has lasting adverse effects on the individual's functioning and mental, physical, social, emotional, or spiritual well-being" (paras. 1 and 2). Trauma has a profound impact on the brain, body, nervous system, and emotional mind, often disrupting their natural functions and leading to long-term consequences. Neurobiologically, trauma can alter the brain's structure and function, particularly in the areas responsible for memory, emotional regulation, and stress response, such as the hippocampus, amygdala, and prefrontal cortex (Porges, 2017; Dana & Porges, 2018). These changes can result in heightened anxiety, hypervigilance, and difficulty regulating emotions.

The body may manifest trauma through physical symptoms like chronic pain, gastrointestinal issues, and cardiovascular problems, as it remains in a state of heightened arousal (Oberlander et al., 2008; Perroud et al., 2011). The autonomic nervous system becomes dysregulated, making it difficult for individuals to return to a state of calm after experiencing stress (Porges, 2017). Emotionally, trauma can lead to persistent feelings of fear, shame, and helplessness, which further exacerbate the physiological and psychological impacts (Centre for Addiction and Mental Health, 2021). Together, these effects create a cycle of trauma that affects every aspect of an individual's well-being, requiring comprehensive and empathetic interventions to address both the immediate symptoms and the underlying causes of trauma.

Benjet et al. (2016) reported that 70% of the general population has been exposed to trauma. Trauma exposure can pertain to crime, natural disasters, accidents, illness, violence, sexual abuse, and other violations (Quiros & Berger, 2013). In delving deeper into understanding the feminist perspective on trauma, it is crucial to recognize how trauma can profoundly impact one's emotional and psychological well-being. The high prevalence of traumatic experiences in society can lead to the polarization of either developing strong resiliency or having long-lasting traumatic effects (Quiros & Berger, 2013). Russin and Stein (2022) analyzed the impact of adult trauma on families and found that there are multi-level impacts that include the

> individual-level (i.e., quality of psychological health, burden, secondary traumatic stress, quality of physical health, and positive impacts), interpersonal and environmental level (i.e., quality of relationships with survivors, navigating environment, maltreatment and safety, and social impacts), and other experiences (i.e., social roles, needs, coping strategies, and sociocultural context). (p. 1288)

Russin and Stein (2022) also found that secondary trauma can lead to "physical, emotional, cognitive, behavioral, social, safety, and relational impacts" (p. 1288).

## Feminist Intersectional Perspectives on Trauma

From the fourth-wave contemporary feminist perspective, trauma is further defined as the enduring impact of systemic oppression, manifesting across psychological, physical, and emotional realms. It recognizes the compounded effects of intersecting identities, viewing trauma not just as an individual experience but as a collective consequence of entrenched societal inequalities. Therefore, if one person is impacted by trauma, we are all impacted by trauma.

Colonialism and capitalism have had profound and enduring impacts on societal trauma, particularly through the lenses of supremacy and exploitation (Bhattacharyya, 2018). Contemporary feminist intersectional theory emphasizes the need to understand trauma not just as an individual experience but as a collective consequence of systemic oppression. Colonialism and capitalism, driven by supremacist ideologies, have perpetuated cycles of violence, exploitation, and dehumanization, resulting in widespread trauma across marginalized communities (Coulthard, 2014). This trauma is not merely an emotional or psychological wound; it is deeply entrenched in the historical and ongoing structural inequalities that shape society.

The patriarchal society has traditionally managed traumatic events from an authoritarian, top-down approach (Mosurska et al., 2023). Managing trauma focuses on immediate symptom relief, helping clients cope with the distressing effects through techniques like grounding, mindfulness, or manualized intervention processes. Managing trauma addresses the surface-level manifestations of the response, enabling clients to function day to day. Society must acknowledge that marginalized groups have limited resources, experience more disasters due to greater loss, and are presented with more barriers to the trauma recovery process (Pyles, 2007). Feminist practitioners have the obligation to pause and reflect on how social frameworks influence traumatic environments and affect people while cautioning society against putting too much emphasis on the natural disasters themselves and not enough importance on the surrounding social environments (Wisner et al., 2003), which impact the development and expression of a client's traumatic response. In contrast to the management of trauma, healing trauma involves an immeasurable, transformative process that seeks to understand and disrupt the systemic roots of trauma. Healing is centered on empowering individuals to reclaim their narratives, confront the underlying sources of pain, and nourish resilience within the context of their intersecting identities. From a feminist perspective, healing might also mean challenging and changing the societal structures that perpetuate trauma, aiming for long-term, systemic transformation.

Feminist practitioners, drawing on the critical awareness of intersectionality (Crenshaw, 1989) and the politics of care (Tronto, 1993), are called to respond to trauma from a bottom-up and inclusive process to include the perspective of the community. Feminist trauma-informed strategies prioritize the recognition of how power, privilege, and oppression intersect in the client's lived experience. This style of intervention is unlike traditional, manualized approaches to trauma treatment, which typically place the focus of intervention on symptom management in isolation. The feminist intersectional approach necessitates a shift from merely treating trauma as an isolated event to understanding it as a manifestation of systemic violence and recognizing community members as the experts in disaster management, crisis, and trauma response. In this way, an equitable approach to healing trauma centers the voices and experiences of those most affected by the legacies of colonialism, capitalism, and patriarchy (hooks, 2000).

# Feminist Intersectional Trauma-Informed Strategies

Distinguishing feminist strategies within trauma treatment is rather challenging due to the influence of early pioneers in trauma work who were also feminists (Brown, 2019). Mental health professionals serving survivors of gender-based violence contributed significantly to the current body of trauma literature, coining terms such as *rape trauma syndrome* (Burgess & Holmstrom, 1974) and *battered women's syndrome* (Walker, 1979). Influential feminist therapists such as Judith L. Herman and Christine Courtois shaped the early exploration of sexual abuse and violence issues. The feminist intersectional therapy lens offers feminist perspectives on trauma healing for diverse client groups by outlining the following areas: (a) strategies for reflexive trauma practice, (b) strategies for working with communities, (c) strategies for working with clients, and (d) the Feminist Intersectional Trauma Disruption Model.

## Strategies for Feminist Intersectional Therapists for Self-Development

### Feminist Humility

Cultural humility is a pivotal aspect of multicultural orientation within the helping professions, emphasizing curiosity and critical examination of cultural knowledge over competency (Hook et al., 2013; Zhu et al., 2023). Han and Lee (2023) expand on cultural humility to offer *feminist humility*, which recognizes clients as experts in their own lives with exceptional coping skills. Practitioners who adopt feminist humility display attributes of respecting clients' decisions, strengths, and coping skills. Feminist practitioners approach clients with genuine curiosity and a willingness to understand their trauma narratives. To disrupt trauma, feminist practitioners could embrace a stance of genuine curiosity about clients' unique experiences, histories, and cultural contexts. These strategies align with the feminist principles of empowerment and egalitarian relationship-building between practitioners and clients.

## Critical Examination of Cultural and Systemic Factors

Reducing the overall impact of trauma requires practitioners to engage in ongoing critical self-reflection and examination of cultural knowledge. By understanding the broader cultural and systemic factors that contribute to a client's trauma, practitioners can offer more nuanced and effective interventions. This strategy moves beyond a simplistic competency model and toward an approach rooted in feminist humility.

## Self-Awareness of Trauma by Clinician

Trauma exposure is common among helping professionals, often referred to as "wounded healers" (Fear, 2022), indicating that many practitioners have faced traumatic experiences before entering the field. This personal history can enhance their ability to empathize and support clients. Research shows that helping professionals, including counselors, child service providers, and direct support workers, report higher rates of adverse childhood experiences (ACEs) than the general population (Han & Carrola, 2024; Esaki & Larkin, 2013). In feminist clinical practice, it is crucial to consider a professional's own trauma history to foster egalitarian therapeutic relationships. Reflective practice, grounded in cultural humility and feminist consciousness, is essential to prevent perpetuating power imbalances and harming clients. Feminist clinicians must be aware of how their own trauma histories may influence the helping relationship, especially when working with clients who have experienced oppressive relationships (Reynolds, 2020; SAMHSA, 2014).

## Regular Reflective Supervision

Feminist practitioners should engage in regular reflective supervision sessions, during which they can openly discuss their own trauma histories, biases, and emotional responses with a supervisor who also uses an intersectional ecosystem context. This practice encourages self-awareness and helps clinicians recognize how their personal experiences might impact their interactions with clients.

## Consciousness-Raising Groups for Feminist Helping Professionals

Participating in or facilitating consciousness-raising groups with other feminist practitioners can be a powerful intervention. These groups provide a space for professionals to explore and discuss the intersections of their identities, trauma histories, and the broader systemic forces at play. This collective reflection enhances self-awareness and helps practitioners prevent unintentional harm in their work with clients.

## Mindful Self-Reflection Practices

Incorporating mindfulness and self-reflection exercises into daily practice can help feminist clinicians stay attuned to their emotional states and potential triggers. Regularly setting aside time for journaling, meditation, or other reflective practices allows practitioners to process their own experiences, ensuring they approach client interactions with a clear, unbiased, and compassionate mindset.

# Strategies to Use with Communities

## *Nurturing Community Resilience*

Community trauma, which disproportionately impacts Black, Indigenous, and People of Color (BIPOC) (Hardy, 2023; Mullan, 2023; Weisner, 2020), is deeply rooted in systemic inequalities such as racism, discrimination, and poverty. Historical trauma, compounded by the legacies of war, imperialism, colonization, domination, and enslavement, is perpetuated across cultural, political, racial, and ethnic lines over time (Hübl, 2020; Brave Heart, et al., 2011). Communities impacted by systemic inequities face heightened psychosocial disparities and mental health challenges. These challenges are exacerbated by a fragmented mental health system that predominantly serves White, middle-class norms and expectations (Hardy, 2023; Mullan, 2023).

Addressing community trauma requires a multifaceted approach that includes recognizing the impact of structural racism, strengthening social networks, facilitating access to culturally relevant mental health services, and empowering collective change. Feminist theory expands the understanding of trauma to include the intersectional effects of Eurocentric, Christian-dominant, heteronormative, and patriarchal systems on trauma responses. This broader perspective underscores the value of community participation in the healing process, fostering community resilience by empowering individuals and groups to collectively address and heal from the systemic traumas that affect them.

## *Facilitating Community-Based Healing Circles*

Establishing community-based healing circles can be a powerful feminist intersectional intervention to disrupt trauma and reconnect clients with their communities. These circles create brave, inclusive spaces where individuals can share their unique intersectional experiences, validate each other's narratives, and build collective resilience. Healing circles help to counteract the isolation and fragmentation often caused by trauma, reinforcing community ties and shared strength.

# Strategies to Use with Clients

## *Fostering Empowerment Through Feminist Humility*

Feminist practitioners can reduce trauma by approaching clients as the true experts of their own experiences, respecting their decisions, strengths, and coping mechanisms. This strategy encourages clients to reclaim their power and agency, fostering an environment where they feel validated and supported in their healing journey. When practitioners prioritize clients' narratives and view them as active collaborators in the therapeutic process, they disrupt the disempowerment that trauma often perpetuates.

## *Promoting Culturally Relevant Mental Health Resources*

Feminist practitioners can work to disrupt trauma by connecting clients to culturally relevant mental health resources that resonate with their lived experiences. This might involve partnering with local organizations, community leaders, or cultural practitioners who understand the unique challenges faced by BIPOC communities. Practitioners can help clients in their intersectional identities feel seen and supported, strengthening their connection to their community by ensuring that mental health services are both accessible and culturally attuned.

## *Empowering Collective Action and Advocacy*

Encouraging clients to engage in collective action or community advocacy can be a transformative intervention that disrupts trauma. Whether through organizing around issues of structural inequality, participating in community-building activities, or advocating for systemic change, clients can reclaim their agency and contribute to the resilience of their communities. This sense of purpose and collective empowerment can be a vital component of healing, as it shifts the focus from individual trauma to community recovery and empowerment.

# Feminist Intersectional Trauma Disruption Model

The Feminist Intersectional Trauma Disruption Model is a framework that is centered on the client narrative. During each stage of the model, feminist clinicians must reflect on their biases and positionality within the client's situation, ensuring that they approach the client's narrative with sensitivity and an awareness of power dynamics. The Feminist Intersectional Trauma Disruption Model is nonlinear and is nondirective. This model explores a different approach to trauma intervention and may require more time spent with the client to attend to the principles of fourth-wave feminist intersectional theory.

## Reduce Trauma Response

Like all therapists, the feminist clinician focuses on calming, soothing, and regulating the client's trauma response. The clinician engages the client in a discussion surrounding their physical safety and emotional vulnerabilities. If safety is at risk, clinicians follow their agency's safety protocols immediately. The goal is to create a brave and collaborative space where the client feels secure without pushing them beyond their window of tolerance. The goal is to help the client achieve a state of calm and regulation, grounding them in the present moment.

## Honoring Client's Narrative

The feminist clinician fully embraces the belief that the client is the expert in their own life, regardless of the circumstances. Feminist practitioners validate and normalize the client's experiences, employing feminist humility to foster a relationship built on transparent egalitarianism. This involves supporting the client as they explore their feelings and circumstances, facilitating insight, growth, and a deeper understanding of trauma while looking for narratives of power or disempowerment. The clinician and client collaboratively explore the client's narrative, including their social locations and the broader contexts of their traumatic experiences.

## Increase Feminist Trauma Literacy

The feminist clinician seeks to balance the power differential between the client and practitioner and between the client and their community. The clinician supports the client in building agency and autonomy within their social, cultural, and political context. Together, they develop language around the client's trauma experiences and explore how these narratives intersect their identities and roles with various forms of oppression. This is also a stage for consciousness raising, where the impact of trauma on the whole person (body, mind, and spirit), interpersonal relationships, and communities is examined.

## Disrupt Trauma through Advocacy

The feminist clinician and the client engage in collaborative efforts to facilitate social transformation and disrupt the trauma. This includes enhancing coping skills based on the client's strengths, acknowledging and celebrating client resilience, and empowering the client to become an advocate for themselves and perhaps their communities. On a broader scale, this stage focuses on nurturing community resilience, networking, and challenging oppressive policies at local, state, and federal levels. If desired by the client, both clinician and client can work together to address and dismantle systemic inequities.

# Feminist Intersectional Example of Roberta: From Crisis to Trauma Transformation

Roberta has come back to the agency for more long-term support due to physical and emotional symptoms connected with ongoing fears of Juan's incarceration, possible deportation of the family, and the onset of panic attacks. A feminist Spanish-speaking clinician familiar with Guatemalan culture has been assigned to work with Roberta. This feminist practitioner is grounded in the recognition of intersectional privilege and oppression. She is familiar with working with undocumented families and has contacts with programs that help provide legal counsel and other necessary services (educational, health care, transportation, etc.). By anticipating the oppressive barriers to treatment and helping to find a local solution, the clinician can provide Roberta with culturally appropriate therapeutic services. The clinician has reviewed the records from Roberta's crisis and intake sessions to avoid retraumatizing Roberta by repeating information already given to the agency.

As a feminist clinician, advocating and removing barriers became an initial focal point. Since childcare is an issue for Roberta, the clinician has worked with a local nonprofit to provide Spanish-speaking childcare for Roberta's children, reducing one primary barrier to the intervention process. Because of this, Roberta is more likely to engage in therapy consistently. The agency was able to use community resources to help Roberta in the past, including finding a way to engage with social services that encouraged a consistent and supportive relationship. The feminist clinician listens to and honors Roberta's narrative about her fears her children will be taken by the government. Due to Roberta and her families' undocumented status, the clinician advocates with local nonprofits to help support Roberta in acquiring necessities, including food and shelter for her and the children. The clinician, in cooperation with Roberta, displays trustworthiness to create a brave therapeutic space. The practitioner is aware and conscious of her own biases and status as a Latina American with full citizenship.

To reduce Roberta's trauma-related symptoms of anxiety and panic, the clinician starts the session with a basic breathing or grounding technique. The clinician explains each step of the mindfulness practice to ensure that Roberta is comfortable, is willing to try these techniques, and can use these techniques whenever she feels dysregulated. As a primary caregiver herself, the practitioner is also aware that if she can support Roberta to be less reactive, she can help Roberta support the emotional regulation of her children.

Once Roberta is grounded, the clinician performs an agency routine safety check. The practitioner also inquires how things are going between Roberta and her husband, knowing that there is a history of IPV. The practitioner exercises feminist humility in how she labels things, as Roberta has not named the domestic challenges between her husband and herself as physical abuse. Roberta is supported by the clinician in describing incidents between herself and her husband.

Once immediate safety concerns are discussed and a client narrative is established, the practitioner moves into increasing Roberta's trauma literacy. It is important to note that the availability of a culturally appropriate therapist and a history with the agency allows the initial stage to move more quickly than in other situations. The feminist therapist places emphasis on language outlining oppression, patriarchy, and violence as it intersects with trauma. This includes psychoeducation for Roberta around oppressive systems (immigration, criminal justice, health care, etc). The therapist helps Roberta become empowered in her narrative and examine her trauma through her intersectional identities and roles. She continues to evolve and becomes more encouraged to assert herself within the therapeutic space. Roberta continues to be encouraged to explore how her body stores and processes trauma and how that can manifest as physical health-related issues.

The clinician also helps Roberta understand how internalized oppression can manifest in trauma symptoms in herself and her children, including sleep disturbances, behavioral issues, and somatic challenges. The feminist practitioner and Roberta practice having Roberta check in with herself and her body for an indicator on how she is reacting to the trauma within her circumstance. Roberta is also encouraged to teach her children how to check in with their bodies when they are experiencing challenging emotions or behaviors. The clinician supports Roberta in gaining autonomy over her feelings.

Once the foundation for understanding trauma and oppression is laid, the feminist practitioner and Roberta can move on to disrupt her trauma. During this stage, the feminist clinician focuses on Roberta's strengths and provides resources to develop the skills to reframe her trauma, adding ecosystemic oppressions as a contributor to her trauma to help address symptoms. The practitioner uses examples of Roberta's strengths to acknowledge her resiliencies and, if appropriate, that of her ancestors. This stage focuses on building the client up and ensuring she is supported and engaged in community healing. Roberta can learn to be an advocate for herself, her family, and others in similar situations.

Feminist intersectional therapy is a new model of intervention that adds a systemic community lens and related privileges and oppressions to the clinical process. To disrupt her trauma, the feminist clinician actively seeks to connect Roberta to community resources that link her with other undocumented people who share her fears and are actively advocating for change.

The feminist practitioner recognizes their own intersectional privileges and oppressions. The final stage of the model necessitates that the clinician challenges oppressive and patriarchal norms that are harmful to both Roberta and society. Personal and political issues may become an ongoing central part of the final healing process. This model asserts that while trauma may not be entirely eradicated, perspectives can be shifted surrounding the intersectional privileges and oppressions, and the pervasive impact of trauma can be actively disrupted for the benefit of clients and communities alike.

# Closing Thoughts

Crisis counseling and trauma work through a feminist intersectional clinical lens showcase the intricate link between individual crises, multiple oppressions, and systemic disparities. It also critically examines the subjective essence of crises, emphasizing how intersectional, personal, and societal influences shape perceptions of events as dangerous, harmful, or opportunistic. Feminist intersectional approaches to clinical practice contest oppressive structures and systems and encourage clinicians to consider these strategies as opportunities for applying feminist intersectional therapy to clinical practice while supporting client and community healing. This positive endorsement of feminist practices is a powerful call to action for feminist clinicians, encouraging them to leverage these strategies in developing transformative change and healing with clients and communities.

# What If?

What if every crisis intervention incorporated a feminist lens that recognized the intersectional nature of each client's experience?

What if practitioners prioritized creating brave spaces in every therapeutic encounter, allowing clients to feel both seen and heard?

What if crisis counseling always included a component of community engagement to empower collective resilience and healing?

What if trauma literacy became a foundational element in all therapeutic practices, equipping clients with the language to articulate their experiences?

What if the mental health system was restructured to serve marginalized communities with the same efficacy as it does White, middle-class populations?

What if feminist humility guided every therapeutic interaction, fostering deeper client-practitioner relationships rooted in mutual respect and empowerment?

What if the role of the practitioner extended beyond the therapy room to include advocacy against oppressive policies that impact clients?

# References

American Psychiatric Association (APA). (2022). *Diagnostic and statistical manual of mental disorders* (DSM-5TR) (5th ed., rev.). American Psychiatric Association.

Benjet, C., Bromet, E., Karam, E. G., Kessler, R. C., McLaughlin, K. A., Ruscio, A. M., . . . Koenen, K. C. (2016). The epidemiology of traumatic event exposure worldwide: Results from the World Mental Health Survey Consortium. *Psychological Medicine, 46*(2), 327–343. https://doi.org10.1017/s0033291715001981

Bhattacharyya, G. (2018). *Rethinking racial capitalism: Questions of reproduction and survival.* Rowman & Littlefield.

Brave Heart, M. Y. H., Chase, J., Elkins, J., & Altschul, D. B. (2011). Historical trauma among Indigenous peoples of the Americas: Concepts, research, and clinical considerations. *Journal of Psychoactive Drugs, 43*(4), 282–290.

Brown, L. S. (2018). *Feminist therapy*. American Psychological Association.

Brown, L. S. (2019). *Feminist therapy* (2nd ed.). American Psychological Association.

Burgess, A. W., & Holmstrom, L. L. (1974). Rape trauma syndrome. *American Journal of Psychiatry, 131*(9), 981–986. https://doi.org/10.1176/ajp.131.9.981

Centre for Addiction and Mental Health (CAMH) (2021). *Trauma.* https://www.camh.ca/en/health-info/mental-illness-and-addiction-index/trauma

Coulthard, G. S. (2014). *Red skin, white masks: Rejecting the colonial politics of recognition.* University of Minnesota Press.

Collins, P. H. (2000). *Black feminist thought: Knowledge, consciousness, and the politics of empowerment* (2nd ed.). Routledge.

Collins, P. H., & Bilge, S. (2020). *Intersectionality.* Polity.

Crenshaw, K. (1989). Demarginalizing the intersection of race and sex: A Black feminist critique of antidiscrimination doctrine, feminist theory and antiracist politics. *University of Chicago Legal Forum, 1989*(1), 139–167.

Crenshaw, K. (1991). Mapping the margins: Intersectionality, identity politics, and violence against women of color. *Stanford Law Review, 43*(6), 1241–1299.

Crenshaw, K. (2017). *On intersectionality: Essential writings.* The New Press.

Dana, D., & Porges, S. W. (2018). *The polyvagal theory in therapy: Engaging the rhythm of regulation.* W. W. Norton.

Esaki, N., & Larkin, H. (2013). Prevalence of adverse childhood experiences (ACEs) among child service providers. *Families in Society: The Journal of Contemporary Social Services, 94*(1), 31–37. https://doi.org/10.1606/1044-3894.4257

Fear, R. M. (2022). *A psychoanalytic study of the wounded healer: Life stories, myth and reality* (1st ed.). Routledge. https://doi.org/10.4324/9781003316503

Greenstone, J. L., & Leviton, S. C. (2011). *Elements of crisis intervention: Crises and how to respond to them.* Cengage Learning.

Han, E., & Carrola, P. (2024). Adverse childhood experiences, work-related stress, and trauma-informed care among novice counselors. *Journal of Counselor Preparation and Supervision, 18*(3). 10.70013/508qkr18

Han, E., & Lee, I. (2023). Empowering women in counseling by dismantling internalized sexism: The feminist-multicultural orientation and social justice competencies. *Journal of Mental Health Counseling, 45*(3), 213–230. https://doi.org/10.17744/mehc.45.3.03

Hardy, K. V. (2023). *Racial trauma: Clinical strategies and techniques for healing invisible wounds.* W. W. Norton.

Herman, J. L. (1992). *Trauma and recovery.* Basic Books/Hachette Book Group.

hooks, b. (2000). *Feminist theory: From margin to center.* Pluto Press.

hooks, b. (2015). *Feminism is for everybody: Passionate politics* (2nd ed.). Routledge.

Hook, J., Davis, D., Owen, J., Worthington, E., & Utsey, S. (2013). Cultural humility: Measuring openness to culturally diverse clients. *Journal of Counseling Psychology, 60*(3), 353–366. https://psycnet.apa.org/doi/10.1037/a0032595

Hübl, T. (2020). *Healing collective trauma: A process for integrating our intergenerational and cultural wounds.* Sounds True.

James, R. (2008). *Crisis intervention strategies.* Thomson Brooks/Cole.

James, R. K., & Gilliland, B. E. (2017). *Crisis intervention strategies.* Cengage Learning.

Mosurska, A., Clark-Ginsberg, A., Sallu, S., & Ford, J. (2023). Disasters and indigenous peoples: A critical discourse analysis of the expert new media. *Environment and Planning E: Nature and Space, 6*(1), 178–201. https://doi.org/10.1177/25148486221096371

Mullan, J. (2023). *Decolonizing therapy: Oppression, historical trauma, and politicizing your practice.* W. W. Norton.

Oberlander, T. F., Weinberg, J., Papsdorf, M., Grunau, R., Misri, S., & Devlin, A. M. (2008). Prenatal exposure to maternal depression, neonatal methylation of human glucocorticoid receptor gene (NR3C1), and infant cortisol stress responses. *Epigenetics*, *3*(2), 97–106.

Perroud, N., Paoloni-Giacobino, A., Prada, P., Olie, E., Salzmann, A., Nicastro, R., et al. (2011). Increased methylation of glucocorticoid receptor gene (NR3C1) in adults with a history of childhood maltreatment: A link with the severity and type of trauma. *Translational Psychiatry*, *1*(12), e59.

Porges, S. W. (2017). *The pocket guide to the polyvagal theory: The transformative power of feeling safe*. W. W. Norton.

Pyles, L. (2007). Community organizing for post-disaster social development: Locating social work. *International Social Work*, *50*(3), 321–333. https://doi.org/10.1177/0020872807076044

Quiros, L., & Berger, R. (2013). Responding to the sociopolitical complexity of trauma: An integration of theory and practice. *Journal of Loss and Trauma*, *20*(2), 149–159. https://doi.org//10.1080/15325024.2013.836353

Reynolds, V. (2020). Trauma and resistance: "Hang time" and other innovative responses to oppression, violence and suffering. *Journal of Family Therapy*, *42*, 347–364. https://doi.org/10.1111/1467-6427.12293

Russin, S. E., & Stein, C. H. (2022). The aftermath of trauma and abuse and the impact on family: A narrative literature review. *Trauma, Violence, & Abuse*, *23*(4), 1288–1301. https://doi.org/10.1177/1524838021995990

SAMHSA's Trauma and Justice Strategic Initiative. (2014). *SAMHSA's Concept of trauma and guidance for a trauma-informed approach*. Retrieved on September 12, 2023, from https://ncsacw.acf.hhs.gov/userfiles/files/SAMHSA_Trauma.pdf

Sokoloff, N. J., & Dupont, I. (2005). Domestic violence at the intersections of race, class, and gender. *Violence Against Women*, *11*(1), 38–64.

Substance Abuse and Mental Health Services Administration. (2014). *Trauma-informed care in behavioral health services*. SAMHSA – Substance Abuse and Mental Health Services Administration.

Substance Abuse and Mental Health Services Administration. (2024). *What is trauma?* https://www.samhsa.gov/trauma-violence

Sue, D. W. (2016). *Counseling the culturally diverse: Theory and practice*. John Wiley & Sons.

Tronto, J. (1993) *Moral boundaries: A political argument for an ethic of care*. Routledge.

Walker, L. E. (1979). *The battered woman*. Harper & Row.

Weisner, L. (2020). *Individual and community trauma: Individual experiences in collective environments*. https://icjia.illinois.gov/researchhub/articles/individual-and-community-trauma-individual-experiences-in-collective-environments

Wisner, B., Blaikie, P., Cannon, T., & Davis, I. (2003). *At risk: Natural hazards, people's vulnerability, and disasters* (2nd ed.). Routledge.

World Health Organization. (2012). *World health statistics 2012*. World Health Organization.

World Health Statistics. (2018). *Monitoring health for the SDGs, sustainable development goals*. World Health Organization. License: CC BY-NC-SA 3.0 IGO.

Zhu, P., Luke, M. M., Liu, Y., & Wang, Q. (2023). Cultural humility and cultural competence in counseling: An exploratory mixed methods investigation. *Journal of Counseling & Development*, *101*(3), 264–276. https://doi.org/10.1002/jcad.12469

# 10

# Feminist Intersectional Career Theory

## Carol Klose Smith, Darcie Davis-Gage, Janine Rowe, and Olivia Turner

*As people develop their career aspirations and goals, embedded patriarchal social, cultural, and political hierarchies, stigmas, and definitions of success affect career possibilities and choices based on people's intersectional identities.*

The North American perspective of work has been shaped, in part by the industrial and post–World War II eras. Major career counseling theories were developed to explain the career choice and development of Eurocentric, heteronormative men in the workforce. These theories focused predominately on career choice and career transitions, specifically on explaining the White, middle-class male experience, generally excluding such intersectional considerations as socioeconomic status, culture, race, gender, gender identity, and marginalized individuals (Blustein et al., 2019). In recent years, feminist perspectives have significantly influenced the field of career counseling, offering a critical lens through which to understand and address the complexities of career development (Enns & Niles, 2013). A feminist career counseling perspective offers more inclusivity and broader possibilities and examines choices of career counseling theories with freedom from the existing patriarchal constructs of career.

Feminist career therapists must consider the various ways in which individuals make meaning from work, their intersectional identity, the importance given to work, and the realities of their placement on Maslow's Hierarchy (Maslow, 1943). For some, work is a way to meet needs. It is transactional and a necessity for survival. Other individuals may view work as a way to maximize their personal self. They see work as a part of themselves. They may even define themselves by what they do. Still others may see work as a calling (Duffy et al., 2018). Feminist theory uniquely contributes to assisting individuals in navigating the complexities of career development in a diverse society. Social, cultural, and political considerations are essential when assisting individuals in their career development.

# Feminist Intersectional Career Theory Basic Principles

Feminist intersectional career theory is a postmodern approach to career and vocational development. As a postmodernist theory, the focus is on the subjective intersectional experience of the individual (Sampson, 2009). Understanding an individual's life includes focusing on any privileges and oppressions they experience and the patriarchal systems they navigate; this is a cornerstone of the feminist approach. In the past, many patriarchal, Eurocentric, Christian-dominant conceptualizations of career were seen as linear pathways, beginning at the bottom of a hierarchy, and through solid effort and a good work ethic, one would rise through the ranks to ever-increasing responsibility, increasing salary and increasing prestige. This ethos also implied that sacrificing time with family was necessary for success. Hardy (2023) suggested that normative beliefs like the American dream and the myth of meritocracy often left oppressed people with internalized devaluation. Hardy (2023) said, "It creates an exhausting, psychologically and emotionally taxing condition in which people of color are constantly wondering whether they are doing enough, educated enough, and working hard enough and, the deeply buried unconscious sentiment, whether they are good enough" (p. 125). Yet, many of these social constructs and normative cultural beliefs still exist in today's society and are a part of the unspoken expectations to get ahead (Duarte, 2017). As the world has gone through significant changes in how one interacts with the world of work, the broadening acceptance of who is qualified for traditionally gendered or cultural jobs, the conceptualization of work, and being successful at work are ever-changing.

Many of the career theories of the 20th century have focused on early career choice by matching career with the skills and interests of the individual. These early career theories did not consider intersectional identities, including gender, lack of socioeconomic opportunities, and experiences of oppression or discrimination (Betz, 2023). For a postmodernist feminist intersectional career approach, the evolving social, cultural, and political context of society and the consideration of interlocking oppressions have implications for career or work life. This approach allows for a greater understanding of how one interacts with society and the privileged and oppressive realities in the world of work. It involves identifying career choices and understanding the ongoing concerns arising from a client's interaction between work and life. In short, feminist intersectional career counseling involves a holistic approach that encompasses one's analysis of an ecosystem, recognizing privilege and oppression, understanding one's personal development and life satisfaction, recognizing that people have different cultural priorities, and having a fluid understanding of the ever-elusive "life–work balance."

Feminist Intersectional Career Theory provides clients an opportunity to explore their career development and also assists clients in raising consciousness, making choices free of social and cultural mandates, and encouraging authentic self-examination around personal privilege and oppression. A core element is to examine the relationship between the individual and their ecosystem. This approach highlights understanding the "meaning-making" clients assign to the struggles they face (La Guardia, 2023). As such, the theory has several tenets essential to feminist career counseling: early socialization of intersectional identities, intersectional identities and career decisions, the feminist therapeutic relationship, and feminist intersectional conceptualizations.

## Early Socialization of Intersectional Identities

Socialization of gender roles and intersectional identity formations begin early in life. However, to understand the importance of this socialization, first, one must identify the complex nature of sex, gender, gender roles and how they interact with race, socioeconomic status, abilities, educational opportunities and all other relevant ecosystems. Gender and race are understood to be socially constructed (Obach, 1999) and in third-wave feminist clinical theory, these and other intersecting identities can carry multiple oppressions. For example, a White female child and a Black female child likely have very different experiences with society, school systems, opportunities, and future wages (Fouad & Burrows, 2023). Additionally, a neurodivergent child of color may have a different experience than a neurodivergent White child. The feminist view offers a detailed understanding of each person's unique intersectional developmental experiences, recognizes and honors their oppressions, and understands that all identities have unique challenges toward goals of empowerment.

Career influences begin in childhood. Children may begin to distance themselves from occupations that do not align or are socially unacceptable to their developing sense of self (Gottfredson, 2005). While one may wish to believe that children are isolated about how their intersectional identities interface with the world of work, this is a myth. Even first- and second-grade children can often identify an occupation by gender, socioeconomic status, or even racial/ethnic minority societal views. Over time, career choices may be categorized by jobs that the individual may find acceptable, such as gender, prestige level, or interests (Gottfredson, 2005). Individuals may reject specific careers based on perceived social desirability and economic potential, sometimes resulting in individuals picking not their best-fit career but one that is acceptable based on their intersectional privileged and oppressed experiences. Eurocentric, heteronormative, Christian-dominant, patriarchal constructs around career might limit career choices and fulfillment during this developmental process. Learned helplessness, internalized devaluation, poverty, abuse, and so on all may have an impact on this selection or rejection of potential careers.

## Gender Roles, Intersectional Identities, and Career Decisions

Although intersectional identities cannot be separated from gender, it is worth reviewing some career research on gender. Gendered perceptions of work affect how men and women approach and navigate their career choices (Betz, 2023; Bourne & Ozbilgin, 2008). Fouad et al. (2023) found that among women and adolescent girls; more traditional career aspirations were related to a stronger emphasis on family, implying that while great strides have been made, some women feel the need to choose careers that are seen as "family-friendly," which often have lower career aspirations and lower economic potential. Gendered career choice and prejudice can be traced as a contributor to persistent gender inequalities at work and home (Betz, 2023; Miche & Nelson, 2006), as well as the positivity of work experiences and finding satisfaction and meaning in their work (Fouad & Burrows, 2023). For example, although women are entering the professional workforce in mass numbers, they are, for the most part, largely underrepresented in high-earning prestige occupational positions when compared to men (Nadeem & Khalid, 2018).

However, the disparity is not just about gender but also intersectionality (Fouad & Burrows, 2023). BIPOC women (Black, Indigenous, and people of color) hold only 13% of top executive positions compared to 20% of White women (McKinsey & Company, 2021). In part, this can be due to the intersection of cultural values in BIPOC communities, sexism, and the patriarchal influence these components have on BIPOC women (Miville, 2013). Nadeem and Khalid (2018) note that traditional gender roles persist despite urbanization, the push for higher education, technological advances, and increased media exposure to many different cultures. In addition, these perceptions persist within society and within the workplace (Bourne & Ozbilgin, 2008). Traditional patriarchal gender roles and stereotypes create the expectations that women are meant to be subservient, docile, and inferior to men in almost all the avenues they pursue, including occupational domains.

## Feminist Therapeutic Relationship

One of the core concepts of feminist theory is the creation of an egalitarian therapeutic relationship (Brown, 2018; Evans et al., 2011). The career counseling relationship by its very nature has a power differential; career counselors who work without an egalitarian approach are often seen as experts, which places a client in a less powerful position. Therefore, feminist career counselors recognize the inequalities experienced by client's openly and consciously work to empower clients (Indelicato & Springer, 2007). This is done through recognizing the client as an authority in their own life and providing empathic regard to the client. This sharing of power and creating a relationship of equals may seem a minor consideration, but the influence on the therapeutic relationship is considerable (Brown, 2018; Evans et al., 2011).

Feminist counselors view the client as the expert of their lives (Brown, 2004, 2018). The career counselor's role is to assist the client in explorations and analysis of themselves and to assist in their growth. This is a collaborative process in which a working relationship is fostered with the client to establish therapeutic goals, "an exploration of meaning-making and being fully and consistently reflective" (Ballou & West, 2000, p. 286). The purpose of an egalitarian relationship from a feminist perspective is to partner with clients in exploring their identities, gaining higher consciousness, and becoming empowered with full awareness and autonomy of choices for career paths despite societal constraints.

## Feminist Intersectional Career Therapists: Self-Reflection

Fundamental to feminist therapy is an understanding of oneself. As humans we do not enter a therapeutic relationship value or bias free. Thus, the feminist therapist has a need to consistently explore, acknowledge, and monitor our own biases, power, assumptions, and values. In the context of engaging in career counseling, feminist therapists must explore their own assumptions about work, work values, and views on socially and culturally embedded career beliefs such as work ethic, work–life balance, unemployment, gender role socialization, parenting and work conflicts, and so on. In short, a career counselor needs to be aware of how conscious and unconscious automatic thoughts, developmental embedded messages, and other social, cultural and political norms shade their views of privilege and oppression in the world of work.

## Feminist Intersectional Career Conceptualization

Feminist intersectional career therapists view clients from a strength-based perspective. Instead of focusing on what is wrong with the client, this approach embraces the idea that behaviors and feelings indicate clients' lived experiences (Brown, 2018; Evans et al., 2011). The process of career counseling naturally focuses upon the strengths of an individual within their work lives, acknowledging their values, abilities, and interests. Some clients, depending on their previous experiences of privilege and oppression, rewards and punishments, or successes and failures, may struggle with learned helplessness, self-doubt, and other insecurities when venturing into novel career situations. A feminist therapist strives to assist clients in developing an understanding of the connections between their past and current experiences, highlighting resilience in the face of discrimination and oppression, and assisting clients in examining choices and options that are available to them.

Feminist intersectional career conceptualization begins with understanding the client's presenting goal, which may include exploring feelings, thoughts, beliefs, and the sociocultural context in which they live. Exploring the early socialization of intersectional identities, career values, and any internalized assumptions is important. These internalized assumptions may be outside the client's awareness. In some cases, the client may need to explore their identity before the career work can begin. Oppression, rejection, and discrimination may have deflated willingness to move forward toward one's hopes and dreams. Fear of trying, fear of failure, and suppressing hope may be the residues of the client's sociocultural context.

## A Feminist Intersectional Career Counseling Model

The application of a fourth-wave feminist career model highlights power, privilege, and oppression within and among intersectional identities in both the world of work and the larger society. Modern career theory needs to encourage exploration of what work means given the context of clients' lives. The following Feminist Intersectional Career Model is updated from Jodry's and Armstrong's (2010) original feminist model of career and employment counseling. While the model implies a linear process in how it is presented, one may find a more circular process helpful for the client, at times returning to previous topics of conversations from earlier stages. It is also important to note that good career work is just good therapeutic work (Lent & Brown, 2013). While the topics may be focused on career choice, vocational concerns, and work–life balance, foundational feminist therapy principles apply.

# A Feminist Intersectional Career Model: The Personal Is Political

## Exploring the Presenting Concern: Personal Narrative

As mentioned earlier, an egalitarian relationship is essential in feminist therapy, with particular attention paid to therapeutic power monitoring. The focus of this phase of the process is the client/clinician relationship and creating a safe and supportive space to engage in the necessary exploration of what brings them to career work. It is also during this phase that clients are invited to express their goals. The empowering egalitarian therapeutic relationship supports the client's desired goals, offering additional possibilities for them to choose from during goal formation. It should be noted that a feminist intersectional career approach implies that career and work-related goals will be surrounded by a holistic examination of other areas of their lives, such as life tasks, goals, and the ecosystems of the client.

## Exploring Intersectional Identities: Conscious Knowledge of Self

This stage is focused on assisting the client in exploring their intersectional self and how their interlocking identities are perceived and valued by society. This will include self-reflection and examination of the self within the social, cultural, and political contexts of their unique lived experiences. It may be both uncomfortable and also empowering to uncover inner beliefs, analyze their development, and contextualize which have Eurocentric, heteronormative, Christian-dominant patriarchal roots. Given that traditional patriarchal career norms have often been internalized as "truth," clients may not have questioned their beliefs or assumptions about the world of work (Jodry & Armstrong, 2010). Feminist intersectional exploration techniques may be useful in this phase.

It is also important for the career therapist to explore past jobs/education and careers and examine why the previous choices were made. Are there familial or social pressures? Are there any patriarchal-embedded messages that inform the choices that need to be further explored? How did clients form their career thoughts, both positive and negative? It is also important to explore if any patriarchal system injuries, especially in the education system, may have circumscribed and/or compromised previous career exploration.

## Patriarchal Differentiation: Owning Choices

Patriarchal differentiation is adapted from Bowen's concept of differentiation from the family of origin (Bowen, 2006; Jodry & Armstrong, 2010). The client can critically examine all aspects of their life, including socially, culturally, and politically embedded expectations, definitions of success, and so on. With full consciousness of how they arrived at their current beliefs, the client can keep or change them. Either way, after the differentiation process, the client takes full responsibility for their decisions. Exploring how an individual may have passively accepted, assimilated, compromised or circumscribed occupational choices early in life may be valuable to help the client raise consciousness and critically analyze. Children are often less constrained and more open to exploring early occupational hopes and dreams before learning societal mores. It may be helpful to examine the evolution of what happened to those early ideas. While taking a pragmatic approach to career decision-making is not to be discounted, examining the context of how a client made past career choices is valuable.

## Supporting Goals: Empowerment

Within society, many individuals may have experiences of oppression and discrimination that have shaped their perceptions of the world of work. Exposure to traditional patriarchal employment expectations may also have shaped the clients' career development in the choices they made and may have reduced possible choices. Exploring these can set the stage for moving beyond previous career choices. The client's power can also be gained through understanding and managing any oppressive parts of the ecosystem and employment environment. The feminist career counselor empowers the client to explore any and all goals, especially nontraditional ones, that have been diminished and discouraged by oppressive systems (Jodry & Armstrong, 2010).

## Vision Expansion

At this point in the process, clients are encouraged to explore various possibilities and consider their new options. In addition, it is important to include the client's differentiated values, interests, education, and natural skills, which are free from patriarchal or oppressive messages (Jodry & Armstrong, 2010). It is important for the empowerment process that the client directs and conducts the exploration. Exercises in feminist intersectional career techniques might aid counselors in encouraging clients to think critically about options that may not have been available to them previously.

## Real Freedom of Choice

Ideally, this phase highlights differentiated, critically analyzed beliefs and allows a client to determine pathways forward that align to who they are as an individual rather than societally derived expectations based upon intersectional privilege and oppression and social, cultural, and political bias or prejudice (Jodry & Armstrong, 2010). Clients at this phase of the process use their new higher consciousness and knowledge of self to decide a pathway that is authentic to themselves and can fully embrace their choices. Empowering clients to explore both the gains and challenges that exist with various decisions about their future is foundational to feminist career work. This phase also acknowledges the genuine barriers that may be encountered by those individuals who may choose a less than societally acceptable pathway. While a choice may be professionally fulfilling, certain choices may have a personal cost (Conlin et al., 2021). Exploring anticipated challenges and barriers is essential, especially for those who may encounter opposition. It is important to note that clients may choose not to make any changes and maintain their status quo. The important aspect is allowing the client the social and psychological freedom to explore and make their own decisions from a fully informed lens. All choices are equal.

Another important consideration at this phase is for clients to realize that they have the power to change decisions and plans. Decisions made can change. Career development and choice are fluid processes in which one adapts to new knowledge and opportunities. It is impossible to consider all potential obstacles or opportunities that may occur in the future, but empowering the client with resiliency will help with any future challenges.

# Feminist Intersectional Career Applications

Traditional career theories often overlook diverse experiences and challenges faced by individuals at the intersections of multiple marginalized identities. Intersectionality highlights the complexity of career development and underscores the need for tailored interventions that address the dimensions of clients' identities from a feminist perspective (Collins, 2015). Feminist intersectional career counseling interventions empower individuals to navigate their career paths with agency, resilience, and authenticity. Drawing upon feminist principles of equity, social justice, and intersectionality, feminist clinical applications are offered as tools when working with career counseling to provide counselors with practical strategies for promoting greater equity and empowerment in the realm of career development. By centering intersectional experiences and voices of marginalized individuals and challenging systemic barriers to career success, feminist intersectional career applications hope to offer transformative pathways toward more inclusive and just career futures.

## Gender Intersectional Analysis

In feminist intersectional career counseling, both *power* and *gender role analysis* serve as critical tools for understanding and addressing the dynamics of power and privilege that shape individuals' career experiences. *Gender analysis* in feminist career counseling underscores the need to recognize the gendered nature of career development experiences, advocating for an intersectional perspective that acknowledges how gender intersects with other social identities. During sessions, counselors can engage in reversal questioning, which involves examining career concerns from other genders, which assists the client in expanding their perspective of the concern (Degges-White et al., 2013). This framework encourages clients to challenge traditional gender notions and explore alternative narratives (Worell & Remer, 2003).

## Intersectional Power Analysis

A *power analysis* involves examining how structures and systems of power, such as gender, race, class, sexuality, and ability, intersect to influence career opportunities, access to resources, and experiences of discrimination and oppression (Han & Lee, 2023). Feminist career counselors may apply a four-step process by helping clients to identify the power dynamics within the context of their career aspirations and experiences, consider how intersecting identities contribute to their experiences of power and privilege in the workplace, recognize and challenge any internalized beliefs or messages that may perpetuate feelings of inferiority or limitation based on their social identities, consider how their actions can contribute to broader social change, and identify opportunities for advocating for structural change within their organization or industry.

Another way of clinically applying a power analysis is by having the client understand interpersonal power. A client may list everyone in their lives, separated by gender or in an ecosystem model, to examine their proximity to the client. The client then determines which person holds more power in each relationship. A deep examination may include analyzing who will sacrifice more for the relationship, who cares more about the relationship existing, and so on. A clinician can use a Likert scale to help the client determine the continuum of power. Together, the clinician and client see if there are patterns that arise with certain types of people and how powerful or powerless they feel.

## Intersectional Self-Analysis

An intersectional self-analysis moves beyond gender and allows clients to explore all identities (e.g., race, gender, nationality, abilities, sexuality, education, socioeconomic conditions, etc.). The client weighs how much each identity impacts them socially, culturally, and politically related to privilege or oppression and how important each identity is to the client's sense of self. Also critical is which combinations of identities are irreducible. A clinician can create a "card sort" to help move through the analysis and connect identities to career choices (Jodry & Armstrong, 2010). How much do intersectional identities need to be considered to be congruent and authentic?

## Conscious Raising

Consciousness raising (CR), a foundational feminist intervention, is a powerful tool in career counseling by fostering a deeper self-awareness, critical reflection of social cultural and political influences, and hopes of ultimate empowerment among clients. Kawano (2011) emphasizes the importance of culturally relevant practices within CR groups for optimal effect. In a career counseling setting, a counselor might utilize CR interventions to help clients recognize the influence of Eurocentric, heteronormative patriarchy on their career aspirations, choices, and experiences. CR sessions in career counseling can involve discussing how traditional patriarchal norms shape perceptions of suitable career paths for men, women, LGBTQ+ individuals, BIPOC individuals, people with different abilities, people of different ages, and so forth. Clients may be prompted to reflect on their own passively embedded internalized beliefs about types of people and work, as well as the external pressures they face from family, peers, culture, politics, and society. Through this process, clients can gain insight into how these influences may have impacted their career decision-making and explore alternative narratives that align with their authentic selves and aspirations.

One way to explore this is a collaborative examination of *What careers/jobs have I never considered due to* _____. In the exercise, a client lists five jobs that were never considered due to gender and/or other identities, five jobs that were never considered due to resources, five jobs that were never considered due to lack of ability, and five jobs they were afraid to consider because they would probably fail. This gives the therapist a fruitful place to explore the potential influences the cultural, social, and political norms have had on this client. This allows not only consciousness raising but also more freedom in future career choices.

## Promoting Career Self-Efficacy

Self-efficacy is focused on answering the question "Can I do this?" However, another central question is "If I do this, what will happen?" This has been termed outcome expectations (Lent & Lopez, 2002). Both an individual's perception of their abilities and the potential outcome influence self-efficacy beliefs. From a feminist perspective, another factor to consider is societal and other systemic messages and expectations. Developing self-efficacy beliefs and outcome expectations is a lifelong process that often begins in childhood and is intertwined with embedded societal and patriarchal messages about careers and capabilities.

Feminist career examinations and explorations that influence career self-efficacy and outcome expectations may be adapted for age and developmental levels. They can also be adapted as collaborative strategies to transparently explore patriarchal influences and impacts on career aspirations and paths. One of the primary interventions is finding and creating relationships with role models. The adage "if you can see it, you can be it" certainly applies to career development. A role model can communicate about the pathway they took, the challenges encountered, and the education and skills they needed. Role models, in short, provide evidence that one can succeed and are even more important for marginalized individuals (Thiem & Dasgupta, 2022).

Another aspect that may influence self-efficacy is the social support of others. The role of family, peers, and teachers in career self-efficacy is an important predictor (Jemini-Gashi, 2021). Social support should be explored with the client and in the absence of social support the counselor is encouraged to intentionally instill hope and provide encouragement (Subotnik et al., 2010).

## Examination of the Imposter: Raising Congruence

Imposter syndrome is an individual's innate fear of being uncovered as a fraud or of not deserving their achievements or career opportunities (Bravada et al., 2020). Ironically, this feeling is persistent despite one's accomplishments and achievements. Imposter syndrome is more common among women and underrepresented racial, ethnic, and religious minorities (Bravada et al., 2020) and is connected to feeling as if one does not belong. Pursuing a nontraditional career pathway may make one more vulnerable to imposter syndrome. Additionally, those who experience imposter syndrome may also experience a cycle of overachievement, perfectionism, and potentially burnout (Bravada et al., 2020).

The cycle begins with feelings of inadequacy and the need to overcompensate so as not to be seen as a fraud. Hard work and effort are generally rewarded with high grades and opportunities to move forward, but the fear of being discovered as a fraud continues, leading to more overcompensation, continued work, and, over time, a sense of reduced job satisfaction (Vergauwe et al., 2015). A feminist career clinician can help clients assess if they feel like imposters and then explore any connections to oppressive or biased career messages, external, internal, or both. Counselors and clients can collaborate on ways to track when imposter syndrome occurs and to challenge any disempowering systemic and internal messages that are experienced.

## Life Role Analysis: Timeline of Changing Roles and Influences

Examining life roles, professional obligations and work–life balance is important since these competing demands may be causing challenges. Life role analysis is a process that assists the client in examining an individual's various roles within their life (e.g., worker, parent, family member, learner), the values one holds, and societal expectations (Brott, 2005). Exploring life roles is a strategy that explores priorities and expectations the client may hold of themselves and others. In order to facilitate life role analysis, several techniques are possible, such as a narrative approach, a timeline, and a career genogram. Whichever approach is more helpful for the client, the feminist clinician and the client can collaborate on identifying pivotal career moments or events, systemic impacts on career paths, previous career choices, and/or patterns of occupation in the family.

## Definition of Success: How Did I Decide This?

Cultural values and norms have a significant influence on how clients may define success. How an individual defines their vocational success may be an extension of their cultural values and the accompanying cultural norms (Benson et al., 2020) and may be shaped by patriarchal definitions of success (for example, money, prestige, fame, or power). A feminist therapist can first help clients identify their definitions of success (Jodry & Armstrong, 2010). After this, they can explore where the definitions came from. How did the client learn what success means? Who are role models of success? How do these align (or not) with the client's values? Part of this exploration can be examining any systemic impacts on the definitions of success. With awareness about definitions and their origins, a client can choose to endorse current definitions of success or consider refining definitions.

## The Role of Advocacy in Career Choice

Feminist career counseling transcends the "traditional" helping role that counselors embrace. More traditional approaches uphold the status quo that overtly reinforces White supremacy and the patriarchy (Lewis et al., 2011). Counselors who embrace a feminist career counseling approach integrate the role of advocacy into career choice to combat oppressive forces.

Incorporating advocacy into career choice entails helping clients define their career priorities, find a support network, and work with clients to accumulate resources that foster growth (Hirschi, 2020). This approach demands a more holistic view of career counseling.

Advocacy in career exploration helps highlight and minimize oppressive barriers. As showcased by the social justice counseling paradigm, advocacy work addresses conditions (e.g., social, political, and economic) that negatively impact personal and career development (Lewis et al., 2011). Counselors can advocate with and for clients, with clients' permission. If a client is not interested in advocacy, a feminist clinician can still do their professional advocacy related to removing career barriers and widening career options for all.

## Feminist Intersectional Career Client Example

The client is a 32-year-old transgender female (pronouns: she/her) who has been struggling with relationships at work. The client has worked as an automobile mechanic since completing technical school after high school. She said being a mechanic has been a good choice; she enjoys the challenge of fixing cars and the camaraderie with the other individuals at the garage. Fixing cars has provided a sense of satisfaction. However, lately, as the client has begun socially transitioning and embracing a more stereotypical female expression and appearance, her work relationships have changed. The client was not naive in assuming that relationships would not be impacted but was hopeful that somehow it would work out because of the already existing coworker relationships. The client explains that she has felt more isolated at work during lunch and break times, that the easy-going conversations enjoyed previously are missing, and that things feel more tense. There are a few individuals who noticeably avoid her, but most people are politely distant. While there has not been any outward sign of blatant discrimination at work, the client worries that it could happen at any moment. She feels particularly on edge when using the bathroom at work.

The client lives in a mid-sized mid-western city. The environment within the city has been LGBTQ+ friendly. However, some of the more rural areas within the region have been less welcoming to LGBTQ+ community. Recently, reports of discrimination and harassment have occurred within the region. They worry that the friendly nature of their community could change and what that could mean for themselves and their friends. The client does not want to leave her employment and start over somewhere else. The current employment offers excellent health insurance, which has been important for the client pre-transition and will continue to be important for the client should she want to engage in any form of medical transition. The client is hoping to navigate this transition smoothly and stay employed at their current job.

## Feminist Intersectional Application

A feminist clinician working with this client should first consider analyzing their thoughts, feelings, and biases regarding gender minorities, specifically individuals who are transgender, and make sure that they will be able to effectively create an inclusive and welcoming therapeutic environment for this client. An egalitarian therapeutic dynamic is especially pertinent in this case as the client has been invalidated and discriminated against in the workplace setting, where they are navigating a male-dominated space as a transgender woman. Co-creating this egalitarian relationship would occur in the Exploring the Presenting Concern: Personal Narrative stage through compassion, transparency about the therapeutic process, and informed consent.

In the Exploring Intersectional Identities: *Conscious Knowledge of Self*, the feminist therapist would work with this client to examine her intersectional identities and how they are affecting her presenting concern. Doing an *Intersectional Self-Analysis* could facilitate this process. Being a transgender female has been identified as the most salient social identity in the situation. However, age, race, economic class, or other identities may also be important to consider, along with potential life roles beyond the job setting. This job was selected while the client identified as male; now, as a female, being a mechanic is a somewhat nontraditional occupation. Exploring that could be fruitful. This could lead to *Patriarchal Differentiation: Owning Choices* where the client could examine her career beliefs and early career decisions and decide now, with full awareness about how patriarchal norms and messages could have impacted her earlier, whether she wants to refine any career beliefs. As part of this exploration, a gender analysis might be helpful. She is socially transitioning to a female. Considering how gender impacts her, including beyond the job, might deepen the exploration. Is she experiencing different dynamics in relationships beyond those at work? Where is her gender being affirmed?

The Supporting Goals: *Empowerment* is an important stage for this client. She has already identified having an oppressive, rejecting experience at work. To stay in her present workplace, she will need to decide how she wants to become more empowered, if any. If she were to go to a different garage, what might be different there? What might be similar? Does her satisfaction with her work provide enough sense of empowerment to give her meaning in her job? Does she want to choose, with awareness, to navigate her workplace as a transgender female? Does she want to try to work on relationships with her current coworkers?

This client has been happy with being a mechanic and may choose to stay in that occupation. In the *Vision Expansion*, the feminist therapist can ask if the client has any interest in exploring other occupations, or not. Either way, in *Real Freedom of Choice*, the client can take all the material she has processed and any new awareness she has gained and make a conscious decision about what to do now. This could be a good time to *Promote Career Self-Efficacy*. Are role models available to help this client see potential roadmaps to success? The feminist clinician could try to find potential role models if the client cannot identify any. Also in the stage, advocacy might be important. The client is aware of local, recent discrimination of the LGBTQ+ community. If the client is interested in doing advocacy, the therapist could support that or help the client consider options for advocacy. If the client is not interested in advocacy, the therapist could explore their advocacy to support the LGBTQ+ community, separate from their counseling, and not betray confidentiality.

## Ethics and Possible Pitfalls

Several ethical considerations are pertinent regarding feminist approaches to career counseling, including embracing a reflexivity of self-as-therapist and critical integration of career assessments. Career counselors adopting a feminist approach to career counseling, involving critical and liberatory perspectives of the status quo, may question whether this approach is equivalent to imposing their views upon the client (Dik et al., 2012). Traditional career training emphasizes focus on individual client behaviors, experiences, and attitudes, giving less attention to oppressive systems that perpetuate injustices among workers. Career work's theoretical roots have long focused on individuation in their focus on adjustment, adaptability, and compromise as markers of career maturity (Prilleltensky & Stead, 2012) with less attention to the important work career counselors can do to challenge oppressive and marginalized systems. Feminist integrative career counseling eschews myths of counselor neutrality and encourages counselors and clients to embrace the explicitly intertwined connections between career satisfaction and sociopolitical conditions (Conlin et al., 2021). Counseling is inherently value-laden and occurs within an ecological context and invokes ethical responsibility to explicitly outline positions of non-neutrality and beneficence. Feminist career counselors work with clients to both cope with and challenge oppressive systems simultaneously (Prilleltensky & Stead, 2012). Failure to do so can result in inadvertent compliance with the societal status quo through failure to meet ethical values of beneficence.

Feminist career counselors consider intersectional identities at all stages of the counseling process. The assessment stage is particularly at risk for errors of omission, which underestimate or distort the internalized constraints and societal barriers experienced by minoritized individuals. A comprehensive exploration of these barriers involves assessment, however, and sex bias in career assessment presents ethical concerns and challenges for feminist career counselors. Extant literature reveals psychometric manifestation of gender bias in career assessments, as most commonly used career assessments are based on hegemonic ideals of career satisfaction (Hackett & Lonborg, 1993). Career therapists attempting a "gender-neutral" view of career assessment inadvertently reinforce gender role stereotypes and fail to recognize the burden of societal expectations operating throughout the client's life.

Psychometrically "sound" career assessments with robust reliability and validity may still fail to consider social pressures, resulting in the potential for adverse effects for the client (Cole, 1981). For example, career aptitude tests may measure developed or encouraged abilities, and career interest tests may identify socialized experiences and pressures rather than genuine interests (especially in traditionally masculine areas, including science, math, and mechanical abilities). Cognitive assessments may misattribute sacrificing beliefs as cognitive distortions instead of reflections of role conflict or socialized self-efficacy expectations (Hackett & Lonborg, 1993). Qualitative career assessments, such as genograms, career lifelines, career autobiographies, card sorts, and occupational daydreams, proactively engage a holistic view of career concerns, facilitating the integration of intersectional identities into career planning (McMahon, 2008).

# What If?

The world of work has always reflected the values of our society. The patriarchal society in which we live has often placed differential prestige and pay for various occupational positions. Work that is valued is seen as prestigious and is better paid. In a society that defines the individual by the work they do one begins to wonder—what if we valued the individual for who they are and not what they do for a living? The patriarchal lineage that established the middle class in America was founded in a way that rewarded a work ethic that sacrifices time from family and other pursuits. Valuing the worker would involve honoring the work–life balance and providing time to explore other pursuits. Embracing the notion of working to live. Thus allowing individuals to construct their sense of what work means to them.

# References

Ballou, M., & West, C. (2000). Feminist therapy approaches. In M. Baggio & M. Hersen (Eds.), *Issues in the psychology of women* (pp. 273–297). Kluwer Academic/Plenum.

Benson, G. S., McIntosh, C. K., Salazar, M., & Vaziri, H. (2020). Cultural values and definitions of career success. *Human Resource Management Journal, 30*(3), 392–421. https://doi. org/10.1111/1748-8583.12266

Betz, N. E. (2023). Self-efficacy theory and the career behavior of women. In W. B. Walsh, L. Y. Flores, P. J. Hartung, & F. T. L. Leong (Eds.), *Career psychology: Models, concepts, and counseling for meaningful employment* (pp. 193–212). American Psychological Association. https://doi. org/10.1037/0000339-010

Blustein, D. L., Kenny, M., Autin, K., & Duffy, R. (2019). The psychology of working in practice: A theory of change for a new era. *The Career Development Quarterly, 67,* 236–254. https://doi. org/10.1002/cdq.12193

Bourne, D., & Ozbilgin, M. F. (2008). Strategies for combating gendered perceptions of careers. *Career Development International, 13*(4), 320–332. https://doi.org/10.1108/13620430810880817

Bowen, M. (2006). The use of family theory in clinical practice. *Comprehensive Psychiatry, 7*(5), 345–374. https://doi.org/10.1016/S0010-440X(66)80065-2

Bravada, D. M., Watts, S. A., Keffer, A. L., Madjusudhan, D. K., Taylor, K. T., Clark, D. M., . . . Hagg, H. K. (2020). Prevalence, predictors, and treatment of imposter syndrome: A systematic review. *Journal of General Internal Medicine, 35*(4), 1252–1275. https://doi.org/10.1007/s11606-019-05364-1

Brott, P. E. (2005). A constructivist look at life roles. *The Career Development Quarterly, 54*(2), 138–149. https://doi.org/10.1002/j.2161-0045.2005.tb00146.x

Brown, L. S. (2004). Feminist paradigms of trauma treatment. *Psychotherapy Theory, Research, Practice Training, 41,* 464–471.

Brown, L. S. (2018). *Feminist therapy* (2nd ed.). American Psychological Association.

Cole, N. S. (1981). Bias in testing. *American Psychologist, 36,* 1067–1077.

Collins, P. H. (2015). Intersectionality's definitional dilemmas. *Annual Review of Sociology, 41,* 1–20. https://doi.org/10.1146/annurev-soc-073014-112142

Conlin, S. E., Douglass, R. P., Moradi, B., & Ouch, S. (2021). Examining feminist critical consciousness conceptualizations of women's subjective well-being. *The Counseling Psychologist, 49*(3), 391–422. https://doi.org/10.1177/0011000020957992

Degges-White, S. E., Colon, B. R., & Borzumato-Gainey, C. (2013). Counseling supervision within a feminist framework: Guidelines for intervention. *Journal of Humanistic Counseling, 52*(1), 92–105. https://doi.org/10.1002/j.2161-1939.2013.00035.x

Dik, B., Duffy, R., & Steger, M. (2012). Enhancing social justice by promoting prosocial values in career development interventions. *Counseling and Values, 57.* https://doi.org/10.1002/j.2161-007X.2012.00005.x

Duarte, M. E. (2017). Career counseling research-practice disparities: What we know and what we need to know. *South African Journal of Education, 37*(4). https://doi.org/10.15700/saje. v37n4a1486

Duffy, R. D., Dik, B. J., Douglass, R. P., England, J. W., & Velez, B. L. (2018). Work as a calling: A theoretical model. *Journal of Counseling Psychology, 65*(4), 423–439. http://dx.doi.org/10.1037/cou0000276

Enns, C. Z., & Niles, S. G. (2013). Feminist career counseling: Empowering diverse women. *Journal of Career Development, 40*(1), 38–53.

Evans, K. M., Kincade, E. A., & Seem, S. R. (2011). *Introduction to feminist therapy: Strategies for social and individual change.* SAGE.

Fouad, N. A., & Burrows, S. G. (2023). Gender and ethnic/racial disparities in the workplace. In D. L. Bluestein & L. Y. Flores (Eds.), *Rethinking work.* Routledge. https://doi. org/10.4324/9781003272397

Fouad, N. A., Kozlowski, M., Schams, S., Weber, W., Tapia, W. D., & Burrows, S. (2023). Why aren't we there yet?: The status of research in women's career development. *The Counseling Psychologist, 51*(6), 786–848.

Gottfredson, L. S. (2005). Applying Gottfredson's theory of circumscription and compromise in career guidance and counseling. In S. D. Brown & R. W. Lent (Eds.), *Career development and counseling: Putting theory and research to work* (pp. 71–100). Wiley.

Hackett, G., & Lonborg, S. D. (1993). Career assessment for women: Trends and issues. *Journal of Career Assessment, 1*(3), 197–216. https://doi.org/10.1177/106907279300100301

Han, E., & Lee, I. (2023). Empowering women in counseling by dismantling internalized sexism: The feminist-multicultural orientation and social justice competencies. *Journal of Mental Health Counseling, 45*(3): 213–230. https://doi.org/10.17744/mehc.45.3.03

Hardy, K. V. (2023). *Racial trauma: Clinical strategies and techniques for healing invisible wounds.* W. W. Norton.

Hirschi, A. (2020). Whole-life career management: A counseling intervention framework. *The Career Development Quarterly, 68*(1), 2–17. https://doi.org/10.1002/cdq.12209

Indelicato, N. A., & Springer, S. H. (2007). Feminist therapy. In J. Archer & C. J. McCarthy (Eds.). *Theories of counseling and psychotherapy: Contemporary applications* (pp. 310–339). Pearson Prentice Hall.

Jemini-Gashi, L., Duranku, Z. H., & Kaltrina, K. (2021). Associations between social support, career self-efficacy, and career indecision among youth. *Current Psychology, 40*, 4691–4697. https://doi.org/10.1007/s12144-019-00402-x

Jodry, J., & Armstrong, K. (2010). The personal is political: Using feminist theory as a model of career and employment counseling. *Ideas and Research You Can Use: Vistas*, 1–9. http://counselingoutfitters.com/vistas/vistas10/Article_06.pdf

Kawano, K. (2011). Consciousness-raising activities and Japanese women's psychology. *Feminism & Psychology, 21*(4), 503–509. https://doi.org/10.1177/0959353511422693

La Guardia, A. C. (2023). Feminist approaches. In S. V. Flynn & J. J. Castleberry, J. J. (Eds), *Counseling theories and case conceptualization: A practice-based approach* (p. 77–102). Springer.

Lent, R. W., & Brown, S. D. (2013). Understanding and facilitation career development in the 21st century. In S. D. Brown & R. W. Lent (Eds.), *Career development and counseling: Putting theory and research to work* (2nd ed., pp. 1–26). Wiley.

Lent, R. W., & Lopez, F. G. (2002). Cognitive ties that bind: A tripartite view of efficacy beliefs in growth-promoting relationships. *Journal of Social and Clinical Psychology, 21*(3), 256–286. https://doi.org/10.1521/jscp.21.3.256.22535

Lewis, J. A., Ratts, M. J., Paladino, D. A., & Toporek, R. L. (2011). Social justice counseling and advocacy: Developing new leadership roles and competencies. *Journal for Social Action in Counseling & Psychology, 3*(1), 5–16. https://doi.org/10.33043/jsacp.3.1.5-16

Maslow, A. H. (1943). A theory of human motivation. *Psychological Review, 50*(4), 370–396. https://doi.org/10.1037/h0054346

McKinsey & Company. (2021). *Leadership roles remain out of reach for many women of color.* https://www.mckinsey.com/featured-insights/sustainable-inclusive-growth/chart-of-the-day/leadership-roles-remain-out-of-reach-for-many-women-of-color

McMahon, M. (2008). Qualitative career assessment: A higher profile in the 21st century? In J. A. Athanasou & R. Van Esbroeck (Eds.), *International handbook of career guidance.* Springer. https://doi.org/10.1007/978-1-4020-6230-8_29

Miche, S., & Nelson, D. L. (2006). Barriers women face in information technology careers: Self-efficacy, passion and gender biases. *Women in Management Review, 21*(1), 10.

Miville, M. L. (2013). *Multicultural gender roles: Applications for mental health and education.* Wiley.

Nadeem, F., & Khalid, R. (2018). The relationship of gender role attitudes with career aspirations and career choices among young adults. *Pakistan Journal of Psychological Research, 33*(2), 455–471.

Obach, B. K. (1999). Demonstrating the social construction of race. *Teaching Sociology, 27*(3), 252–257. https://doi.org/10.2307/1319325

Prilleltensky, I., & Stead, G. B. (2012). Critical psychology and career development: Unpacking the adjust–challenge dilemma. *Journal of Career Development, 39*(4), 321–340. https://doi.org/10.1177/0894845310384403

Sampson, J. P. (2009). Modern and postmodern theories: The unnecessary divorce. *Career Development Quarterly, 58*, 91–98.

Subotnik, R. F., Edmiston, A. M., Cook, L., & Ross, M. D. (2010). Mentoring for talent development, creativity, social skills, and insider knowledge: The APA catalyst program. *Journal of Advanced Academics, 21*, 714–739. http://dx.doi.org/10.1177/1932202X1002100406

Thiem, K. C., & Dasgupta, N. (2022). From precollege to career: Barriers facing historically marginalized students and evidence-based solutions. *Social Issues and Policy Review*, 16(1), 212–251. https://doi.org/10.1111/sipr.12085

Vergauwe, J., Wille, B., Feys, M., De Fruyt, F., & Anseel, F. (2015). Fear of being exposed: The trait-relatedness of the impostor phenomenon and its relevance in the work context. *Journal of Business Psychology*, 30(3), 565–581.

Worell, J., & Remer, P. (2003). *Feminist perspectives in therapy: Empowering diverse women*. Wiley.

# 11

# Feminist Intersectional Theory and Spiritual Philosophies

## *Joanne Jodry, Ann M. Callahan, and Ashley Krompier*

*Spiritual lives are often constructed on Christian-dominant, Eurocentric, heteronormative patriarchal established views, which can restrict and limit people from exploring and experiencing other spiritual paths.*

## Feminist Spirituality

Spirituality, religions, existential meaning, and other life philosophies have played and continue to play a role in healing human suffering physically, psychologically, and emotionally (Jones et al., 2015; Koenig, 2012; Li et al., 2016; Shafranske, 1996). Many therapists have integrated spirituality into their clinical practices and been supported by their clinical communities, as evidenced by specific divisions for spiritual concerns in various mental health professional organizations (e.g., American Psychological Association, Div-36; American Counseling Association [ASERVIC]; The Society for Spirituality and Social Work, etc.).

Although many forms of religions and spiritual practices exist, the United States is a Christian-dominant society, with 70.6 % identifying as Christian (Pew, 2024). Between 2007 and 2014, the Pew Research Center (2024) surveyed 35,000 Americans in all 50 states; results suggested that Americans identified as 70.6% Christian, 22.8% religiously unaffiliated, 5.9% non-Christian, and 6% did not know This historical and current Christian-dominant faith infiltrates and influences other U.S. social, cultural, and political systems and sets norms and policies for everyone despite individual personal beliefs. For example, although it is written in the U.S. Constitution that there can be no government-established religion (U.S. Constitution, Amendment I), cultural norms and social behaviors have not fully embraced that concept. This is evidenced by many public schools following the Christian calendar for holiday breaks, a repetitive push for prayers in school, calls to put the Ten Commandments from the Bible in public locations, and so on. No matter what spiritual traditions a person is raised with in the United States, they are exposed to the ecosystem where the majority Christian beliefs influence norms around what makes a successful life, concepts of sin or evil, moral sexual behaviors, and so on. As with other cultural and social norms, the majority thought can serve to oppress those who do not fit the collective views of "right," "good," or "normal."

Feminist spirituality recognizes that although exploring spirituality, religions, and other existential issues offers many therapeutic benefits for some clients, other marginalized, oppressed, and rejected clients may become injured by this area of life (Jodry & Levitt, 2023). As with most social, cultural, and political systems, the religious/spiritual social constructs contribute to the collectively accepted ideas of "normal" and "right" ways of behaving and living. Like the other systems, religious and spiritual constructs are also developed and understood through a Eurocentric, Christian-dominant, heteronormative patriarchal lens. If a person embraces the dominant accepted view of spiritual "norms" and finds religious or other vehicles to spirituality, they may experience no discomfort or need for spiritual discernment. Others whose lived experiences, biological existences, or critical thoughts do not fit into the religious dogma or embedded spiritual collective understandings may experience psychological or spiritual injuries. Jodry and Levitt (2023) also discuss how some patriarchal religious constructs (PRC) might serve to injure a person spiritually and stunt further spiritual growth by alienating some identities and/or deeming some organic natural behaviors as "sin."

## Feminist Spiritual Conceptual Underpinnings

Definitions can create strict constructs, possibly resulting in an inability to be inclusive, expand, and evolve. However, for clear understanding and spiritual application to feminist intersectional clinical practice, *spirituality will be defined as a worldview and a process that helps people cope with questions about life's meaning and purpose and understand the mysteries of human existence.* Additionally, spiritual exploration, contemplation, and practices may bring about experiences of alignment, awareness, congruence, enlightenment, and the opportunity to cultivate meaningful development.

For many, religion involves a belief system that informs a method for expressing one's faith. While the practice of religion is not necessarily the same as the experience of spirituality, religious institutions often contextualize the experience of spirituality. Whether a polytheistic religion like Hinduism or a monotheistic religion like Christianity, Islam, or Judaism, all theistic religions share a belief in some form of existence of a G-d-like being or higher power that is beyond the natural world. Most people said they were certain (63%) or fairly certain (20%) in the existence of God(s) (Pew, 2024; Lipka & Gecewicz, 2017;). Additionally, according to Gallup (Jones, 2023), while 47% of Americans identify as religious, 33% identify as spiritual but not religious. This leaves a wide range for exploring the complex understanding of individual spiritual perspectives, which a feminist therapist must examine to understand the client's worldview intertwined with intersectional identities.

### The Ego and Spirituality

The ego has been described as "enabling the individual to adapt to the concerns of reality" (Safran, 2012, p. 31). If the ego creates a conscious reality that the person constructs to define and defend their truths of reality, where does the mystical part of life fit in the ego?

Despite the concrete, conservative, reformed, or liberal beliefs people have about universal mysteries of life and death, purpose or nihilism, and/or earth's place in the universe, there are no proven truths about why humans have higher consciousness than other species. However, the ego might find that a very uncomfortable place since the ego's purpose is to organize and categorize new information coexisting with current realities, as well as mitigate the desires of the id and superego (Safran, 2012). Could the ego stifle spirituality in a rush to satisfy the need for reality?

### Embedded Images of God

The feminist therapist can explore and understand how religion and/or spirituality factor into each client's intersectional life experience, if at all. Clients may have been exposed to many conscious and unconscious spiritual images and, based on their intersectional identities, may have perceived them with a unique lens. Throughout their lived experience, people are exposed to art, music, and other influential images they may not even be aware of consciously. For example, with the influence of European art, the image of God became represented as a White man—despite the origins of Western religions in the Middle East. The *Head of Christ*, a famous popular painting of Jesus as a blue-eyed White man, has been reproduced over 500 million times (Newsweek, 2007). This may have contributed to many people in the West seeing Jesus, God the Father, Moses, or Abraham as White. Rizzuto (1979) suggested that these images of a White male may affect marginalized peoples' psyches and ultimately impact their experiences of God. On any conscious and unconscious level, women and people of color who visualize a White man as God and the ultimate superior being may have implications around how they see themselves and their power in the hierarchy and meaning of life. Conversely, perhaps White men who relate to the White image of God may see themselves as more powerful. Howard and Sommers (2019, 2015) suggested that these images may also promote a sense of individual and collective White superiority.

# Feminist Spiritual Development

It might be helpful for a feminist therapist to understand how their clients' spiritual beliefs may have evolved. Fowler's (1995) stages of faith, which integrated Piaget's study of logic, Selman's perspective-taking, and Kolberg's moral judgment, among others, into his model, is used as a loose guide to underscore a feminist perspective of faith/spiritual development and can serve as a tool to aid a feminist therapist in understanding the intersectional complexity of individual beliefs.

## Pre-Stage: Undifferentiated Faith

A child is born into an existing macrosystem that has established embedded cultural, social, political, and spiritual traditions, beliefs, and norms. The primary relationship is with the caregiver(s) who helps the child maintain life. The caregiver(s) has an intersectional identity and has adapted to their environment, and that sense of adaptation influences caregiving, beliefs around lifestyle, and parenting. The infant's ego process of deciding whether the environment can be trusted begins (Erikson, 1980, 1997). If the environment meets the child's needs, cognitive associations with safety in that environment possibly begin to embed into the child's sense of "normal," "truth," and "good" as a "schema of object permanence"

(Fowler,1995, p. 120). This might be when primal images, smells, sounds, and the like, become embedded as a comforting understanding of safety that later becomes known as truth. A feminist therapist might try to examine what these early images and experiences may have been.

## Stage 1: Intuitive-Projective Faith

As a preschool child cannot yet think abstractly (Fowler, 1995), this stage is experienced concretely. The child begins to understand the world through the familial and environmental experiences and all levels of the Eurocentric, Christian-dominant, heteronormative, patriarchal-driven micro and macro exposure the child has to rituals and religious activities. A child is also directly told by the adults and the systems around them what is right and wrong. Comfort and/or fear of God or a religious environment could begin to embed in the child's ego based on exposures surrounding spiritual matters. For example, the image of a wounded, bleeding White man dying on a cross or the concept of the purity of virgins in white as the highest form of the mother may also begin to develop in the mind concretely. Additionally, for some Christians, associating childhood fantasies (Santa Claus, Easter Bunny, etc.) with sacred holidays might have a potential cognitive schematic spiritual impact on later spiritual development for realities. A feminist therapist might attempt to understand a client's memories of early cognitive associations in their spiritual development and collaboratively see if they are helpful to their current beliefs.

## Stage 2: Mythic-Literal Faith

A child in this stage begins to be exposed to the larger interpersonal community through educational systems, organizations, group activities, and perhaps religious teachings specific to their age. All these systems stem from patriarchal history and have existing legacies that serve as an underpinning for "normal." During this time, a child may attend or know other children who attend religious education (Confraternity of Christian Doctrine or "CCD" in the Roman Catholic Church; Hebrew classes, etc.). If they are in public schools, many children will follow a Christian calendar of holiday schedules (Christmas and Easter holidays). This is also the stage when they are exposed to larger groups of others and different thoughts (Fowler, 1995).

Symbols become more multidimensional and gain power (Fowler, 1995). Faith and spirituality become stories that are being told and the rituals that are being practiced in traditional systems born in patriarchy. Like much of world history, religious/spiritual stories have a selective bias often chosen and interpreted by people with their own intersectional identities within a patriarchal system. The storyteller is often assimilated to the norms based on what they were exposed to in their spiritual background. As mentioned, children are often exposed to images and learn about the fantasies that society has collectively created as competing stories around rituals and spiritual holidays (Santa Claus, etc.). At this stage, these may have a more conscious impact on spiritual development because meaning begins to become attached to them. A feminist therapist might explore the meaning that clients have associated with images, and fantasy connections to spiritual topics. It might be helpful to discover and explore how the client's developmental experiences impacted their current views of spirituality.

## Stage 3: Synthetic-Conventional Faith

This stage in which abstract thought is more developed often occurs in adolescents (Fowler, 1995). During this stage, the teen begins to understand the norms, privileges, or oppression of their family's spiritual beliefs. They may begin to critically analyze some of the previous religious or spiritual beliefs they have been exposed to, looking for logical explanations. Some religious traditions have ceremonies for adolescents to become spiritual "adults" welcomed as fully confirmed religious group members (confirmation, bar/bat mitzvah, etc.). For some, committing to such a life decision may be challenging so early in their development; for others, it may not be an issue.

As teens continue to develop, their alignments with spiritual beliefs may begin to shift from the authority of religious leaders or parents to friends and social influencers, who are also couched and assimilated into patriarchal norms. Many older teens shift their focus to their personal identity development and finding a hierarchy for the ego/self (Erikson, 1980). The quest for ego identity in the teen years is often influenced by patriarchal hierarchy ideals, capitalism, power (desire for privilege and rejection of oppression), and achievements. This identity quest might be conflated with spiritual development unless other influences exist to understand societal norms that may or may not be congruent with spiritual beliefs. A feminist therapist may want to examine the intersectional influences of identity development and how they influence the client's spiritual beliefs.

## Stage 4: Individuative-Reflective Faith

In young adulthood, critical thinking often develops more, and people might question and analyze what they have been told and previously experienced spiritually. Past authority figures may be questioned, and people may begin to decipher between perceptions and truths. This might be when a feminist therapist can collaboratively examine a person's spiritual beliefs with a patriarchal lens in an ecosystem context. The examinations have no direction or agenda. The goal is to allow for increased consciousness and freedom in conscious decision-making. Conversely, this might be when a person differentiates from their family's spiritual beliefs and patriarchal society's influence and becomes more invested in spiritual life. It is essential that feminist therapists, consciously or unconsciously, do not play a role in influencing the client from a feminist perspective.

## Stage 5: Conjunctive Faith

Although some people do not reach this stage, this is a stage of self-awareness, reflection, and exploration (Fowler, 1995). This is a stage when a person might begin an intentional quest to understand the many life philosophies, spiritual practices, world religions, and so on, to understand the meaning of life better and create a broader frame of spirituality. This stage might challenge a client's existing beliefs from a feminist perspective because it must also include an examination of the Eurocentric, heteronormative, patriarchal influences that have driven many decisions and reactions in one's life. Properly examining one's existence, meaning, and purpose does not mean rejecting all that one has known because of its sources. A true examination of spirituality is understanding all aspects and having a fully conscious choice, instead of an embedded unconscious automatic reaction, of the beliefs that will guide their life.

## Stage 6: Universalizing Faith

This is a stage of life that few people might reach because it moves into acceptance of not knowing the answers to life's mysteries. This stage might allow a person to become more congruent and authentic in their understandings and worldviews of life. In this stage, a person comes to understand that all spiritual experiences and beliefs are equally valid. For the feminist therapist, this resonates with the clinical applications of therapy. Honoring intersectional differences, believing people's experiences, and putting all others in high esteem equally are feminist principles as well as recognizing that the majority view is not correct; it just holds the most social power. This frame allows people to understand their intersectional oppression and how it might hold people back from becoming their fully authentic selves. Although Fowler (1995) suggests that this stage is often great world teachers (e.g., Gandhi, Mother Teresa, etc.), a feminist therapist might see this as an advocating stage to help others raise their consciousness to live the most fully functioning authentic lives possible.

# Feminist Intersectional Therapeutic Relationship Conditions and Spirituality

Feminist therapeutic relationship principles stress the importance of maintaining process transparency, flattening the expected social hierarchy between the therapist and client, and acknowledging, analyzing, and consistently monitoring the power differential within the therapeutic relationship. When working with spiritual issues, additional therapeutic considerations may be necessary. Many intersectional variations of spiritual beliefs and understandings may conflict with the feminist values of the therapist. As with all feminist therapy, feminist values cannot be imposed on the spiritual therapeutic process, or that is just another form of oppression to the client. Callahan (2009) suggested that spiritually sensitive clinical work must involve conveying respect for another person's inherent value and dignity through "I-thou" communication (Buber, 1970). Feminist therapists must accept all spiritual ways of knowing, even if they view them as oppressive systems.

One method often considered by feminist therapists in attempts to flatten hierarchies is therapeutic self-disclosure. There are many intersectional complications to consider when deciding whether spiritual self-disclosure will be therapeutically helpful. Often, using language or labels to describe spirituality cannot adequately express the complications of spiritual beliefs. For example, if someone discloses that they are Roman Catholic, what does that mean? If the therapist were also to reveal that they are Roman Catholic, that might imply the beliefs are the same. The range of beliefs, the intersectional identities, and cultural and geographic influences on the "Catholic" might mislead clients into thinking of greater similarities where they may not be. Conversely, the feminist therapist may have vastly different spiritual ideologies than the client, and that, too, can be misleading to the client, who might assume there would be a lack of understanding or respect for their spiritual positioning. Therefore, feminist therapists must discern deeply when considering self-disclosure and working with feminist spirituality.

In addition to each clinical mental health discipline having an ethical code that sets forth guidelines for clinical practices, many also provide details on what defines spiritual competency (ACA, NASW, etc.). In accordance with the mental health discipline's ethical code and the state's legal licensing requirements, each feminist therapist must remain competent within their scope of practice and avoid dual relationships. For example, for a pastoral counselor, the scope of practice may include more religious context and interventions than for a psychologist.

# Feminist Intersectional Spirituality Model

# (Adapted and updated from Jodry and Levitt, 2023)

Feminist therapists working with spiritual issues might find it challenging when working with clients who feel marginalized, oppressed, excluded, or even rejected by a religious/ spiritual group that shares a majority of collective beliefs that conflict with their own human existence, critical beliefs, or behaviors. From a feminist intersectional lens, a person's intersectional spiritual identities, including their past or present religious traditions, developed critical thoughts around spirituality, specific cultural influences on spirituality, and potential past spiritual injuries, must be examined to understand possible levels of privilege and oppression they may be experiencing. Feminist therapists collaboratively explore the client's unique experiences, with or without spiritual injuries, to further their move toward higher consciousness to make choices, empowerment to resist validation, and create meaning in their lives.

To remain competent when working with spiritual issues, a feminist therapist should self-examine their own spiritual experiences and intersectionality of beliefs continuously. Feminist therapists take full responsibility for their personal beliefs, examining any patriarchal religious construct (PRC) injuries that must be realized and understood to maintain awareness and competency (Jodry & Levitt, 2023). Although some feminists reject or view religion as oppressive, therapist's own PRCs or any biased views against religious beliefs must not be included in the therapy. As with any feminist therapy, the goal is to raise consciousness, examine all aspects of spirituality, and make room for freedom of a fully conscious choice. This feminist intersectional spiritual model is not necessarily linear in the application. The creativity of the feminist therapist and the direction that the client chooses can change the therapeutic process. This is a collaborative client-led process.

## Stage 1: Spiritual Patriarchal Differentiation

In this step, the client will do an intersectional examination of their spiritual and existential beliefs regarding the meaning of life. They will examine how they came to believe or not believe what they do about mystical life questions. They will review who or what influenced their beliefs. They will also acknowledge any of society's levels of oppression or privilege regarding their beliefs. This step is designed to help the client understand their past embedded social, cultural, and political messages related to spirituality, examine the influence of the oppressive ecosystem on their experiences, and explore the current impact on their beliefs. This step does not devalue any beliefs or faith a client may find comfort in or may want to embrace because of its patriarchal roots. Consciousness raising is the goal, so the client is able to make a conscious choice that is differentiated from the patriarchal influence.

## Step 2: Spiritual Intersectional Examination

Clients all bring unique intersectional identities to therapy, which never allows for just one form of therapeutic intervention. In this step, the client examines their intersectional identities beyond but including their religious or spiritual identities and acknowledges related oppressions, privileges, and experiences associated with them. Special attention is paid to their spiritual beliefs and how society, their families, and the community would accept any potential changes if desired. This may also be a time to consider ancestors and those spiritual legacies. For some populations, specific religions were forced upon them for survival. A client might want to look past their current beliefs and examine their ancestral beliefs. Additionally, the client should examine how any sense of inclusion, rejection, or praise associated with spiritual experiences is woven into their identities and how that shaped their beliefs.

## Step 3: Spiritual Exploration for Consciousness Raising and Existential Freedom

This step may or may not happen, depending on the client's commitment to spiritual exploration, fear of change, use of defense mechanisms, or other understandable resistances. In this step, clients work to understand different beliefs they have yet to be exposed to. This can be done by attending rituals in other faiths, reading philosophical and spiritual books, conversing with friends who are also interested in spiritual endeavors, and so forth. This could also include interviewing spiritual leaders and beginning new practices such as contemplation, yoga, or meditation. It is solely up to the client to choose the journey. However, it is up to the feminist therapist to be familiar with the many different spiritual philosophies that exist so that they can be competently discussed with the client. This process of self-education allows the client to make fully conscious, differentiated, informed choices about their spiritual future with autonomy.

## Step 4: Spiritual Empowerment

Once the client has been able to examine the influence of social, cultural, and political constructs, understand their intersectional existence around their spirituality, and explore other philosophies and beliefs (if desired), the client begins to take responsibility for what they believe. Existential freedom dictates that one can make conscious choices, know the consequences, and take responsibility for one's choices. Faith, rituals, community, lifestyle, life purpose, belief in God, and spiritual advocacy are all choices. Therapeutic consciousness raising allows them to make all examined decisions actively instead of reactively. Clients can then decide that these are "their" truths. This is an ongoing, lifelong process that clients can continue if they desire. A growing openness of the client's ability to change their minds and add new spiritual thoughts in the future can be part of this process.

## Step 5: Spiritual Behaviors and Advocacy

Once a client decides on a spiritual construct that works for them, the next step is what to do with those beliefs. This might involve finding a community to support or encourage critical thinking around those beliefs (e.g., religion, group of friends, online groups, places of retreat, etc.), creating a consistent ritual to maintain the ongoing decisions (e.g., mediation, daily prayer, drumming, create an altar in house, daily devotion to self or others, etc.), create a plan for continued exploration (e.g., visit holy sites, reading lists, etc.), and consider service to others (e.g., serving the community and those suffering, involvement in or creating a nonprofit, etc.). This would not be a feminist spiritual model if we did not mention advocacy. However, advocacy comes in many forms. It could range from praying for yourself and others to marching to change oppressive legislation. If advocacy is involved with the client's process, it has to be entirely up to them and be congruent with their spiritual decisions.

# Feminist Intersectional Therapeutic Applications

Regardless of the therapeutic approach, some of the following techniques or clinical applications might be helpful tools for feminist clinicians working with issues of religion and spirituality. Callahan (2010) developed a relational spirituality model based on research that provides a foundation for addressing religion and/or spirituality concepts and activities throughout the clinical intervention. This model may inspire feminist therapists to use these collaborative therapeutic relationship-building activities while maintaining congruence, power monitoring, and transparency. For example, individual spiritual coping activities include meditation, prayer, and the like, which a feminist therapist can support as self-interventions. On an interpersonal level, the feminist therapist can create a respectful, supportive, empowering environment for clients to discuss their religions and/or spirituality and can also help connect clients to others around these topics. Lastly, therapists can try to arrange their spaces to include contemplative elements.

Below, distinctly feminist techniques will all aim to examine the following collaboratively: help the client identify their current belief system rooted around values, roles, and spirituality; reveal and address any adopted or learned beliefs that create inner conflict and barriers to spiritual wellness; identify where beliefs originated and how they impact daily functioning; identify areas where the client can live in spiritual congruency to aid in healing; and identify the process that the client will use to move through life in a responsible, empowered, existential congruence, honoring their intersectional identities and beliefs.

Feminist therapists might work with the client to invite possibilities of empowerment, alignment, congruency, awareness, and fully conscious choices. The client might explore what it means to live their life by acknowledging choices that can actively be made versus living life in a reactionary, disempowered state. Doing creative activities such as creating a vision board in session allows the client a moment to use their hands, their mind, and their spirit to craft a life for themselves. Any tool, technique, or activity that visually enables clients to create and choose a vision of a life they desire or is representative of their life gives the client the awareness to acknowledge their power in creation within their life. It places the responsibility and opportunities that come with taking responsibility, such as freedom and empowerment, back into the client's hands. At no point do feminist therapists function as spiritual or religious leaders or guides, or pressure clients in any way concerning their religious and spiritual choices.

## Spiritual Development and Religious, Spiritual, and Patriarchal Construct Injuries

The feminist therapist will use the feminist intersectional spirituality model to examine the moments of spirituality the client remembers and how it has evolved. This might include religious activities they have been involved in as well. The client will be invited on a journey through what moments and memories they recall having, where they recall going, what they recall doing, and how they felt about the experiences with curiosity, sensitivity, and exploration of the connected emotion. Next, the feminist therapist might shift to a here-and-now awareness—pondering how the previously excavated periods of experiences impacted them and how that shows up in their present spiritual beliefs and behaviors. Through collaborative exploratory questioning, the client and therapist can understand and identify what barriers, impasses, and other obstacles are related to their spiritual identity and worldviews.

This technique could be used to construct a spiritual timeline in session. The timeline would highlight events noted as significant to the client from birth through the present. These important events would include any happy or conflicting memories stemming from spiritual ceremonies, rituals, traditions, sin's role in their levels of esteem rooted in beliefs, and so forth. The feminist therapist would note particular times of conflict or any discomfort the client is experiencing and address those memories immediately. Once a timeline is established, the feminist therapist might begin to help the client contextualize the patriarchal constructs that may be associated with their memories. Once the context is understood, discussion around conscious choices can begin.

## Ancestral Exploration, Spiritual Genogram

The feminist therapist might use ancestral exploration to dive deeper into understanding the client's perspectives, experiences, and current experience of their intersectional identities in a spiritual context. Collaboratively, the client and therapist might investigate and explore the client's ancestral lineage of spirituality. The therapist will follow their lead in discussing any spiritual injuries that the client was born into and those that were passed down from parents and any other ancestors. This journey may bring the client to a narrative investigation of family knowledge outside of the session, where knowledge from their findings could then be brought back to session to further deepen the client's awareness of their spiritual history. The feminist therapist will explore what current spiritual traditions are followed today and when and if there was ever a time when these traditions were not a part of their family's experience. This may serve to be comforting and healing and/or may uncover more spiritual injuries to be addressed.

This technique can use genograms as a tool to visually represent the family tree, including detailed information on relationships, connections, and any spiritually relevant information, patterns, and feelings that can be recalled and highlighted. The genogram can be used as a reference point for deeper session exploration. It is important to note that some cultures, mainly Eastern cultures, believe in reincarnation; genograms might be a tool that would allow a client to represent an ancestral family line of returned souls. Feelings such as joy and pride may arise, and emotions such as shame and anger may also occur in session. The feminist therapist must always be conscious and present to help empower clients through this process.

## Feminist Existentialism Exploration and Choices

The feminist therapist and client might leverage existential thought to explore the meaning of life, explore a sense of purpose, and understand the responsibility of making choices (Yalom, 1980). The goal is to uncover the roots of the client's belief system and to put social, cultural, and political contexts around them. The feminist therapist helps the client evaluate their spiritual beliefs' oppressive or privileged nature and identify beliefs that empower or drain power from the client's lived existence. Making different choices might encourage a different frame of higher consciousness; any potential consequences of new choices must be analyzed. The goal is to understand that power exists in one's life to make spiritual choices, take responsibility for those choices, and accept the consequences. The goal is to make decisions with a higher awareness of embedded spiritual messages and to consciously make choices instead of unconsciously reacting. The final stage of this clinical application might be for the client to consciously choose to own the messages within them and thus consciously create their own internal guiding compass.

Questions that might be helpful in this process include: *When did I learn ___? What are the foundations of my beliefs around what I can be/say/do ___? Where did these messages come from? Are these messages mine? If these messages are not mine, whose are they? As an adult, do I still choose to believe these?*

## Feminist Intersectionality of Spiritual Oppression Analysis

The feminist therapist can focus on exploring all of the interlocking intersectional identities of a client. Intersectional identities often evolve with lived experiences and sometimes go unexamined. The important identities may vary by client, but some areas worth exploring for a spiritual undertaking might be geography, socioeconomic status, religious values and beliefs, family culture, in addition to identities of age, race, affectional orientation, gender, ability, and so on. After these identities are examined, it will be necessary for the client to identify which parts they feel are oppressed and which are privileged by society, culturally and politically. The client can even rank which identities they are most and least connected to or representative of themselves and which identities society recognizes and attributes to them. Additionally, how these identities and related oppressions of a person's life have impacted the client's sense of self, autonomy, capabilities, and identity related to spirituality might be explored. This can help the client and therapist understand what is most important to the client's self-concept and what they face in the larger culture. The goal is to raise consciousness around their intersectional identities and understand where these elements of identity, points of oppression, and privilege impact their sense of spirituality and ability to make meaning in their lives.

## Feminist Reconciliation: Deconstruction of "Sins"

"Sin" is a religious construct that permeates into society's sense of right and wrong. Often, "sin" is defined spiritually, but it can be interchangeable with secular, social, cultural, and politically unacceptable norms. The concepts of absolution, confession, and reconciliation are prominent in Western Christian religions. When a client presents as having "sinned," the feminist therapist has an opportunity to deconstruct and possibly reconstruct what "sinning" means as a social construct, how it has historically been determined, and the Eurocentric heteronormative Christian-dominant patriarchal influences that defined what a "sin" is. The client may want to redefine what a "sin" is to them without the patriarchal influences, which may lead to a path of awareness, consciousness, and spiritual healing. Here are some points that may be explored: *What are sins? Who decided what a sin is? How have they impacted you? How has society's definition of the things it has labeled as sins impacted your spirituality?* The goal is to use a concept like sin, understand what it means for the client, and understand if it has embedded itself in the client's identity. The therapist must hold no power over the client, emphasizing that the client is encouraged to choose what is right and what is wrong for themselves. The goal of the feminist therapist is to aid the client in understanding that the central point to healing is a choice held within themselves that can be free of the social cultural and political constructs.

## Soul Path, Dharma Path

Often in Eastern culture, "dharma" describes one's life journey, and in Western culture, "soul" describes the spiritual part of human existence. Dharma can also be viewed as a soul's purpose or path while on this earth. These terms can be interwoven to conceptualize helping clients become or remain mindful of the purpose of their human existence. Clients can decide what they would like their spiritual or psychological guiding forces to be: everyday reactions to transactions, activities that intend to create less personal suffering, service to others, and so on. Once they collaboratively explore their options, the feminist therapist empowers the client to decide what thoughts might remain at the forefront of decisions. Discussions, then, might explore how to live out their choices. It could be conceptualized that when one is true to their dharma, they are living their truth, taking aligned action, and are consciously awake to the active role they play in their life. In other words, they are congruent. Creating alignment and congruency with their decided paths is the goal here. The feminist therapist might help the client learn ways to advocate for themselves within their lives, honor their truths, and use assertive communication skills to align themselves with found decisions.

## Feminist Intersectional Therapeutic Example

Grace comes into counseling for the first time, identifying as a heterosexual, cisgender, Black, Jewish female. Grace shares that her mother identifies as White and Jewish, and her father, Black and Baptist, though more spiritual than religious, and that these elements are important to her story. Grace is 27 and has been living back at home for one year since completing both an undergraduate and graduate program. She comes to therapy desperately seeking to understand what is "wrong" with her, having reported that she is having a hard time finding and keeping a job and just had a breakup. Grace feels she lacks direction and meaning in her life and is always questioning her own spiritual history and beliefs.

As the feminist therapist sits with Grace, the feminist intersectional spirituality model is used to aid in navigating and understanding their time together. In stage one, the therapist explores spiritual patriarchal differentiation with Grace. The therapist uses a spiritual timeline technique in session to formulate an overview of any injuries that have occurred and to further help establish where Grace's beliefs came from, what they are, and how this shaped her present sense of meaning in life. Grace shares that she attended Hebrew school, had a bat mitzvah, and that she and her mother followed the Jewish faith conservatively attending Shabbat services every Friday and twice a year for the high holidays until Grace left for her undergraduate degree at age 19. Grace has described that early on, support within her home and in the Jewish community was present and felt comforting. She recognizes that her mother and father shaped her spiritual, Black, and Jewish identities for her. And although she had gone away to college and had new experiences, Grace began to feel that she never claimed who she was or what she believed in for herself as an adult. This understanding sparked fear and curiosity in Grace, which was processed in session.

As sessions continued, stage two brought about a spiritual intersectional examination. Through exploration, it became clear to Grace that through the large Jewish community in her town, her Jewish identity felt approved of and privileged, while her Black identity felt oppressed. During her college years, Grace went to a four-year HBU (historically black university) where her Jewish identity felt oppressed and marginalized, and her Black identity suddenly felt like one with more empowerment and privilege. Here, Grace discovers a deeper inner strain that had existed, one that dictated who she was based on her surroundings instead of who she felt and chose to be. At home, Grace felt influenced by her mother's spiritual and religious Jewish nature, and at school, she felt included by her predominantly Black classmates and those in the sorority she joined. But Grace realized she never felt that she could decide her truth for herself.

Grace begins to dig deeper and becomes curious about herself by exploring her ancestral lineage on both sides of her family. Grace creates a genogram and discovers new information, including information about her mother. In session, the therapist and Grace process the connections Grace made from the information gathered on the genogram and how they connect to her current situation in life. Grace reveals that many people on her mother's and father's side were spiritual; they did not attend religious gatherings but had a strong community. Additionally, Grace's mother tells her that when Grace was eight, both she and her mother were accused of "not being Jewish enough" by a woman at the temple. Though Grace didn't consciously recall this experience, she did remember a time when she and her mother went from socializing to rarely speaking with anyone at the temple. Grace began to piece together moments where she heard suppressed contempt for Judaism bubble up in conversation at home. Grace processes how this discovery played a large role in her inner dialogue, her feeling like something was wrong and that she was not good enough. She began to see that she had an internalized resentment and conflict about who she was and her sense of not belonging to society because of this experience's impact on her and her family.

Grace's desire for change and inner peace was heightened. She felt lost and was curious to find herself. She found that she was not drawn to attend temple any longer and found solace in her discoveries about her lineage of spiritual pursuits that brought great comfort to her life. Stage three is a spiritual exploration of consciousness raising and exploring existential freedom. Grace reads many philosophical and religious texts and finds herself drawn to read about Jewish and Black spiritual practices and Eastern spirituality. The feminist counselor explores these topics in session with Grace and finds that she really enjoys the calming effects of meditation. She soon chooses to attend yoga classes on Fridays and reports feeling connected to herself through her newfound spiritual practice.

After some time in session, Grace moves into stage four, spiritual empowerment. Concepts such as existential thought are openly discussed in session, and Grace acknowledges her attachment to outdated parts of herself. Her newfound interest in spiritual practices like yoga and meditation allows Grace the space to feel empowered and more firmly rooted in something meaningful to her day to day. She identifies with her spirituality, occasionally goes to temple, and feels more connected to a universal whole. At this point, in sessions, Grace digs deeper into what things she grew up believing, where those beliefs came from, and what she believes today. Grace works toward accepting what she finds in her exploration and takes responsibility for the choices she is now making toward a more empowered and autonomous identity.

Step 5 involves spiritual behaviors and advocacy. Grace wants to form a community and uses social media platforms to gather others locally to join her in her meditation practice. Grace has a goal of becoming a certified yoga instructor and chooses to teach at her temple's Hebrew school once a week to make some money. Grace feels empowered to teach young people the importance of spirituality in religion. Grace decides it's important for her to create opportunities to share the lessons she has learned and because of her experiences feels called to allow people a space where they feel welcomed and safe. Grace leaves therapy feeling grounded in a sense of existential freedom, and empowerment in the unique ways she's begun to create an aligned life consciously with newfound purpose and autonomy.

## Special Considerations with Feminist Spirituality

### Sexual/Affectional Orientation and Gender Identity Minorities

One population that is at risk of being marginalized, oppressed, and rejected by religious/ spiritual groups may be the LGBTQIA+ community. Although some welcoming spiritual communities exist, variations of oppressive dogmas are found throughout different religious beliefs that are often influenced by geographic locations. While religion and spirituality can support people who are suffering, a punitive religious stance and/or microaggressions toward people who are LGBTQIA+ can lead to psychological distress and clinical mental health issues (Cole, 2023; Jodry & Levitt, 2023; Lomash et al., 2019). Okrey Anderson and McGuire (2021) suggest that there is a risk for long-term distress regardless of whether individuals stay in their faith communities or are disaffiliated. Nevertheless, religion/spirituality can still be a desired resource for some. Feminist therapists may want to pay special attention to any spiritual injuries from past experiences that may be impacting the client's spiritual growth in the present (Jodry & Levitt, 2023). Feminist therapists can help by learning about safe, affirming faith communities and religious beliefs (Coburn & McGeorge, 2019). Affirming communities can support healing and the joy of belonging with "like-minded" people (Gandy et al., 2021).

## Hospice Care and Spirituality

Based on a qualitative study of hospice workers, Callahan (2012) found that it is affirming to convey spiritual sensitivity by recognizing personhood, therapeutic touch, being present, listening, singing, reframing, affirming, using self-disclosure, normalization, and advocacy. Callahan's (2013, 2015, 2017) relational model for spiritually sensitive clinicians further suggested that systemic factors, such as the clinician's level of expertise and the client's spiritual needs, create the conditions for relational spirituality. A clinician's level of expertise is defined by the capacity to facilitate meaningful relationships. Enhancing life meaning through relationships is considered a universal spiritual need. Therefore, spiritually sensitive clinicians are a process and a product. It entails a therapeutic relationship that facilitates enhanced life quality through meaningful relationships or relational spirituality. In palliative care, it is suggested that the purpose of spiritually sensitive clinicians is to help people experience meaningful relationships (Reese et al., 2022). A feminist therapist might want to consider adding conversations around empowerment to those served by hospice, creating space for clients to find power in their situations no matter how limited their capacity. Choices might include those around eating, socializing, solitude, and so on. It is important, wherever not dangerous and possible, to allow the hospice client to find agency in their decisions.

## Challenges of Feminist Intersectional Theory and Spirituality

Inviting critical thinking about anyone's spirituality and faith may be difficult. Particular natural resistances can be encountered depending on where the client is in their faith development. Challenging images of God can also be threatening to a person who feels a personal relationship has been established with that image. The feminist therapist must remember that the client's desire leads any of these explorations and the feminist therapist has no agenda for the client to change religious or spiritual beliefs.

As with any feminist therapeutic process, power and hierarchies are acknowledged and monitored. How do discussions around God or "Higher Power" (who some think has ultimate power) interact with therapeutic power, client empowerment, and flattening hierarchies? The feminist therapist must address these concerns transparently, honoring the client's intersectional identities and therapeutic desires.

One of the greatest self-monitoring challenges as a feminist therapist is unintentionally imposing values. When clients are injured by the dominant majority's religious or spiritual views, the therapist must empower the client without input. Imposing values is what the dominant majority does; it would be contraindicated for a feminist therapist to do it as well. For example, those who identify within the LGBTQIA+ are often marginalized for their affectional and gender orientations and may be seen to embrace communities that do not embrace them. The choice needs to be fully conscious; then there is complete freedom in decision-making.

# What If?

What if the dominant image of God in the United States was not a White man but a woman of color? Would that change cultural, social, and political norms?

What if a true image of Christ was visualized as a Middle Eastern man during prayer? Would that change anything?

What if we did not start spiritual conversations with children until they could think abstractly in their teens? Would spirituality be different individually or collectively?

What if the United States was not a Christian-dominated country? Would the social, cultural, and political norms be different? Or not?

# References

Buber, M. (1970). *I and thou* (W. Kaufmann, Trans.). Touchstone. (Original work published 1923)

Callahan, A. M. (2009). Spiritually-sensitive care in hospice social work. *Journal of Social Work in End-of-Life and Palliative Care*, 5(3-4), 169–185.

Callahan, A. M. (2010, November). *Exploring the relational aspects of spiritually-sensitive hospice care*. Audio conference for the North American Association of Christians in Social Work.

Callahan, A. M. (2012). A qualitative exploration of spiritually sensitive hospice care. *Journal of Social Service Research*, 38(2), 144–155. https://doi.org/10.1080/01488376.2011.619425

Callahan, A. M. (2013). A relational model for spiritually-sensitive hospice care. *Journal of Social Work in End-of-Life and Palliative Care*, 9(2-3), 158–179. https://doi.org/10.1080/15524256.2013.794051

Callahan, A. M. (2015). Key concepts in spiritual care for hospice social workers: How a multidisciplinary perspective can inform spiritual competence. *Social Work & Christianity*, 42(1), 43–62.

Callahan, A. (2017). *Spirituality and hospice social work*. Columbia University Press. http://cup.columbia.edu/book/spirituality-and-hospice-social-work/9780231171731

Coburn, K. O., & McGeorge, C. R. (2019). What do Christian clergy say? Advice from Christian pastors to family therapists about working with LGB clients. *Contemporary Family Therapy*, 41, 236–246. https://doi.org/10.1007/s10591-019-09490-0

Cole, M. (2023). Psychological effects of Christian teaching about sin and hell. *Mental Health, Religion, & Culture*, 26(8), 736–754. https://doi.org/10.1080/13674676.2023.2261412

Confucious. (2022). *The analects of Confucious* (J. Legge, Trans.). King Solomon Publishing.

Erikson, E. H. (1980). *Identity and the life cycle*. W. W. Norton.

Erikson, E. H., & Erikson, J. M. (1997). *The life cycle completed*. W. W. Norton.

Fowler, J. W. (1995). *Stages of faith*. Harper Collins Publisher.

Gandy, M. E., Natale, A. P., & Levy, D. L. (2021). "We shared a heartbeat": Protective functions of faith communities in the lives of LGBTQ+ people. *Spirituality in Clinical Practice*, 8(2) 98–111. https://doi.org/10.1037/scp0000225

Howard, S., & Sommers, S. R. (2015). Exploring the enigmatic link between religion and anti-Black attitudes. *Social and Personality Psychology Compass, 9*, 495–510. https://doi.org/10.1037/rel0000144

Howard, S., & Sommers, S. R. (2019). White religious iconography increases anti-Black attitudes. *Psychology of Religion and Spirituality, 11*(4), 382–391. https://doi.org/10.1037/t03889-000

Jodry, J., & Levitt, R. B. (2023). Feminist counseling theory and spirituality: Beyond patriarchal religious constructs. *Counseling & Values, 68*(1), 18–37. https://doi.org/10.1163/2161007X-68010003

Jones, A., Cohen, D., Johnstone, B., Yoon, D. P., Schoop, L. H., McCormack, G., & Campbell, J. (2015). Relationships between negative spiritual beliefs and health outcomes for individuals with heterogeneous medical conditions. *Journal of Spirituality in Mental Health, 17*, 135–152. https://doi.org/10.1080/19349637.2015.1023679

Jones, J. M. (2023). *In U.S., 47% identify as religious, 33% identify as spiritual.* Gallup. https://news.gallup.com/poll/511133/identify-religious-spiritual.aspx

Koenig, H. G. (2012). Religion, spirituality, and health: The research and clinical implications. *International Scholarly Research Network*, 1–33. https://www.ncbi.nlm.nih.gov/pmc/articles/PMC3671693

Li, S., Stampfer, M. J., Williams, D. R., & VanderWeele, T. J. (2016). Association of religious service attendance with mortality among women. *Journal of American Medical Association Internal Medicine, 176*(6), 777–784. https://pubmed.ncbi.nlm.nih.gov/27183175

Lipka, M., & C. Gecewicz, C. (2017). More Americans now say they're spiritual but not religious [web log comment]. https://www.pewresearch.org/fact-tank/2017/09/06/more-americans-now-say-theyre-spiritual-but-not-religious

Lomash, E. F., Brown, T. D., & Galupo, M. P. (2019). "A whole bunch of love the sinner hate the sin": LGBTQ microaggressions experienced in religious and spiritual context. *Journal of Homosexuality, 66*(10), 1495–1511.

Newsweek Staff. (2007, June 6). Have you seen this man? *Newsweek.* https://www.newsweek.com/have-you-seen-man-102285

Okrey Anderson, S., & McGuire, J. K. (2021). "I feel like God doesn't like me": Faith and ambiguous loss among transgender youth. *Family Relations: An Interdisciplinary Journal of Applied Family Studies, 70*(2), 390–401. https://doi.org/10.1111/fare.12536

Pew Research Center. (2024). *Religious landscape study.* https://www.pewforum.org/religious-landscape-study

Pew Research Center. (2020). *Religious landscape study: Religions.* https://www.pewforum.org/religious-landscape-study

Reese, D., Nelson-Becker, H., & Callahan, A. M. (2022). Spirituality and social work practice in palliative care. In T. Altilio, S. Otis-Green, J. Cagle, & R. Brandon (Eds.), *Oxford textbook of palliative social work* (pp. 201–213). Oxford University Press. https://doi.org/10.1093/med/9780199739110.003.0019

Rizzuto, A. M. (1979). *The birth of the living God: A psychoanalytic study.* University of Chicago Press.

Safran, J. D. (2012). *Psychoanalysis and psychoanalytic therapies.* American Psychological Association.

Shafranske, E. P. (1996). *Religion and the clinical practice of psychology.* American Psychological Association.

Yalom, I. (1980). *Existential psychotherapy.* Basic Books.

# 12

# Feminist Intersectional Therapy and Sexuality

## *Kathleen McCleskey, Valerie Stolicker, and Janys Murphy Rising*

*Concepts of sex, sexuality, and gender are socially, culturally, and politically framed from a Eurocentric, Christian-dominant, heteronormative, patriarchal lens and often serve to restrict and oppress intersectional expressions of the sexual self.*

For many therapists, sexual issues are a part of the spectrum of concerns that clients bring to therapy, so they must be ready to work with clients on those issues in an empowering manner. Clients may come to therapy specifically to discuss sexual concerns, or these issues can emerge while working on other issues. Feminist clinicians will approach sexual content as they will other kinds of client concerns—by taking a broad, systemic view that includes how Eurocentric, heteronormative, Christian-dominant patriarchal messages and systems impact clients and their well-being. From a feminist perspective, distress and pathology can be either the result of oppression or can be exacerbated by it (Brown, 2018), and this is true in all therapeutic areas, particularly sexuality. It is important to note that, historically, there have been disagreements within feminism regarding some sexual topics. During the 1980s, opposing perspectives emerged from lesbian feminists regarding patriarchal influences on sexuality (Ferguson, 1984). Radical feminists espoused that pornography, sadomasochism, and any sexual practices that recreated or reinforced male domination over females should be rejected. In response, "pro-sex" feminists asserted that radical feminists were oppressing sexuality and that sexual liberation and agency was the goal, for women and others to be able to practice whatever sex was pleasurable with consenting adults.

## Sex Positivity

The term "sex positivity" emerged from the "pro-sex" feminists' views on sexuality. Sex positivity is used as an umbrella term to frame sexuality as a normal human experience that recognizes a wide spectrum of sexual attitudes, identities, and behaviors that can add to a person's life (Good Vibrations, 2019). Sex positivity incorporates consent as a key component. It also is a nonjudgmental perspective with the understanding that no one needs to participate in sexual behaviors that do not work for them; at the same time, it is important to not judge others for practices that one is not attracted to. In other words, as is colloquially said, "Don't yuck anybody's yum" (Nagoski, 2015, p. 173). A sex-positive stance is one of inclusivity, not one of oppression.

Sex positivity has laid the groundwork to depathologize sexuality, particularly for women, sexual minorities, people of color, and sex workers (Fahs, 2014) The sex-positive movement has frequently focused on celebrating and validating sexual identities, values, behaviors, and practices that have previously been judged, criticized, and oppressed. Through this lens, sex positivity can be seen as primarily expanding "freedom to" options for sexual liberty (Fahs, 2014). Fahs (2014) notes that true freedom does not exist unless there is both "freedom to" make choices and also "freedom from" having choices imposed on us. "Freedom from" examples of sexual liberty could include not feeling pressured to have sex, not engaging in certain kinds of sexual behaviors, or not being seen as a sexual object or sexual stereotype. If clients are experiencing any of these or other sexual limitations or oppressions, a feminist therapist could help clients to become empowered to add positive freedom and reduce negative freedom, all of which can be impacted by patriarchal systems and social norms.

# Societal and Cultural Impacts on Sexuality

Societal and cultural influences on sexuality can be viewed through the umbrella of patriarchal impacts. Patriarchal messages about sexuality can reinforce gender and other norms, power imbalances, and harmful stereotypes (Nógrádi, 2018). These messages manifest in various areas of society, including media representation, sexual education, and interpersonal relationships, and can include sexual objectification, double standards, victim blaming, and heteronormativity. This can often serve to oppress, shame and hurt people who do not fit these sexual social constructs. Social messages can also promote sexual stereotypes and fetishization of people according to race or ethnicity (see, e.g., Zheng, 2016). Feminist therapists recognize and address the impact of societal norms, gender roles, identity intersections, and power dynamics on individuals' experiences and choices and their areas of privilege and oppression.

Intersectionality is a key concept as of third-wave feminist theory that emphasizes the interconnectedness of various social categories (Dill & Kohlman, 2012). Individuals experience multiple forms of oppression and privilege simultaneously. It is evident that individuals' experiences are shaped by factors such as gender, race, class, age, religion, disabilities, sex, body type, and affectional orientation, and so forth. Understanding the intersectionality of different identities, both visible and invisible, guides the feminist therapist to understand and honor the unique experiences and oppressions experienced by individuals with multiple marginalized identities. For instance, a Black lesbian woman may face a particular set of challenges that are distinct from those faced by a White heterosexual woman or a Black transgender man. By taking an intersectional approach, a feminist therapist can more adequately address the complexities of individual experiences. It also helps contextualize the need for advocacy to create an inclusive and equitable society for all. Examples of specific identities related to sexuality follow, but this is simply a sampling of the vast number of potentially intersecting identities.

# Gender

Societal gender norms and expectations influence the development of an individual's sexuality, often resulting in the perpetuation of inequality, discrimination, and repression (Mikkola, 2023). Gender roles are seen as societal constructs that often reinforce unequal power dynamics and the suppression of women's and nonbinary individuals' agency. These roles dictate expectations and behaviors that align with traditional views of binary masculinity and femininity, creating a patriarchal message that places cisgender men in positions of power and authority while cisgender women are expected to be submissive, nurturing caretakers (Lai & Hynie, 2011).

Masculine sexuality is often perceived as being assertive, dominant, and aggressive, while feminine sexuality is portrayed as passive, submissive, and focused on pleasing their partner. Women may face scrutiny for openly expressing sexual desires or for being sexually assertive, which is not the dominant perception or norm. In contrast, men are often encouraged to express their desires and only face scrutiny when their desires are outside the heteronormative structure (homosexuality, submissive acts, etc.). These societal expectations perpetuate inequalities, hindering authentic sexual expression for both genders by restricting the range of acceptable behaviors.

Transgender persons have rarely had their sexuality celebrated. Transgender individuals have often been seen as asexual, and medical providers have not incorporated sexuality concerns within medical care (Fielding, 2021). Frequently, when transgender people have been studied, it has been in relation to oppressions, comorbidities, or negative outcomes. Taken together, these have kept trans people marginalized and oppressed in their sexuality. Gender-expansive persons' sexuality is also marginalized. For example, dating apps may not have options for nonbinary identifications or searches (Jas, 2020), rendering individuals invisible and overlooked.

One of the central gendered concepts in feminist theories of sexuality has been the "male gaze." Coined by feminist film theorist Mulvey (1975), the male gaze refers to the way in which media and society often depict females as objects of male desire, reducing them to passive objects to be looked at. Objectification theory explains that when women and other marginalized genders are portrayed as objects of desire, it can lead to their worth being reduced to their physical appearance and sexual appeal (Lefebvre, 2020; Moradi & Huang, 2008). They may feel a large amount of pressure to fit into the beauty standards placed on them by patriarchal standards in their community. When these individuals feel as if—or are told—they do not meet these standards, it can lead to low self-esteem, reduced cognitive performance, and body image concerns (Moradi & Huang, 2008). Gay males have also been found to experience body objectification, as have lesbian women (Massey et al., 2020) and transgender women (Lefebvre, 2020). While the male gaze is most often examined in terms of its impact on females, it is important to note that males are socialized into developing it, and internalizing that embedded behavior also impacts males negatively (see, e.g., Goldin, 2022).

Feminists view gendered norms and expectations as restricting not only cisgender females, nonbinary, transgender, and sexual minority persons but also restricting cisgender males as well. Patriarchal culture reinforces male power, and it also provides narrow scripts of gendered expectations, including sexual scripts (Daniels et al., 2002). Cisgender males may find themselves unwilling or unable to conform to these scripts, and they may face consequences. Feminist therapists strive for a more inclusive and equitable understanding of gender and sexuality, emphasizing the importance of respecting and acknowledging the diverse ways in which individuals experience and express their sexuality, regardless of their gender identity or assigned sex, and also emphasizing ways that all genders are restricted from being their authentic sexual selves.

## Specific Race, Ethnicity, and Gender Intersections

Specific sexual stereotypes of race and ethnicity form intersections of oppression that injure clients around their sexuality. Sexual stereotypes have long existed about African American females (e.g., a temptress/Jezebel) and African American males (sexually aggressive, especially with White women); these stereotypes date back to enslavement and were used to justify the rape of enslaved females and fear of enslaved males; other stereotypes sexualize African American bodies (large penises for males, large bottoms for females) and behavior (promiscuity) (Rosenthal et al., 2020). Latinas have been stereotyped as being either hypersexual or asexual (Vargas, 2009), being curvy, having children at a young age, and being more likely to have STIs (Rosenthal et al., 2020), whereas stereotypes of Latinos include the passionate Latin lover (Newcomb et al., 2015; Vargas, 2009) and the rapist (Rosenthal et al., 2020). People of Asian descent have also been sexually stereotyped; Asian women have been viewed as feminine and submissive, and Asian men are perceived as softer and more feminine than men of other races or ethnicities. (Zheng, 2016) All of these stereotypes can impact people's internally embedded sexual identities as well as their interpersonal sexual experiences.

## Class

The social location of class creates a complex framework where social and economic hierarchies both reinforce and limit expressions of sexuality (Taylor et al., 2010). Patriarchally created class dynamics perpetuate traditional gender norms and expectations. Economic disparities can restrict access to education, healthcare, and resources, which in turn limits the agency and choices related to sexual experiences. Individuals from lower classes may feel greater financial pressure to conform to patriarchal societal norms for survival. These pressures may limit alternative forms of sexual expression and freedom to explore and define sexuality more authentically. For example, working-class lesbians in one sample had little geographic mobility and this continued proximity to people who knew them was an inhibiting factor for them to freely explore affectional identity (McDermott, 2010). In contrast, middle-class lesbians' "mobility through social spaces" (p. 204) outside where they grew up allowed them more freedom to come out as lesbians.

## Religion

Feminist therapy offers a critical lens to consider the ways in which religion can be used to control and restrict people's sexual autonomy and seeks to dismantle the oppressive dynamics. Religion can be a complex factor in many clients' lives. For some, religion provides spaces for community, self-reflection, and spiritual growth. For others, it is conflictual, oppressive, and rejecting. And for many others, it is both. Some feminist theologians have sought to reinterpret religious texts and narratives in ways that challenge traditional notions of gender and promote more egalitarian and inclusive understandings of sexuality (Vuola, 2016). However, religion has often been used as a means to control and regulate women's bodies and sexual behavior (Baumeister & Twenge, 2002) as well as to restrict behaviors, attractions, contraception, and pornography use (Litam & Speciale, 2021). Patriarchal religious constructs serve to inhibit sexual autonomy, exploration, and self-expression while maintaining Eurocentric, Christian-dominant, heteronormative patriarchal norms that reinforce gender roles and other dictates that cause spiritual wounds (Jodry & Levitt, 2023). People may be expected to conform to heteronormative and monogamous dogma, which can turn to embedded internalized shame and psychic injuries (Jodry & Levitt, 2023). Additionally, religious teachings that promote abstinence-only education or condemn contraception and abortion limit women's access to reproductive healthcare and perpetuate harmful stereotypes about female sexuality (Baumeister & Twenge, 2002).

## Age

Feminist theory challenges the notion that a person's sexuality diminishes over time and that society should devalue sexual expression based on age. Patriarchal norms and messages overlook or dismiss the sexual desires and needs of older individuals, perpetuating the assumption that sexual desires and experiences decline with age (Taylor & Gosney, 2011). Pejorative prejudices include that sex among older people may be considered repulsive or comedic. Society generally portrays older individuals as asexual, but there is actually a range of importance placed on sex in later life, which can be impacted by health and partner availability as well as by individual desire to remain sexually active (Gott & Hinchliff, 2003). Older adults are among the most overlooked potential client populations in terms of sexuality counseling.

## Ability

Individuals with disabilities face their own unique challenges and inequalities that can significantly affect sexuality (Addlakha et al., 2017). They often face discrimination, stigmatization, and exclusion in various aspects of their life, including their expression of sexuality. Access to comprehensive sexual education, healthcare, and sexual expression is limited for disabled individuals due to social barriers and ableist attitudes. In addition, societal beliefs of binary femininity and masculinity are often bolstered, which adds to the marginalization of individuals with a disability, particularly those who do not conform to traditional expectations (Cheng, 2009). Patriarchal expectations of bodies and cultural histories of bodies are important areas to explore (Garland-Thomson, 2002). These multiple oppressions can impact all areas of sexuality for people with any sort of disability, whether visible or invisible.

## Affectional Orientation

Affectional orientation also plays a crucial role in shaping and influencing one's sexuality. Feminist theory recognizes that human beings are socialized into binary gender norms, where heterosexuality is often assumed as the default orientation (Evans et al., 2011). This assumption perpetuates heteronormativity, where society expects and favors heterosexual relationships and desires. Consequently, individuals who do not conform to heterosexuality may face marginalization, discrimination, oppression, and even rejection. Queer people have faced stigma, oppression, and discrimination both individually and as members of queer communities (Ginicola et al., 2017). They have been treated as one community despite distinct identities and subgroups within the larger community. Queer people have also been historically oppressed by the mental health community with non-heterosexuality being pathologized (ALGBTIC LGBQQIA Competencies Taskforce, 2013). Minority stress theory focuses on the negative impact on LGBTQ individuals from living in a society that is hostile to their identities; it has been illustrated that some queer persons commonly experience hypervigilance in both private and public spaces because of the anticipation of bias or discrimination (Rostosky et al., 2022).

## Bodies

Body type does not inherently determine one's sexuality. However, society often promotes certain body types as more desirable, perpetuating unrealistic beauty standards and objectification of women, in particular (Raja, 2023). Traditional notions of sexuality have long been dominated by cisgender, heterosexual, and androcentric narratives, often excluding or stigmatizing individuals whose bodies and desires fall outside of these parameters (Fielding, 2021). Fielding (2021) describes "erotic privilege" as having a body that is deemed worthy of both having desire and being desired (p. 17). There are particular challenges faced by people with bodies outside the margins of erotic ideals, which include but are not limited to transgender bodies, older bodies, overweight bodies, or disabled bodies. In other words, bodies that do not fit the patriarchal ideals are marginalized and devalued. An extension of that dynamic can be the professional minimization of having erotic desire—for example, medical providers (or even therapists) may not attend to the sexuality concerns of these marginalized persons.

# Sexuality in Therapy

Many common sexual issues can have an element of shame, and shame can be connected to systemic messages about the self, about sex, and about sexual behaviors (Litam & Speciale, 2021). In addition, the stigma around candidly discussing sexual matters can impact both clients and clinicians. As with all issues, it is imperative that feminist therapists do their personal work to be comfortable with professionally working with sexual matters. As noted by Buehler (2021), clinicians have grown up in the same culture as many of their clients and are therefore not immune from feeling shame or embarrassment when openly discussing sex. Examining potential countertransference is imperative.

It is also important to note that there is special training and certification for anyone interested in becoming a sex therapist—the American Association of Sexuality Educators, Counselors, and Therapists (AASECT) is the credentialing body for that certification. Not all therapists may be interested in pursuing certification as a sex therapist, but all clinicians should be able to discuss sexual issues with clients in a professional and ethical manner.

The DSM-V-TR, which the patriarchal medical model system requires many feminist clinicians to use, continues to have a gender binary, medicalized, and deficit-based description of sexual problems and concerns, which can be an uncomfortable framework for feminist practitioners to use (Pukall, 2023). A feminist therapist will want to collaboratively and with transparency provide context to clients about diagnosing, in general, and also specifics of any sexual diagnoses. Diagnosis can be a shared activity between the client and feminist therapist reviewing criteria together. Finding a diagnosis can be a positive experience for clients who may be relieved to know that their concern has a name and treatment options, or it may be a challenging experience to receive a negative label that frames a problem as a physical or psychological dysfunction.

# Feminist Intersectional Conceptualization With Sexuality

From a feminist perspective, an overall goal is to help clients raise their consciousness, allowing them to move toward freedom, to be authentic, and to assert personal autonomy. This is also true when dealing with sexual issues. Most often, bringing up sexual concerns is a vulnerable experience. Most people want to be sexually "normal" and want reassurance that whatever is going on with them does not make them abnormal (Nagoski, 2015). In contextualizing "normal," feminist therapists can help clients to reframe perspectives by situating problems within the greater Eurocentric, heteronormative, Christian-dominant patriarchal culture and systems. Clinical feminist practitioners can expand patriarchal-embedded social and cultural frameworks through consciousness-raising explorations. Clients often internalize disempowering and disaffirming messages and feminist therapists will want to listen for these external and internal impacts as clients share their stories and process concerns with them.

As an example, if a client presents with difficulty feeling arousal, persons of any gender may think there is something wrong with them personally. Depending on the genitals they have, they may feel failure to perform, failure to respond, or both. A medical perspective may point to medical interventions (or not), and for some problems, a medical screening is helpful. A feminist therapist, however, will also consider how patriarchal messages, norms, and expectations impact the problem. How is the problem being experienced based on gender, age, affectional orientation, partner status, ability, and the like, and in terms of intersections of these? If there is a consistent lower libido, is that being labeled as abnormal? What socially constructed messages about arousal may apply? Do messages differ based on the person's genitals? What do partners express about the client's arousal? How does the client define the arousal experience? Feminist therapists consider external, oppressive forces from the dominant patriarchal culture as well as from other systems which may include family-of-origin systems or partner systems. All these systems can provide disempowering or disaffirming messaging to clients regarding sexual issues.

# A Feminist Intersectional Model for Working with Sexual Concerns

## Normalizing Sexuality as a Holistic, Wellness-Oriented Topic

In this first stage in this model, feminist therapists can use a sex-positive approach in terms of pre-intake paperwork, during intake, and in sessions. Presenting sexuality as a positive and universal part of development and life can create an environment where clients may be more comfortable engaging in discussions of sexual concerns. Actively asking about sexual issues normalizes that these are valid concerns to discuss. Clinicians can create and maintain an inclusive and affirming posture, showing their comfort with discussing sexual topics.

## Inquiring/Broaching about Framing Sexuality within Systemic Frameworks

Once clients have introduced sexual topics, feminist clinicians can seek permission to explore concerns or issues through a systemic, contextualizing lens to help determine how the patriarchal systems may have impacted the client's beliefs around sex. Because of the sensitive nature of sexual concerns, collaborating on exploration is critical. This models the power-sharing dynamic of the feminist egalitarian relationship. When clients ask for clarity about systems, therapists can identify both individual (family of origin, peers, partner relationships) systems and greater systems (media, religion, culture, etc.) that can be potentially connected to how the problem is defined or experienced.

## Understanding and Identifying Patriarchal Influences on Sexuality

If clients are willing to explore systemic impacts and messages around their sexualities, feminist clinicians can offer psychoeducation about patriarchal influences on sexuality. This stage is where intersectional identities can be examined. Clients can identify the systems that pertain to them, such as cultural, religious, educational, and so on, and the feminist therapist can also offer information about overt and covert messages and norms. The aim here is not to force clients to accept patriarchal frameworks but rather to offer them context for sexual beliefs and any problems associated with it and to help them gain insight.

## Collaboratively Exploring Patriarchal Impacts Today

In this stage, clients and the feminist clinician collaboratively explore embedded conscious and/or unconscious sexuality messages, expectations, and values that the client identified in the previous stage. How do patriarchal norms and assumptions impact these concerns? How do they frame problems, and potential solutions? This stage can include exploration techniques, such as an intersectional power analysis, a feminist q-sort, and so forth, to delve into the client's sexual concerns. As part of these explorations, feminist practitioners want to identify where clients have power, autonomy, and choice and where they do not. These explorations could also include delineating where clients have both "freedom to" and "freedom from" in terms of sexual concerns (Fahs, 2014).

## Assertive Goal-Setting

If the client gained any new insights from the previous stage, the feminist clinician and client will decide if they would like to incorporate new thoughts into action goals. Goal-setting needs to be truly collaborative, with the client identifying and/or endorsing goals they are invested in. A feminist therapist may suggest having an element of empowerment or assertiveness in the goals so as to be able to help the client gain or maintain autonomy. If desired by the client, goals can also include consciousness raising about systemic impacts on the client and their life.

## Feminist Interventions and Goal Alignment

Interventions follow clients' goals and should align with them. A feminist clinician will utilize the egalitarian therapeutic relationship as a primary intervention to empower the client to gain autonomy, and if desired, in working toward change. Change may be focused on the client, on a partner system, and/or greater systems, on exploring areas of sexuality, on exploring intersectional identities, or any combination of these. If the client identifies oppressive societal impacts, then therapists can point out how those impacts are present in change efforts and how they may be rejected or resisted.

## Know When to Refer to Specialists

As stated earlier, counseling for some sexual issues may require medical screening. In addition, there may be other collateral services that would benefit clients (for example, pelvic floor physical therapy). The feminist therapist should collaborate in the community to create and maintain a list of trusted providers and collateral resources. In curating this list, it is important to discern the values of those providers and collateral resources to ensure that they will both aid the client in their healthcare needs as well as provide support that is grounded in anti-oppression. A feminist therapist will consider how referrals to providers can enhance the work the client is doing in therapy or can create potential conflict. If a provider is sharing patriarchal, medical model messages that are counter to what the feminist therapist is exploring, it can confuse the client and must be discussed.

# Possible Feminist Intersectional Applications with Sexual Issues

## Egalitarian Therapeutic Relationship with Issues of Sex

The feminist egalitarian therapeutic relationship has long been a hallmark of feminist therapy and is considered to be a powerful force for healing, as clients can experience in therapy the kind of power-sharing relationship they may not experience outside of it (Evans et al., 2011). Because sexuality issues and concerns can be sensitive areas for clients, this power-sharing approach can help establish that the client is in agreement with areas of exploration, potential interventions, and directions that the therapy is going.

To implement this egalitarian approach with sexual issues, a feminist therapist will be sure to seek permission from clients to explore sexual topics. The therapist will honor clients' comfort levels with sexual topics and can use immediacy to discuss how the process of counseling is consistent or not consistent with clients' goals around sexuality.

## Assertiveness Skill-Building with Sexual Concerns

Building assertiveness skills is another intervention that feminist clinicians often offer to clients (Worell & Remer, 2003). Assertiveness skills can be tied to how clients experience power in many areas of their lives in personal and professional settings including their sexuality. With sexual concerns, clients may or may not feel comfortable and confident in communicating their sexual identities, values, desires, needs, or boundaries. Building assertiveness skills can help clients to learn, in a supportive environment, how to express their personal power in these ways.

It may be helpful to explore societally and culturally based messages about sex and assertiveness, including impacts of intersectional identities. Some clients may have been shamed or ridiculed when asking for what they want sexually, especially if that includes queer or kink desires. Building assertiveness skills with sexual issues may combine and connect with aspects of other techniques, such as a power analysis or psychoeducation.

## Psychoeducation around Sexuality and Sex

In counseling for sex issues or concerns, there are many ways that psychoeducation can be useful to clients; as outlined earlier, many socially constructed identities have had both implicit and explicit patriarchal messaging about sex, oppression, and privilege. It can be helpful to explore these and connect them to client's definitions of problems and solutions. Connected to this, psychoeducation about sex positivity and about body positivity can be helpful. Teaching clients about sex positivity can be both consciousness raising and empowering as it may help clients redefine what is normal and can therefore expand options, values, and autonomy in sexual matters. Educating about body positivity can likewise expand views of what is normal and can help clients to resist patriarchal messages of beauty and sexual attractiveness.

Some clients may also benefit from education about their bodies and about the mechanics of sex. As noted by Buehler (2021), clients may not have received clear and correct information from their upbringing, and they may have been embarrassed to ask medical providers about sexual concerns. Knowing one's own body and knowing about partners' bodies is empowering and can lead to making more empowered decisions about sex. If clients need more education about sex than a feminist therapist is able to provide, the therapist can refer clients to a sex therapist who has had specialized training to do this.

In processing these areas of psychoeducation, some questions to consider for inquiry with the client can include the following: What are the messages you internalize about your sexuality? Are these messages also present in social media or other mediums? What messages do you note in your close circle? What about messages you learned previously? How do those messages impact you now? What does the term "sex positivity" mean to you? Do you agree with the meaning? What would allow you to feel in alignment with your own sexuality, as well as the sexuality you express with partners? What are your thoughts about body positivity? How do you feel about your own body?

## Intersectional Power Analysis about Sex/Sexuality

A power analysis in another foundational technique of feminist therapy (Worell & Remer, 2003). Power analyses help illuminate where, when, and with whom clients feel personal power and where they do not. Different kinds of power can be explored and defined, either by using resources (see, e.g., Evans et al., 2011, and Worell & Remer, 2003 for examples of kinds of power that can be assessed); or the client and feminist therapist could collaboratively name and define different places where power is relevant to the client. A client may easily, for example, be able to identify power within a sexual relationship or context, but may not immediately connect power in terms of their religious background as informing relational power. Power between clients, clients and their families, clients and institutions, clients and peers, clients and the greater society—these could all be relevant for a client in exploring power connected to their sexuality. Part of this analysis can be an examination of where clients may be giving their own power away, and where they want to claim or reclaim power.

One way to implement a power analysis with sexual concerns could be to use Fahs's (2014) framework of "freedom to" and "freedom from." A client could identify all of the aspects of sex and sexuality where they feel "free to," for example, express their sexuality, explore their sexuality, choose partners, participate in specific sexual behaviors, initiate sex, decline sex, suggest a sexual activity, authentically discuss their sexual experiences with partners, ask for what they like sexually, and so on. Next, the client could identify where they are "free from," for example, any kind of coercive sex, having to justify saying no to sex or to specific sexual acts, sexual harassment, sexual violence, no choice of sexual partners, feeling shame around sex, affectional orientation, and so on. This process could occur in one session or over multiple sessions, including between session work if the client wanted to include that.

After creating these lists, the clients and the feminist therapist could examine them both as whole lists. Some questions might then be used to explore these as entire lists could also examine specific items on a list. Questions that might be used for exploration could include these: What do you feel empowered to do sexually? What choices do you feel free to make in terms of pleasure, behaviors, partners, identities, and so forth? What do you feel empowered to resist sexually? What internal or external pressures can you identify related to your sexuality? Are there areas in which you have trouble resisting pressure to conform to expectations from external sources or your own internal expectations? If a broader power analysis seemed warranted, the therapist could collaborate with the client to see if that would be helpful.

## Gender Analysis

As discussed before, a client's gender and gender identity can have great impacts on sexuality issues and concerns. Another foundational technique of feminist therapy is gender analysis (Evans et al., 2011). In doing a gender analysis with sexuality concerns or issues, a feminist clinician could invite a client first to identify their gender and then explore how they have experienced their gender in terms of sexuality.

Areas that could be helpful to explore include sexual messages and values that were received by the client from families of origin, from systems the client directly interacted with (neighborhoods, schools, religious institutions, etc.), and from larger systems such as the media, the legal system, and political systems. Sexual experiences that aligned or did not align with these messages would also be included. The client and feminist therapist could unravel any patriarchal sexual messages that were consciously or unconsciously endorsed or conveyed that may become embedded as "truths." Likewise, clients can examine or messages that they may have rejected from those messages born in patriarchal norms and expectations. After examining any patriarchally-influenced messages and related experiences, clients could consider which sexuality-related messages they want to endorse, which messages they want to reject, and if there are alternative messages, and aligned behaviors, they want to focus on that are affirming to them.

Potential questions for examination could include the following: What are the messages you have received (from different sources) about sexuality and (the client's gender) across your lifespan? What messages have been disaffirming or limiting? Which have been affirming or liberating? Are there messages you have internalized? Do those help you, hinder you, or both? Are there new messages you want to create to affirm and empower you?

## Who Am I as a Sexual Being?

It could be helpful to examine all of a client's roles and identities related to sexuality. This could be done verbally, in written form, or graphically. A client could identify all their intersectional social locations (gender, affectional orientation, ability, race, age, religion or spirituality, etc.) and explore how those identities intersect in matters of sexuality. Which intersections seem most salient when it comes to sexuality?

Life roles might also be examined, as those can also impact a person's sexual life. Those roles could include mother/father, significant other/partner/spouse/singleton, worker, caretaker, student, retiree, athlete, person with health issues, and so on. Also, these roles could be any sexual or affectional identities such as polyamorous partner, BDSM/kink roles (or identities), or any other roles that are important to the client. Examining intersections between and among these identities and roles can help a client explore these complex intersections and connect them to sexual issues or concerns.

## Feminist Intersectional Therapy Example

Nina, a cisgender biracial woman in her late thirties, seeks counseling after experiencing another failed relationship, this time due to her infidelity while being with her boyfriend Clayton. She has had numerous unsuccessful relationships with both men and women, most of which she blames herself for failing, including in relationships with domestic violence. She has only experienced sexual pleasure with one male partner, while having consistently pleasurable encounters with women. She believes she may be a lesbian, but also recognizes that her inability to communicate her desires and needs to her partners may have contributed to her relationship and sexual difficulties. Nina discloses this information in an initial phone consultation and in intake paperwork.

In their initial session, the therapist began by allowing Nina to pose any questions she had. Building on their earlier discussion about informed consent during the phone consultation, the therapist emphasized that therapy would be a collaborative effort, tailored to Nina's pace and comfort level in discussing sensitive topics. She gave an overview of egalitarian relationship principles and made sure that Nina agreed with those. Nina discussed her recent breakup with Clayton, explaining that their relationship had involved experimenting with polyamory, and although Nina continued seeing another woman, Clayton was unaware of this due to poor communication between them. Feeling responsible for the breakup, Nina expressed confusion about her affectional orientation, describing herself as bisexual or possibly gay, and acknowledged struggles with maintaining a healthy sexual relationship. She was visibly emotional throughout the session, frequently crying as she discussed the end of her relationship and past experiences where she had found sexual fulfillment primarily with women. She disclosed never having enjoyed sex with Clayton though she did care for him. The therapist validated Nina's feelings and normalized her concerns about sexuality and communication difficulties. At the conclusion of the first session, the therapist reassessed Nina's comfort with continuing therapy. Nina acknowledged the difficulty of discussing her issues but expressed gratitude for the safe environment the therapist had created.

In subsequent sessions, the therapist maintained a supportive and nonjudgmental environment, encouraging Nina to share more about her past relationships, including experiences of domestic violence and family dynamics. Psychoeducation became a key aspect of their discussions, focusing on the societal influences that shaped Nina's sexual identity, such as negative messages from her father, her parents, her childhood religion, and media representations of homosexuality and bisexuality.

Together, Nina and the therapist established therapeutic goals aimed at empowering Nina to explore her desires, improve her communication skills, and challenge societal expectations.

They did an Intersectional Power Analysis about Sex/Sexuality, using the Freedom From/Freedom To framework from Fahs (2012). Nina identified a few things she felt free to do regarding sex. She felt empowered to initiate sex, she felt free to enjoy sex in the moment, and was able to consistently orgasm with women. She identified having felt disempowered to freely explore her attraction to women (because of guilt that would set in afterward), to say no to some of the sexual activities that Clayton enjoyed, and to immediately leave relationships that were interpersonally violent. Nina reflected on past instances of feeling controlled or silenced, and the therapist helped her recognize patterns of power imbalance and how these affected her ability to express her sexual desires and boundaries. Through these discussions, Nina began to assert herself more confidently in therapy and in her personal life, reclaiming agency over her sexuality and relationships. Nina began recognizing communication breakdowns, and she began to recognize that these breakdowns came from a place of being fearful due to power imbalances. With the therapist's support and collaboration, Nina developed greater assertiveness and confidence in expressing her emotions.

# Additional Topics to Consider

## Consensual Kink

All feminist therapists should have an understanding of the kink community. This community is broad, with varied erotic interests that fall under the umbrella of kink (Kink Clinical Practice Guidelines Project, 2019). These interests, fantasies, and behaviors can include consensual power exchanges that are counter to the normative expectation of egalitarian dynamics in intimate relationships. Individuals in the kink community, as well as the community itself, have been pathologized by the mental health professions for their interests and behaviors even though the existing body or research shows no real basis for this bias (Yates & Neuer-Colburn, 2019). Consent is critically important in kink, and kink activities that have been consented to are not exploitive (Brown et al., 2020). Kink experiences and communities can differ based on affectional orientation and heteronormativity must not be applied (Muzacz et al., 2023). Feminist therapists should learn about kink, in general, and should get specific training and supervision when working with clients around kink.

When coming to therapy, a person in the kink community may want to discuss relational or sexual topics, may want to discuss topics where kink is connected but not central, or may want to discuss areas where their kink has no bearing. It is imperative that feminist clinicians not assume that problems are with, about, or because of the kink. Feminist therapists need to critically examine their reactions to kink, perhaps especially given that uneven power dynamics may appear non-feminist. As with any other marginalized population, feminist therapists do not recreate in therapy oppressive dynamics that clients experience outside of it.

## Consensual Non-Monogamy

Consensual non-monogamy (CNM) is another relational style that feminist clinicians need familiarity with. As the term implies, these relationships include sexual or romantic experiences beyond a monogamous couple, with the awareness and consent of all involved (Matsick et al., 2014). Swinging, open relationships, and polyamory all fall under the umbrella of CNM, and each has different boundaries for encounters or relationships. Polyamory, in particular, has gained attention in recent years. Similar to the kink community, the polyamorous community has been marginalized and stigmatized (Trexler, 2021), and feminist therapists need to ensure that no oppression is recreated within the therapeutic setting regarding any CNM interests or experiences.

As with the discussion on kink, it is possible that a client may want to talk about relationships, values, practices, and the like, related to consensual non-monogamy, or may want to focus on an area connected to relationships or distinct from them. The client must take the lead in identifying and endorsing areas of therapeutic focus.

## Out-of-Control Sexual Behavior

Out-of-control sexual behavior (OOCSB) is another potential area of therapeutic work. There continues to be discussion about whether this behavior is a "true addiction" (Braun-Harvey & Vigorito, 2015; Buehler, 2021). AASECT (2016) does not endorse the addiction perspective and finds inadequate evidence for using that pathologizing therapeutic model. A feminist perspective on this divide is more consistent with the perspective that sexual behavior can be problematic but not an addiction. AASECT suggests using models "that do not unduly pathologize consensual sexual behaviors" (para. 2) and this aligns with feminist thought and sex positivity.

Clients may label themselves as having sexual addiction and seek therapy for that. A feminist therapist can work with a client to understand the client's definition of addiction/OOCSB and to understand the client's concerns about the behavior. In what ways are the behaviors a problem? It is important not to assume that the quantity of behaviors correlates to distress about them; some individuals identifying as internet pornography addicts have reported great distress that is not correlated to their quantity of pornography usage (Grubbs et al., 2019). In these individuals, it appears that the tension between sexual values and sexual behaviors was a factor in both distress and self-labeling as addicts. If clients are experiencing sexual shame, feminist clinicians can help to contextualize how patriarchal messages and expectations can influence those interpretations.

As with all areas covered in this section, further training and supervision would be important for feminist therapists to be best able to help clients conceptualize OOCSB and to identify feminist and aligned techniques to use.

## Sexual Trauma

As stated earlier, sexual trauma is an all-too-common occurrence. Victims of sexual trauma may be children or adults and may be of any gender (RAINN, 2024). Sexual trauma may be the presenting issue for therapy, or it may be an experience that may or may not have been therapeutically processed. Sexual trauma has been found to have many effects, including PTSD, physical changes in the brain, more difficulties with sexual arousal for women, dissociation during sex, concerns about affectional orientation, and concerns about becoming an abuser (Buehler, 2021), and sexual distress and functioning problems (Gewirtz-Meydan, & Lahav, 2020). Treating the trauma may not automatically resolve sexual issues and concerns; sexual trauma violates many relational boundaries and can impact many parts of a survivor's sexuality.

Feminist therapists can help survivors of sexual trauma process the sexual trauma and its legacy through an affirming, non-blaming perspective. Sexual trauma has long been a focus of feminism and feminist therapy. It has been understood, systemically, as a tool of oppression toward women and other marginalized populations (Brown, 2018). Feminist therapy can help survivors place their trauma within the greater patriarchal influences that contribute to these traumas (Ballou et al., 2003). As with all other therapeutic areas, specialized training and supervision, ideally by a feminist supervisor, is advised.

# Challenges of Using a Feminist Intersectional Approach in Sexuality Counseling

There can be some challenges to using a feminist approach with clients when doing therapeutic work with clients who have sexual concerns or issues, or indeed, with any concerns. The first challenge is that clients may not be interested in the feminist perspective. This can be a challenge because a feminist therapist honors client autonomy but, at the same time, could feel less effective if unable to contextualize problems within systems of oppression. This partnership might still work, however, if the therapist and counselor could agree to look at multiple lenses through which to interpret issues, even though they individually endorse differing perspectives and, through the egalitarian relationship, feel free to disagree at times (which one hopes would happen regardless, being free to disagree).

If clients do not like the term "feminist" but are interested in including a systemic analysis of their problems, then the feminist therapist can decide if they are comfortable using feminist techniques and lenses but not identifying them as such to the client. This, however, does not honor the transparency of the egalitarian relationship. For clients who simply do not want to work with a clinician once they discover they are a feminist, appropriate referrals to other practitioners would be made.

If a client did not want to have an egalitarian relationship with their therapist but instead wanted an expert who would diagnose their problem and then tell them what to do, a feminist therapist could try to explain the benefits of the feminist therapeutic approach and see if the client is willing to explore that. The therapist could also explore, with permission of the client, what help-seeking means to them and how they learned that dynamic. Ultimately, if a client required a mode of therapy that the feminist therapist cannot provide, a referral to other potential providers would be indicated.

Self-disclosure can be another challenge for feminist therapists. Self-disclosure is often discussed as one way to help create a more egalitarian therapeutic relationship through the authentic sharing of the therapist's personhood (Brown, 2018). Brown (2018) discusses how allowing oneself to be known to clients reduces the vulnerability load on clients. This does not mean that feminist therapists self-disclose everything; of course—professional boundaries are still critical, and therapeutic focus must remain on the client. Feminist clinicians need to balance how and what to share with clients so that they are knowable and how to track any impacts of what they choose not to disclose to clients. In working with clients on sexuality and sexual issues, feminist therapists need to be cautious and intentional about what, if anything, they share of their own sexuality (for example, affectional orientation, similar history of sexual assault, etc.). Any self-disclosure of personally sensitive material needs to be ethically and theoretically defensible. If clients and therapists belong to similar communities (for example, the kink community), it is recommended to seek supervision, ideally with a feminist supervisor or peer, in navigating self-disclosure boundaries.

Lastly, feminist therapists need to continue (1) their reflexive self-examinations, and (2), their continuing education throughout their careers. Self-reflection is critical to understand one's own internal experiences not only about work with clients but also about living in the patriarchal systems we collectively inhabit. Therapists need to be able to identify how their own intersectional identities are impacted by patriarchal norms, values, and expectations and to be aware of these on an ongoing basis, as these impacts may shift for them over time. Connected to this is the need to remain informed about current trends in patriarchal systems through various formal and informal continuing education. This helps feminist therapists to reflect on impacts they experience as well as helping them have a keener insight into potential impacts on clients.

# What If?

What if no one experienced sexual shame?

What if sex positivity was the norm?

What if all bodies were accepted as equal?

What if there were no discomfort in discussing sex freely?

# References

Addlakha, R., Price, J., & Heidari, S. (2017). Disability and sexuality: Claiming sexual and reproductive rights. *Reproductive Health Matters*, 25(50), 4–9. https://doi.org/10.1080/09688080.2017.1336375

ALGBTIC LGBQQIA Competencies Taskforce, Harper, A., Finnerty, P., Martinez, M., Brace, A., Crethar, H. C., . . . Hammer, T. R. (2013). Association for lesbian, gay, bisexual, and transgender issues in counseling competencies for counseling with lesbian, gay, bisexual, queer, questioning, intersex, and ally individuals: Approved by the ALGBTIC Board on June 22, 2012. *Journal of LGBT Issues in Counseling*, 7(1), 2–43. https://doi.org/10.1080/15538605.2013.755444

American Association of Sexuality Educators, Counselors, and Therapists. (2016). *AASECT Position on sex addiction.* https://www.aasect.org/print/position-sex-addiction

Ballou, M., Hill, M., & West, C. (2003). *Feminist therapy theory and practice: A contemporary perspective.* Springer.

Baumeister, R. F., & Twenge, J. M. (2002). Cultural suppression of female sexuality. *Review of General Psychology*, 6(2), 166–203.

Biefeld, S. D., Stone, E. A., & Brown, C. S. (2021). Sexy, thin, and white: The intersection of sexualization, body type, and race on stereotypes about women. *Sex Roles 85*, 287–300. https://doi.org/10.1007/s11199-020-01221-2

Braun-Harvey, D., & Vigorito, M. A. (2015). *Treating out of control sexual behavior: Rethinking sex addiction.* Springer.

Brown, A., Barker, E. D., & Rahman, Q. (2020). A systematic scoping review of the prevalence, etiological, psychological, and interpersonal factors associated with BDSM. *Journal of Sex Research*, 57(6), 781–811. https://doi.org/10.1080/00224499.2019.1665619

Brown, L. S. (2018). *Feminist therapy* (2nd ed.). American Psychological Association.

Buehler, S. (2021). *What every mental health professional needs to know about sex* (3rd ed.). Springer.

Carbado D. W., Crenshaw, K. W., Mays, V. M., & Tomlinson, B. (2013). Intersectionality: Mapping the movements of a theory. *Du Bois Review: Social Science Research on Race, 10*(2), 303–312. https://doi.org/10.1017/S1742058X13000349

Cheng, R. P. (2009). Sociological theories of disability, gender, and sexuality: A review of the literature. *Journal of Human Behavior in the Social Environment, 19*(1), 112–122. https://doi.org/10.1080/10911350802631651

Comte, J. (2014). Decriminalization of sex work: Feminist discourses in light of research. *Sexuality & Culture 18*, 196–217. https://doi.org/10.1007/s12119-013-9174-5

Conley, T. D., & Klein, V. (2022). Women get worse sex: A confound in the explanation of gender differences in sexuality. *Perspectives on Psychological Science, 17*(4), 960–978. https://doi.org/10.1177/17456916211041598

Daniels, K. C., Zimmerman, T. S., & Wieland Bowling, S. (2002). Barriers in the bedroom: A feminist application for working with couples. *Journal of Feminist Family Therapy, 14*(2), 21–50. https://doi.org/10.1300/J086v14n02_02

Dill, B. T., & Kohlman, M. H. (2012). Intersectionality: A transformative paradigm in feminist theory and social justice. *Handbook of feminist research: Theory and praxis, 2*, 154–174.

Evans, K. M., Kincade, E. A., & Seem, S. R. (2011). *Introduction to feminist therapy: Strategies for social and individual change.* SAGE Publications.

Fahs, B. (2014). "Freedom to" and "freedom from": A new vision for sex-positive politics. *Sexualities, 17*(3), 267–290.

Ferguson, A. (1984). Sex war: The debate between radical and libertarian feminists. *Journal of Women in Culture and Society, 10*(1), 106–112. https://www.jstor.org/stable/3174240

Fielding, L. (2021). *Trans sex.* Routledge.

Galupo, M. P., Mitchell, R. C., & Davis, K. S. (2015). Sexual minority self-identification: Multiple identities and complexity. *Psychology of Sexual Orientation and Gender Diversity, 2*(4), 355–364. http://dx.doi.org/10.1037/sgd0000131

Garland-Thomson, R. (2002). Integrating disability, transforming feminist theory. *NWSA Journal, 14*(3), 1–32. http://www.jstor.org/stable/4316922

Gewirtz-Meydan, A., & Lahav, Y. (2020). Sexual dysfunction and distress among childhood sexual abuse survivors: The role of post-traumatic stress disorder. *The Journal of Sexual Medicine, 17*(11), 2267–2278. https://doi.org/10.1016/j.jsxm.2020.07.016

Ginicola, M. M., Smith, C., & Filmore, J. M. (Eds.). (2017). *Affirmative counseling with LGBTQI+ people.* American Counseling Association.

Goldin, D. (2022). A male glance at the "male gaze." *Psychoanalytic Inquiry, 42*(7), 601–610. https://doi.org/10.1080/07351690.2022.2121150

Good Vibrations. (2019, November 27). *Let's talk sex positivity.* https://www.goodvibes.com/good-vibes-buzz/sex-in-culture/lets-talk-sex-positivity-gv

Gott, M., & Hinchliff, S. (2003, May). How important is sex in later life? The views of older people. *Social Science & Medicine, 56*(8), 1617–1628. http://dx.doi.org/10.1016/S0277-9536(02)00180-6

Gross, E. (2013). Conclusion: What is feminist theory? In E. Gross, *Feminist challenges: Social and political theory.* Routledge.

Grubbs, J. B., Perry, S. L., Wilt, J. A., & Reid, R. C. (2019). Pornography problems due to moral incongruence: An integrative model with a systematic review and meta-analysis. *Archives of Sexual Behavior, 48*, 397–415. https://doi.org/10.1007/s10508-018-1248-x

Jas, Y. (2020). Sexuality in a non-binary world: Redefining and expanding the linguistic repertoire. *INSEP–Journal of the International Network for Sexual Ethics and Politics, 8*(SI), 11–12. https://elibrary.utb.de/doi/pdf/10.3224/insep.si2020.05

Jodry, J., & Levitt, R. B. (2023). Feminist counseling theory and spirituality: Beyond patriarchal religious constructs. *Counseling and Values, 68*(1), 18–37. https://doi.org/10.1163/2161007X-68010003

Kink Clinical Practice Guidelines Project. (2019). *Clinical practice guidelines for working with people with kink.* https://www.kinkguidelines.com/_files/ugd/3cd6ea_bea576f57132462fa80265b4524b702d.pdf

Lai, Y., & Hynie, M. (2011). A tale of two standards: An examination of young adults' endorsement of gendered and ageist sexual double standards. *Sex Roles, 64*, 360–371. https://doi.org/10.1007/s11199-010-9896-x

Lefebvre, D. (2020). Transgender women and the male gaze: Gender, the body, and the pressure to conform [Master's thesis]. University of Calgary, Calgary, Canada. https://prism.ucalgary.ca/items/7baa51f4-1a2c-4acc-8feb-a8fa9372bc08

Litam, S., & Speciale, M. (2021). Deconstructing sexual shame: Implications for clinical counselors and counselor educators. *Journal of Counseling Sexology & Sexual Wellness: Research, Practice, and Education, 3*(1), 14–24. https://doi.org/10.34296/03011045

Massey, C. J., Keener, E., & McGraw, J. S. (2020). The role of masculinity and femininity in body objectification: Comparison of heterosexual and gay communities. *Gender Issues, 38,* 180–199. https://doi.org/10.1007/s12147-020-09263-2

Matsick, J. L., Conley, T. D., Ziegler, A., Moors, A. C., & Rubin, J. D. (2014). Love and sex: Polyamorous relationships are perceived more favourably than swinging and open relationships. *Psychology and Sexuality, 5*(4), 339–348. https://doi.org/10.1080/19419899.2013.832934

McDermott, E. (2010). "I wanted to be totally true to myself": Class and the making of the sexual self. In Y. Taylor (Ed.), *Classed intersections* (pp. 199–216). Routledge.

Mikkola, M. (2023, Fall). Feminist perspectives on sex and gender. *The Stanford Encyclopedia of Philosophy.* https://plato.stanford.edu/archives/fall2023/entries/feminism-gender/

Moradi, B., & Huang, Y. P. (2008). Objectification theory and the psychology of women: A decade of advances and future directions. *Psychology of Women Quarterly, 32,* 377–398. https://doi.org/10.1111/j.1471-6402.2008.00452.x

Mulvey, L. (1975). Visual pleasure and narrative cinema. *Screen, 16*(3), 6–18. https://doi.org/10.1093/screen/16.3.6

Mukkamala, S., & Suyemoto, K. L. (2018). Racialized sexism/sexualized racism: A multimethod study of intersectional experiences of discrimination for Asian American women. *Asian American Journal of Psychology, 9*(1), 32–46. https://doi.org/10.1037/aap0000104

Muzacz, A. K., McCleskey, K., & Dorn-Medeiros, C. M. (2023). Queer, kinky social justice counseling and advocacy. *Journal of LGBTQ Issues in Counseling, 17*(2), 146–163. https://doi.org/10.1080/26924951.2023.2155751

Nagoski, E. (2015). *Come as you are: The surprising new science that will transform your sex life.* Simon & Schuster.

Newcomb, M. E., Ryan, D. T., Garofalo, R., & Mustanski, B. (2015). Race-based sexual stereotypes and their effects on sexual risk behavior in racially diverse young men who have sex with men. *Archives of sexual behavior, 44*(7), 1959–1968. https://doi.org/10.1007/s10508-015-0495-3

Nógrádi, N. (2018). *Global gender-based violence against women as a matter for global justice theory: Pervasive patriarchal structures and responsibility for harm* [Doctoral dissertation]. University of Leeds (School of Politics and International Studies).

Pinciotti, C. M., & Orcutt, H. K. (2021). Understanding gender differences in rape victim blaming: The power of social influence and just world beliefs. *Journal of Interpersonal Violence, 36*(1–2), 255–275. https://doi.org/10.1177/0886260517725736

Pukall, C. F. (2023). Sexual issues. In S. Hupp (Ed.), *Pseudoscience in therapy: A skeptical field guide* (pp. 162–178). Cambridge University Press.

RAINN. (2024). *Victims of sexual violence: Statistics.* https://rainn.org/statistics/victims-sexual-violence

Raja, B. (2023). *Perpetuating the ideal: The role of fashion magazines in promoting unrealistic beauty.* https://www.jetir.org/papers/JETIR2303652.pdf

Rosenthal, L., Overstreet, N. M., Khukhlovich, A., Brown, B. E., Godfrey, C.-J., & Albritton, T. (2020). Content of, sources of, and responses to sexual stereotypes of Black and Latinx women and men in the United States: A qualitative intersectional exploration. *Journal Issues, 76,* 921–948. https://doi.org/10.1111/josi.12411

Rostosky, S. S., Richardson, M. T., McCurry, S. K., & Riggle, E. D. B. (2022). LGBTQ individuals' lived experiences of hypervigilance. *Psychology of Sexual Orientation and Gender Diversity, 9*(3), 358–369. https://doi.org/10.1037/sgd0000474

Saulnier, C. F. (2014). *Feminist theories and social work: Approaches and applications.* Routledge.

Simmons, M. (2017). Theorizing prostitution: The question of agency. In B. Dank & R. Refinetti (Eds.), *Sex work and sex workers* (e-book). Taylor & Francis. https://doi.org/10.4324/9781351306683

Taylor, A., & Gosney, M. A. (2011). Sexuality in older age: Essential considerations for healthcare professionals. *Age & Ageing, 40*, 538–543. https://doi.org/10.1093/ageing/afr049

Taylor, Y., Hines, S., & Casey, M. (Eds.). (2010). *Theorizing intersectionality and sexuality*. Springer.

Trexler, B. (2021). When two is too few: Addressing polyamorous clients in therapy. *Sexual and Relationship Therapy, 39*(3), 644–659. https://doi.org/10.1080/14681994.2021.1998424

Vargas, D. R. (2009). Representations of Latina/o sexuality in popular culture. In M. Asencio (Ed.), *Latina/o sexualities: Probing powers, passions, practices, and policies*. Rutgers University Press.

Vowels, L. M., & Marks, K. P. (2018). Strategies for mitigating sexual desire discrepancy in relationships. *Archives of Sexual Behavior, 49*, 1017–1028. https://doi.org/10.1007/s10508-020-01640-y

Vuola, E. (2016). Feminist theology, religious studies and gender studies: Mutual challenges. In L. Gemzöe, M.-L., Keinänen, & A. Maddrell (Eds.), *Contemporary encounters in gender and religion: European perspectives* (pp. 307–334). Palgrave Macmillan. http://dx.doi.org/10.1007/978-3-319-42598-6_14

Worell, J., & Remer, P. (2003). *Feminist perspectives in therapy* (2nd ed.). Wiley & Sons.

Yates, S. M., & Neuer-Colburn, A. A. (2019). Counseling the kink community: What clinicians need to know. *Journal of Counseling Sexology & Sexual Wellness: Research, Practice, and Education, 1*(1). https://doi.org/10.34296/01011007

Zheng, R. (2016). Why yellow fever isn't flattering: A case against racial fetishes. *Journal of the American Philosophical Association, 2*(3), 400–419. https://doi.org/10.1017/apa.2016.25

# 13

# Feminist Intersectional Clinical Supervision and Mentoring

## *Joanne Jodry, Kathleen McCleskey, and Donnette Deigh*

*Supervisors and supervisees both bring their intersectional history and identities laden with privilege and oppression to the supervision experience.*

## Feminist Intersectional Clinical Supervision

"Feminist Supervision" could nearly be considered an oxymoron given the feminist theoretical rejection of hierarchies, feminist mentoring goals of equality, and power sharing, in contrast with the images and constructs of power and judgment in a supervisory role. Brown (2016) said,

> Supervision in the feminist paradigm embodies certain dynamic tensions between general ideals of feminist practice, such as egalitarian relationship and empowerment of the client, and the realities of supervisor practice, such as supervisor legal responsibilities for the work of supervisees and supervisor evaluative power. (p. 13)

The legacy and current expressions of the Eurocentric, patriarchal, Christian-dominant, oppressive systems that infiltrate the social, cultural, and political norms, including the mental health system that feminist therapists must work within, potentially may pose feelings of personal and professional incongruencies. Power and empowerment are at the core of feminist clinical theories and collective supervision.

> Purposeful collaboration between supervisor and supervisee to find solutions to the apparent contradictions between empowerment and evaluation inherent in the feminist

supervisory situation is one of the distinguishing features of feminist supervision, as all parties strive to disrupt dominant culture discourses of what constitutes appropriate use of power in educational and training contexts. (Brown, 2016, p. 14)

A feminist supervisor navigates power, ethics, legalities, and congruencies in supervision while attempting to advocate for personal and systemic equality and social justice.

The importance of a feminist perspective in supervision can serve many purposes. A feminist construct of supervision is intended to empower the supervisee toward professional self-awareness, insight, and clinical excellence. The ideal goal is to empower the supervisee, who empowers clients. Modeling the feminist principles of flattening hierarchies and egalitarianism might allow the supervisee more power, voice, and room for creativity than traditional supervision might offer. Degges-White et al. (2013) suggest several benefits to feminist supervision: (1) removing the rigid hierarchy allows the supervisees to express their own opinions more freely; (2) trust is built in the relationship through open dialogues; (3) shared power might help supervisees to trust themselves; and (4) shared power might encourage the trust of the client's expertise. Szymanski (2003) suggested that a feminist supervisor has four essential foundations: collaboration; continuous power monitoring; conceptualizing with an intersectional, diverse, and social context; and modeling and discussing advocacy and activism. Porter and Vasquez (1997) laid a landscape of feminist supervision, suggesting that the feminist supervision relationship was collaborative with an ongoing analysis of power. They also suggested that there were other characteristics associated with feminist supervision, including keeping a social context that emphasizes personal diversity, maintaining ethical standards, using reflexive actions to regularly self-examine reactions to a supervisee's developmental shifts, and modeling advocacy as an underpinning to the supervisee (Porter and Vasquez, 1997).

Feminist supervision also respects different ways of knowing. Absent or marginalized voices are valued as part of conversations. The feminist perspective encourages challenging any knowledge claims of those in privileged positions (Hesse-Biber, 2012) while honoring oppressed views equally.

## Mentorship

Additionally, the supervisory relationship may include mentorship, contributing to a deeper supervisory bond, given the embedded realities of the supervisor's built-in evaluative role. Lorber (2010) describes a mentor as "[b]eing coached by a protective senior about the informal norms of the workplace" (p. 34). A social construct of a mentor might seem like the supervisor is invested in the supervisee's success versus a supervisor who might seem like the relationship exists only to evaluate their performance. McKibben et al. (2019) conducted a study that found that "[s]upervisees who perceived more feminist behaviors from their supervisors were more likely to rank the supervisory relationship stronger and less likely to report withholding information from their supervisor" (p. 38).

Mentorship can also include behaviors that extend beyond supervision meetings. Feminist mentoring has been found to include, for example, helping a supervisee develop a professional identity (Prouty Lyness & Helmeke, 2008). This could include encouraging attendance at professional conferences, guiding a supervisee through submitting a conference presentation proposal, co-presenting with a supervisee at a conference, introducing a supervisee to other professionals (networking), and in-session role modeling and guidance.

# Feminist Intersectional Supervision Formats

## Individual Supervision

During individual feminist supervision, each session is carefully tailored to address the unique intersectional needs and goals of the person being supervised. This personalized approach is designed to tackle the individual's challenges, consider their intersectional identities and support their personal and professional growth. One-on-one sessions allow for in-depth exploration of personal and work-related issues. The focus is on collaboration and empowerment, creating an environment where deep discussions can occur, and significant progress can be achieved. The supervisee can openly discuss sensitive topics in a safe and confidential space without fearing judgment. Additionally, customized feedback is provided to meet the specific needs of the individual, encouraging self-reflection for personal and professional development.

## Triadic Supervision

In triadic feminist supervision, one supervisor collaborates with two supervisees (Jayne & Purswell, 2017). This structure offers a balance of individualized support and a variety of perspectives. It fosters an atmosphere where participants can observe and absorb insights from their peers while the supervisor is a mentor, power monitor, and model of congruent empowerment. Nevertheless, this model comes with challenges, such as managing time effectively and ensuring that all participants have the opportunity to contribute equally.

## Group Supervision

In group feminist supervision, groups involve multiple supervisees and one or more supervisors (Corey et al., 2021), focusing on egalitarian collective learning and support. This structure emphasizes the diversity of intersectional lived experiences and multiple perspectives while offering peer support and collaborative discussion. It provides a broad range of feedback and insights, empowers group problem-solving, and fosters a sense of an egalitarian collective, collaborative community. Feminist group supervisors must be well versed in group facilitation and supervision and should recognize stages of group development (Corey et al., 2021). One strength of feminist group supervision is that it enables supervisees to lead discussions and the supervision process. Traditional hierarchies are disrupted by giving supervisees turns to facilitate meetings and to provide feedback.

# Feminist Intersectional Supervision Mentorship Developmental Model

Inspired by the developmental models of Erikson (1980), Borysenko (1996), and the feminist models of Brown (2010, 2016), as well as the collective works of countless feminist and intersectional theorists, Jodry and McCleskey (2016) conceptualized a feminist supervision and mentorship developmental model updated and adapted here for more inclusivity, diversity, intersectionality, and conceptual use. This is one modality of conceiving and implementing feminist supervision mentoring, and it is certainly not the right way or the only way. This model is presented as a supervisor working with one supervisee over a period of time, but the model can be adapted for different settings that may include shorter-term supervision as well as beginning supervision with a more seasoned practitioner as a supervisee. This model can also be adapted to work in triadic or group supervision. Although this model is presented as sequential stages, it is not intended to be a necessarily linear model. The first stage is expected to occur with all supervisees; depending on the supervisee's professional and personal lived experiences, they could function in any stage except for those at the very end of the model.

## Bonding–Attachment

This is the supervisory stage where the relationship begins. The feminist intersectional conceptualization of this relationship might include transparency about the supervisor's intersectional identities, theoretical feminist guidelines, conceptualization of supervision, and/or mentorship while creating egalitarian dynamics. The expectation when entering the feminist supervisory environment is having mutual respect and creating an environment where power is shared, and everyone's voice is valued. Supervisors should recognize and minimize potential power dynamics between them and their supervisees while being transparent about the required evaluation of supervisees.

A feminist supervisor can share their intersectional identities, theoretical orientation, and thoughts about conducting supervision so that supervisees have an initial sense of the supervision dynamic. Supervisees can be invited to share their own intersectional identities and experiences, theoretical leanings, and supervisory goals with no supervisor judgment. The supervisor must also describe their ethical and legal constraints and ways to navigate them together, sharing their power with the supervisee. Other egalitarian relational considerations might include having no titles be used and replacing them with first names and, perhaps, appropriate self-disclosure about any stress, intimidation, or other emotion the supervisee or supervisor is experiencing.

Additionally, role induction can include discussing the transparent co-creation of the process, expectations, and responsibilities for both roles, acknowledgments, and decisions on how power will be managed throughout the supervision as a shared responsibility. As part of this early discussion, a feminist supervisor will agree to give the supervisee regular feedback on their development and will ask, in return, for regular feedback regarding their experience of the supervisory process to ensure that the supervisee is encouraged to be an active consumer of the collaborative work.

## Autonomous Points of View—Patriarchal Context

From early in the work, the feminist supervisor encourages autonomy within and outside of the supervisory relationship. A foundational concept of feminist intersectional supervision is examining how social, cultural, and political contexts and any oppressive systems impact clients and their intersectional identities, their problems, and the supervision itself. Recognition of the impact that the Eurocentric, heteronormative, Christian-dominant, patriarchal systems allow the supervisee to conceptualize themselves and clients within the oppressive ecosystem for a broader holistic feminist view of therapy. It is important to note that the supervisor's feminist enthusiasm must be monitored here so as not to overwhelm, intimidate, and, even worse, oppress autonomous thinking by imposing feminist values. This is a navigation of an introduction (or continuation) of critical thinking about the oppressive social, cultural, and political systems and their impact on the psyche. Welcoming resistance and other autonomous thoughts are part of the process of autonomy. This work helps build a common foundation of case conceptualization.

## Empowerment—Encouragement

As the supervision progresses, the supervisor and supervisee carefully monitor the relationship power and ensure that the supervisor is not solely setting agendas or deciding on process or content. Power, influence, and dynamics should be discussed openly and with intention regularly as the supervisory relationship continues. This includes the aforementioned feedback from the supervisee to the supervisor. Modeling feminist principles and behaviors of courage, advocacy, and social justice may help supervisees find their areas of courage. Explorations of fears, social passions, and how to find the courage to create a "fear less" life can be examined as related to self as a professional and clinician.

To help encourage supervisee development, feminist supervisors think carefully about when to give advice and encourage supervisees to discern it for themselves. Supervisees are encouraged to "think out loud" without fear of being shamed if wrong. A safe environment scaffolds growth in autonomy to practice critical thinking skills. The responsibility to generate possible clinical "answers" is appropriately shifted over time to the supervisee to encourage personal autonomy and professional empowerment.

## "Fellow Travelers"—Deciding Meaning/Purpose

As the working relationship becomes settled with high investment by all, meaning and purpose of the supervision can emerge as a topic of consideration. In the spirit of Yalom's (1980) therapeutic conception of fellow travelers, the supervisee and feminist supervisor might discuss and process some pragmatic, existential, and/or coincidental reasons that this supervision is happening, the synchronicity of working together and how the client's experience may benefit from this feminist conceptualization. Additionally, they can discuss how each is growing in this work together. "A hallmark of all good psychotherapy supervision is that all parties in the triad–therapist/trainee, client, and supervisor—are transformed positively by the supervisory experience" (Brown, 2016, p. 4).

There can be discussions around the advantages of feminist clinical theory related to other traditional theories and what could particularly benefit clients the supervisee presents. This also allows room for the supervisee to grow through integrating and adapting other theories into their supervision, perhaps with a feminist lens. Supervisees may generate creative ideas that the supervisor can acknowledge and endorse. Knowledge can also be incorporated, including experiences, feelings, and thoughts. Meaning and purpose can be collaboratively assessed and created; simultaneously, they may be recognized and shared by either supervisee or supervisor. It is important to note that meaning and purpose are decided, not magically understood, and the supervisees' decisions are honored.

## Feminist Identity Formation—Social Justice and Advocacy

Once the supervisee begins to understand and wants to work within feminist case conceptualization, the supervisor and supervisee can discuss professional avenues to continue to grow. This can include discussions around whether the supervisee has had any personal revelations of any embedded beliefs (Downing & Roush, 1985) that have impacted them. Additionally, the supervisee freely discusses how feminist theory is congruent or not with their professional aspirations, clinical growth, and philosophical beliefs.

If a supervisee congruently embraces feminist clinical conceptualizations and theory, the supervisor explores with them possible future directions for their careers, including personal and professional advocacy and social justice. Advocacy and justice come in many forms. There can be discussions of how the supervisees see themselves growing as a feminist clinician in the future—or not. If a supervisee does not identify as a feminist clinician, social justice and advocacy can still be a part of clinical discussion but without the feminist frame.

## Relationship Redefined: Mentor–Colleague

Over time, a supervisee is expected to develop into a more independent practitioner. When the supervisee has reached this point and feels confident and established as a professional, the supervision/mentoring relationship needs to be redefined. Although the supervisory egalitarian relationship will have shared power and reflect equal respect, a clear, transparent discussion might be helpful to flatten the hierarchy even further. At this stage, what supervisees want to work on may be more about refining and solidifying professional identities and expanding their areas of clinical interest with additional training. Often, emotional hierarchies remain due to earlier stages of supervision. This can be discussed with the goal of moving into a new way of relating more as colleagues; transparent discussion and regular checking-in can help if it is difficult to move into these new orientations. Whatever evaluation is still required from supervision will be transparently discussed and clarified.

## Consultant–Friend

During the next feminist developmental phase of supervision, there may or may not be a professional supervision arrangement in place any longer. If there is, the relationship has changed, and supervision is now more of a consultation between peers, though any continued evaluative components must be clear. If supervision is no longer a professional relationship, then the new relationship is one of collegiality. The new relationship allows for consultation in both directions. The hierarchy and power differentials continue to be monitored here, as there may still be a legacy of previous evaluative dynamics; also, power can be monitored in terms of acknowledging either person holding more power in any consultation activities or in any shared professional or social activities. In this stage, the feminist supervisor and supervisee will possibly network, collaborate on research, present at conferences, share advocacy activities, and so forth, and continue to help each other obtain feminist goals, fight oppressive systems, and grow.

## Reflection–Generational Mentoring

The hope is that this feminist supervision and mentoring experience has created meaning and helped each person grow professionally while helping clients heal their psychic wounds from all patriarchal systems of oppression. Occasional reflection and self-evaluations might help mentor the next generation of feminist clinicians. As the supervisees become the supervisors, they need to remain current in new thought and new expansions (e.g., from gender-focused feminist thought to intersectional-focused), be aware of new social, cultural, and political oppressive impacts that are injuring clients, and keep a clinical feminist support system growing intergenerationally.

# Feminist Intersectional Applications in Supervision

The following applications, along with their feminist underpinnings, can be used in any feminist intersectional supervision format. They are given as an example and a starting point but are not the only way to infuse supervision with feminist thought and implementation.

## Radical Transparency

To ensure that these practices are effective, supervisors must establish a safe and inclusive environment that encourages supervisees to openly express their vulnerabilities and engage in discussions about challenging topics without fear of judgment or reprisal within a learning community of trust (Goeke et al., 2011). This transparent environment should foster trust, respect, and empathy, allowing for meaningful and productive interactions between supervisors and supervisees. A powerful beginning to radical transparency is the informed consent process for supervision. Supervisees are given information about the feminist supervisor's approach, theoretical orientation, evaluative components and how those will be handled, meeting times, role expectations, emergency procedures, and so on. Supervisees and supervisors can collaborate on expanding or revising an informed consent agreement. Only when both parties agree on the conditions will each sign it. This radical transparency continues throughout the supervision process.

## Managing Power in Supervision

Feminist supervisors inherently have more power, given the needs and desires of supervisee(s), yet empowerment of the supervisee(s) is the goal (Brown, 2016). In addition, there is often an additional hierarchical positionality between the supervisor and supervisee(s) that causes additive power differentials. For example, there may be concurrent roles as professor/student, employer/employee, or there may be a need for a supervisor for required licensing hours or during a probationary period. A supervisee may also be influenced by a phantom hierarchy, either consciously or unconsciously, that is unknown to the supervisor. Some supervisees may have developed interactions with authority or others with dysfunctional ideals based on their intersectional experiences (e.g., worshipping, rejecting, learned helplessness, people pleasing, etc.) that must be considered based on each supervisee(s) development and intersectional experiences. Each supervisee is unique and must find their clinical power in supervision within their own personal complexities.

Although in supervision there can never be equal positions between supervisor and supervisee, feminist supervisors work to have egalitarian relationships. How does a feminist supervisor move toward flattening the hierarchy? Arczynski and Morrow (2017) investigated the complexities of power dynamics and expression in clinical supervision, which resulted in these suggested six strategies (p. 202): (1) *Bringing histories into the room* might include sharing of every party's intersectional oppression and privilege history and/or how their experiences may have shaped them as a therapist. (2) *Creating trust and openness* is often generated with radical transparency and demystifying all parts of the process and expectations.

(3) *Using a collaborative process* helps the supervisee(s) becomes empowered through experiencing an egalitarian supervisory relationship. (4) *Meeting shifting development (a) symmetries* happens when the supervisor can collaboratively acknowledge supervisee(s) professional developmental stage of becoming a congruent professional. (5) *Cultivation of critical reflexivity* is achieved through a supervisor's self-awareness and consists of monitoring their bias, countertransference, and the like, and limiting any use of unnecessary power with the supervision. (6) *Looking at and counterbalancing the impact of context* can happen as the feminist supervisor models and encourages behaviors of advocacy and challenges to the Eurocentric, heteronormative, patriarchal, oppressive norms and systems that cause personal, social, cultural, and political injuries.

Given the patriarchal medical model systems that mental healthcare is entrenched with, realistically, it may be unavoidable not to have to shift power to the supervisor occasionally to interact with the parochial systems through grades, letters of recommendation, insurance, licensing boards, field sites, and so on. In addition, clinical supervision carries both legal and ethical liability for the supervisor regarding responsibility for the supervisee's clients (Corey et al., 2021). Collaboration and transparency with supervisee(s) in co-creating strategies for these situations will help the supervisor maintain feminist congruency.

## Intersectional Self-Awareness/First Impressions Exercise

A helpful exercise for supervisees is an intersectional self-awareness/first impressions exercise, which involves imagining how clients may create first impressions of them. This is not an exercise about exploring intersectional identities but rather about seeing oneself through a client's eyes and considering what they may perceive. Supervisees can assess their physical presentation, which may include gender, race, ethnicity, age, ability, height, body size, or visible body art; their vocal qualities in terms of tone, rate of speech, accents, and language used, including slang; their clothing/attire; their physical habits; and how they behave when nervous, confused, bored, frustrated, and so on. It can be helpful for supervisees to project what assumptions and impressions a client may have of them based on first interacting with them. This can lead to discussions of changeable (language used, for example) versus unchangeable (gender, for example) aspects of their presentation, if it is desirable to work on changeable aspects, and how to consider potentially broaching with clients about unchangeable aspects. This exercise can also be an introduction to discussing intersectional identities of supervisees, their clients, and the supervisor, who can also share their own insights about first impressions.

## Encouragement

When many think of "encouragement," what comes to mind may be visions of cheerleading, telling people they can do something they want to achieve, or talking people into something they may desire. This is not the type of encouragement that necessarily empowers supervisees clinically. Encouragement in feminist supervision might better be understood as helping supervisees find their own internal and external courage. Adler (1956/1964) suggested that "[t]he amount of threat a person can bear without losing courage may be called psychological tolerance" (p. 243). Psychological tolerance will be different for each individual based on their intersectional identities, developmental experiences, and patriarchal systemic injuries. Therefore, the feminist supervisor may want to explore courage, fears, and psychological tolerance with supervisees and any goals they may have around increasing courage and tolerance as a professional.

## Intersectional Honoring of Each Experience: Self-Disclosure

Self-disclosure is a common way for feminist therapists and supervisors to help create and maintain an egalitarian relationship (Brown, 2016). As part of transparent feminist principles, feminist supervisors may consider sharing their intersectional identities, how these have affected their development as a therapist, and how they may continue to challenge them; supervisee(s) are then encouraged to do the same (Arczynski & Morrow, 2017). This exercise might be especially helpful when there are obvious differences between the supervisor and supervisee; but in any case, this reflective exercise is helpful by potentially increasing supervisee comfort with showing vulnerability, with power sharing, and with introducing intersectional identities.

## Power Analysis of Previous Supervision or Related Experiences

Doing a power analysis of previous supervision experiences can be useful to monitor and discuss power sharing in the feminist supervision relationship. Supervisees can be invited to reflect on how and where power was shared, or not, in previous supervision experiences. If they have not had supervision before, they can use any situation where a person had some authority over them while also trying to help them grow—an employment setting or and educational setting could work for this purpose. A power analysis of the previous relationship dynamic can open discussions of where the supervisee had power, wanted power but did not have it, asked (or did not) for power, and whether there were transparent discussions or negotiations of power. After the supervisee shares this information, the feminist supervisor can open the conversation about how power will be shared in this supervisory relationship, inviting the supervisee to collaborate on framing that. This exercise can help distinguish the feminist power-sharing dynamic from previous supervision and could help normalize continuing power monitoring as feminist supervision takes place.

## Discovering Patriarchal Social, Cultural, and Political Injuries

Beyond sharing intersectional identities, it can be helpful to transparently explore any mistrust, oppression, marginalization, and even rejection that supervisee(s) may have encountered in their history or are experiencing currently. Modeling of this by the supervisor could also be helpful. As part of supervisee explorations, they could discover the level of trust, oppression, inclusiveness, privilege, and so forth, in their workplace or academic setting as well as in other settings. As Hardy (2023) suggested, it is also vital to acknowledge any internalized devaluations based on external injuries and oppressive or rejecting experiences. This is information the feminist supervisor can use to begin to empower the supervisee with strategies for and processing managing any clinical, employment, or social barriers to their success. In addition, this exercise operationalizes using intersectionality in counseling and models how to do that.

## Empowering Language

One of the powerful ways that feminist supervisors can model empowerment is through use of language. There are many examples of oppressive legacies of the medical model, which include using less disempowering language for persons seeking help ("patients" versus "clients," for example) (Szasz, 1988). There have also been dehumanizing marginalizing legacies related to people being referred to or identified by a diagnosis, for example, "schizophrenics," "borderlines," or "bipolars." This language may persist in some clinical systems. From a feminist perspective, any time a person is dehumanized and reduced to a label, it is disempowering, even if the person does not hear themselves referred to as such. The disempowerment may be internalized by the clinician who is using that language and may subsequently view the person (consciously or unconsciously) with less holistic, intersectional honor. These are not values or behaviors that feminist supervisors want to reinforce in supervisees. Similarly, any language (verbal or body) describing clients regarding their intersectional identities, such as gender, race, affectional orientation, ability, and so on, must be genuinely respectful. Client identities should reflect how clients identify themselves whenever possible rather than how therapists or supervisors identify them.

## Modeling Congruent Feminist Principles: The Personal Is Political

As a feminist supervisor, it is essential to maintain currency with environmental changes in the ecosystems of supervisees and clients. At times, a supervisor might want to invite discussions of how current social, cultural, and political changes impact them, their supervisees, and current and potential clients. They might also invite the supervisee to review any personal impacts they may be feeling due to any systemic changes. The supervisor's feminist congruency can also be modeled for supervisees by allowing them to see realistic situations where patriarchal systemic influences impact clinical work. Then choices must be made about how to accommodate and navigate those or how to advocate for change. All choices can be honored as long as they are made with full conscious awareness. Likewise, modeling assertive behaviors may help the supervisee learn to do the same. Navigating conversations of the supervisor's systemic advocacy could occur provided it creates no expectation, guilt, or disappointment in/by the supervisee if they do not participate in similar advocacy themselves. The goal is to empower the supervisee and ensure all choices are equal.

## Imposter No More

Since Clance and Imes (1978) introduced the concept of the "Imposter Phenomenon in High Achieving Women," it has resonated with many people throughout different disciplines; it is defined as

> [a] subjective experience of phoniness in people who believe they are not intelligent capable or creative, despite evidence of high achievement, and are highly motivated to achieve but live in perpetual fear of being "found out" or exposed as frauds. (Colman, 2015, p. 368)

Since its conception, the imposter phenomenon has existed in many different intersectional oppressed groups, in addition to women. Hardy (2023) discusses, "[t]he unconscious internalization of messages about the inherent inferiority of the oppressed, and the corresponding superiority of the oppressor is evitable and predictable" (p. 44). It might be beneficial for a supervisor and supervisee to discuss their intersectional identities and the embedded messages in their stories about their potential imposter feelings related to intellect, competence, and creativity. Sharing known strengths may also be helpful. It can be useful to watch for disempowered body language, "buts" or quick instincts to downplay achievements or character traits, or non-majority agreements of what is "good." Discussions around how their self-concepts evolved, how they are currently maintained, and how to dispel unhelpful aspects of them may help in their professional development.

## Unlearning Helplessness—Advocacy and Social Justice

When reviewing their social, cultural, personal, and professional interactions with supervisees, they may feel helpless or disempowered. Often, problems seem too big and overwhelming to the budding professional therapist, or they have tried to help situations and failed many times. They may also have received disempowering feedback from colleagues or previous supervisors. Feminist supervisors can facilitate discussions of frustrations with systems and how those impact supervisees' perceived power levels. These discussions can generate ideas for action, either internally or externally. Collaboratively, supervisors and supervisees may find small places to address micro-level issues. These can range from continuing to reflect on one's power level, thinking of solutions for a specific client situation, or actively protesting a systemic injustice. It is important that the supervisee feels no pressure to act in ways inconsistent with their conscious and intentional choices; the goal is to think they can act and unlearn their helplessness.

# Feminist Intersectional Supervision Examples

The feminist supervisor is an experienced and empathetic licensed clinical social worker with over 15 years of practice in a public mental health agency. The supervisee is Lynn, a recent graduate who was recently hired at the agency. She returned to school later in life and is older than most recent graduates.

## Session Focus

This is the third session, and Lynn and the supervisor are straddling both the Bonding-Attachment stage and the Autonomous Points of View–Patriarchal Context stage. The supervisor is committed to fostering the advancement of clinical skills while recognizing the influence of personal experiences on professional work. The supervisor is interested in helping Lynn continue to increase her self-awareness and in helping her become more comfortable sharing power in the sessions.

## Session Dynamics

### Shared Power Dynamics

The supervisor asks Lynn to help set the agenda for the meeting. Lynn shares that she is having trouble connecting to a male adolescent client she is working with. The client does not talk much to her and seems "on guard." The supervisor shares how this example seems good to self-reflect on and asks if Lynn wants to try that. Lynn agrees.

## Reflective Practice

The supervisor introduces the intersectional self-awareness/first impressions exercise and asks Lynn to note how this client and others may form first impressions about her. Lynn notes that she is the same race as the client, a different gender, a different generation, dresses conservatively, and that when she is nervous and frustrated, she can become less client-centered and more "bossy." The supervisor self-discloses that she has also had to work on similar behaviors in the past and empathizes with the challenge of working with a client who does not want to engage.

The supervisor asks Lynn to imagine she is the client and talk about how he sees Lynn. After thinking about it, Lynn says he probably sees her as "some old woman" who is telling him what to do, that they seem from different worlds, and that he probably can't see how she could understand his life and his problems.

## Collective Problem-Solving

The supervisor asks Lynn what she thinks could be helpful. Lynn immediately says she does not know. The supervisor says that she does not know either, but they can try to generate some ideas together. After some discussion, they collaboratively decide that broaching age and generational differences could introduce transparency into the next session. Similarly, they agree that Lynn can discuss power sharing with the client to reinforce that she is not "in charge" of their sessions.

## Empowerment

When asked how she felt about the plan, Lynn said that she felt good about it and that she felt more confident. The supervisor asked if Lynn might feel tension about starting a new career at an older age, which Lynn agreed about. They discussed the imposter syndrome and decided to include "Imposter No More" as one item to discuss regularly.

## Intersectionality

The intersectionality exercise started discussions of intersectional identities and experiences that could be built on in subsequent sessions. The supervisor can ask Lynn to reflect more on how she has been and is perceived in terms of her intersectional identities, and also how she perceives herself through this frame.

## Mutual Feedback and Growth

At the end of the session, the supervisor asked if they could give each other feedback on how the session went. Lynn agreed. The supervisor asked if Lynn would go first, to try to both normalize Lynn giving her feedback and also to help empower Lynn to take the lead at times. Lynn shared that the exercise helped them consider how others, not just that specific client, see her. She appreciated the supportive disclosures the supervisor made. The supervisor shared her excitement at seeing Lynn help brainstorm ideas and also at giving her feedback. They ended by confirming the next appointment.

# Supervisee Example 2

A feminist supervisor who is a seasoned psychologist and professor oversees a feminist supervision group consisting of six doctoral students enrolled in a psychology practicum course. The group convenes every other week to delve into in-depth discussions, encompassing a wide range of topics such as their fieldwork experiences, case studies, ethical considerations, and professional growth, all within a feminist framework. The sessions provide a conducive environment for the students to reflect on their experiences and gain insights into applying feminist principles within the field of psychology.

## Group Members

Samantha is currently on a journey of self-exploration, seeking to better understand their own gender-expansive identity and how it contributes to their interactions with clients. Lana often grapples with self-doubt in her role as a leader and frequently finds herself questioning her own abilities and tends to defer to others rather than assert herself. Carlos possesses great enthusiasm for advocacy but is still learning about it and is unsure how to effectively implement it into his work. Fatimah often feels a sense of disconnection as a result of language barriers but is determined to find ways to create meaningful connections with clients. Jasmine is comfortable speaking out and is known for her challenging existing norms and actively advocating for systemic change. Robert's experience is marked by imposter syndrome despite consistently excelling academically and professionally, and he wrestles with feelings of inadequacy and self-doubt despite exceptional performance in his work.

## Session Focus

Not all group supervisees are in the same stage of the Feminist Intersectional Supervision Mentorship Developmental Model. Samantha, Fatimah, and Carlos are all in the Autonomous Points of View–Patriarchal Context stage where focusing on self and client exploration in terms of intersectional identities and issues could help them connect with their own lived experiences and those of their clients. Lana and Robert appear to be in the Empowerment–Encouragement stage and could benefit from gaining empowerment. Jasmine appears to be in either the "Fellow Travelers"–Deciding Meaning/Purpose stage where her passion for social justice can be nurtured to help her create meaning and purpose, or in the Feminist Identity Formation–Social Justice and Advocacy stage, if she identifies as a feminist practitioner.

## Session Dynamics

### Shared Power Dynamics

The feminist supervisor begins the session by asking the group supervisees to help set an agenda of what they would like to work on today in terms of case presentations, skill development, and/or professional growth. The supervisor ensures that all supervisees can contribute their thoughts. Most members gravitate toward case presentations and personal growth with skill development if time permits.

## Intersectionality

Samantha discusses a client who has a similar gender identity to their own. The feminist supervisor asks Samantha to reflect on her intersectional identities and how those connect or do not with her client. Samantha discusses their different racial and socioeconomic status (SES) locations and how they are alike but also ways in which their experiences may have been quite different. The supervisor asks for others to consider their intersectional identities concerning a current client, and each member shares about this. Fatimah shares that she believes her clients sometimes think she is unintelligent because of language barriers. Group members are able to link to this sense of assumptions made by clients based on appearance, language, clothing, and so on. While talking about clients, the supervisor models respectful language around gender, affectional orientations, and mental health diagnoses.

## Empowerment through Peer Feedback

Lana tentatively presents a case. The feminist supervisor uses self-disclosure to share how it took them a while to feel confident describing cases in a group. Other members agree that this can feel vulnerable, and they each give Lana feedback on how she explained the main issues in the case. The supervisor asks Robert, who doubts his abilities, how he might respond to Lana's client, and he gives some ideas, which other members endorse enthusiastically. Carlos presents a case he feels challenged by and admits that he is stuck. Samantha links to that, as does Robert, and there is some discussion about the options to get "unstuck."

## Reflective Practice

To help with self-reflection, the supervisor asks group supervisees to identify an area of their work where advocacy could be helpful, either for clients, with the clients' permission, or on behalf of a client population. After each supervisee has identified a possible advocacy action, the supervisor asks them to reflect on their confidence in following through with this or another advocacy plan. Jasmine shares feeling very competent and describes a recent advocacy effort she led at her site. Carlos and Robert both report feeling intimidated about their plans and hesitancy to implement them. This leads to a discussion about the imposter syndrome and some reflection from Robert connecting his male gender identity to his felt expectations about competency.

## Collective Problem-Solving

The supervisor asks the supervisees to help brainstorm what strategies Robert and Carlos could use to implement their advocacy plans. Jasmine suggests breaking the goals down into smaller subgoals, and the group supervisees offer suggestions about how to do that. When this discussion concludes, both Robert and Carlos have additional ideas to work with.

## Mutual Feedback and Growth

As the supervisor begins to wind down the meeting, they ask everyone to share feedback about the session, the supervisor, and/or each other. Supervisees give each other positive feedback for sharing what they did, especially for those willing to be a focus of discussions. The supervisor agrees with this feedback. Samantha says that she appreciated the advocacy focus. Lana says that she appreciated the supervisor sharing some of their early insecurities. They ended by confirming the next meeting.

# Possible Pitfalls of Feminist Supervision

As with many feminist clinical theories, it is incumbent on the feminist supervisor not to impose their values or push advocacy on the supervisee. This may be even more challenging in supervision than in clinical practice because the supervisor is often a professor or a seasoned feminist clinician, and the supervisee may have sought them out for their expertise in the area. Conversely, in academia, a supervisee may be assigned a supervisor and be exposed to feminist conceptualizations for the first time. No matter the route the supervision has taken, the supervisor must navigate congruency of feminist principles while honoring choices or disbelief.

Another possible pitfall might result from the supervisor or supervisee's lack of self-awareness. Feminist intersectional theory might be more challenging to digest for concrete thinkers who like direction, rules, and specific guidelines. The feminist supervisor is obligated to remain current on the social, cultural, and political landscapes and how they may continue to impact the supervisor while recognizing that every supervisee has their own lived experience with these systems.

Given the hierarchical educational system, cultural misunderstandings about feminism, and divisive political system, it is easy for a feminist supervisor to be seen as incompetent or even unintelligent. In academia, egalitarian relationships are often misconstrued as poor boundaries, sharing power is often misconstrued as being weak, and feminist research that may interpret narrative as valuable, if not better than statistic norms, is often viewed as "less than" within patriarchal established higher education systems where supervision often takes place. Conversely, even the young professional who has been raised in these patriarchal systems may misinterpret the feminist conceptions and methods as weaknesses. The feminist supervisor must be able to hold feminist congruency with and transparent discussions around those potential interpretations.

# What If?

What if all supervisors understood and explored their intersectional identities and their impact on them and their supervision styles?

What if all supervisors monitor and share power in supervision with empowerment goals?

What if all supervisors consider the privilege and oppression within the personal ecosystems of the supervisee(s) and clients before engaging in interventions?

What if advocacy for supervisees and their clients is always considered as part of the treatment plan?

# References

Adler, A. (1964). *The individual psychology of Alfred Adler.* Harper Perennial. (Original work published 1956)

Arczynski, A. V., & Morrow, S. L. (2017). The complexities of power in feminist multicultural psychotherapy supervision. *Journal of Counseling Psychology, 64(2).* 192–205. http://dx.doi.org/10.1037/cou0000179

Borysenko, J. (1996). *The Woman's book of life: The biology, psychology, and spirituality of the feminine lifestyle.* Riverhead.

Brown, L. S. (2010). *Feminist theory.* American Psychological Association.

Brown, L. S. (2016). *The feminist psychotherapy model of supervision.* American Psychological Association.

Brown, L. S. (2018). *Feminist therapy* (2nd ed). American Psychological Association.

Clance, P. R., & Imes, S. A. (1978). The imposter phenomenon in high achieving women: Dynamics and therapeutic intervention. *Psychotherapy: Theory, Research and Practice, 15*(3), 241–247.

Colman, A. M. (2015). *A dictionary of psychology (Oxford quick reference)* (4th ed.). Oxford University Press.

Corey, G., Haynes, R., Moutlon, P., & Muratori, M. (2021). *Clinical supervision in the helping professions: A practical guide.* American Counseling Association.

Degges-White, S. E., Colon, B. R., & Borzumato-Gainey, C. (2013). Counseling supervision within a feminist framework: Guidelines for intervention. *Journal of Humanistic Counseling, 52,* 92–105. http://dx.doi.org/10.1002/j.2161-1939.2013.00035.x

Downing, N. E., & Roush, K. L. (1985). From passive acceptance to active commitment: A model of feminist identity developing for woman. *The Counseling Psychologist, 13*(4), 695–709.

Erikson, E. H. (1980). *Identity and the life cycle.* W. W. Norton.

Goeke, J., Klein, E. J., Garcia-Reid, P., Birnbaum, A. S., Brown, T. L., & Degennaro, D. (2011). Deepening roots: Building a task-centered peer mentoring community. *Feminist Formations, 23*(1), 212–234. https://dx.doi.org/10.1353/ff.2011.0014

Hardy, K. V. (2023). *Racial trauma.* W. W. Norton.

Hesse-Biber, S. N. (2012) Feminist research: Exploring, interrogating, and transforming the interconnections of epistemology, methodology, and method. In S. N. Hesse-Biber (Ed.), *The handbook of feminist research: Theory and praxis* (2nd ed., pp. 1–25). SAGE.

Jayne, K. M., & Purswell, K. E. (2017). Triadic or individual? Developmental considerations for clinical supervision. http://www.pacounseling.org/aws/PACA/asset_manager/get_file/160704?ver=3210.

Jodry, J., & McCleskey, K. A. (2016, March). *The personal is political: Using feminist theory as a model of supervision and mentoring.* Workshop presented at the meeting of the Association for Women in Psychology, Pittsburgh, PA.

Lorber, J. (2010). *Gender inequality: Feminist theory and politics.* Oxford University Press.

McKibben, W. B., Cook, R. M., & Fickling, M. J. (2019). Feminist supervision and supervisee nondisclosure: The mediating role of the supervisory relationship. *The Clinical Supervisor, 38*(1), 37–57. http://doi.org/10.1080/07325223.2018.1509756

Porter, N., & Vasquez, M. (1997). Covision: Feminist supervision, process, and collaboration. In J. Worell & N. G. Johnson (Eds.), *Shaping the future of feminist psychology: Education, research, and practice* (pp. 155–171). American Psychological Association. https://doi.org/10.1037/10245-007

Prouty Lyness, A. M., & Helmeke, K. B. (2008). Clinical mentorship: One more aspect of feminist supervision. *Journal of Feminist Family Therapy, 20*(2), 166–199. https://psycnet.apa.org/doi/10.1080/08952830802023318

Szymanski, D. M. (2003) The feminist supervision scale: A relational/theoretical approach. *Psychology of Women Quarterly, 27,* 221–232. https://doi.org/10.1111/1471-6402.00102

Szasz, T. (1988). *The myth of psychotherapy.* Syracuse University Press.

Yalom, I. D. (1980). *Existential psychotherapy.* Basic Books.

# PART THREE

# Specific Populations and Feminist Intersectional Therapy

# 14

# Feminist Intersectional Therapy with BIPOC People

## *David Julius Ford Jr., Sedaria LaNora Williams, Takeesha Hawkins, and Nicole Jackson Walker*

*BIPOC experiences were historically marginalized by feminist theory. Honoring intersectionality and any associated social, cultural, and political oppression toward Black and Brown people cannot be marginalized in feminist theory again.*

## Historical Context of Feminist Theory and BIPOC: Exclusion and Inclusion

Feminist theory has been challenged about its generalizable application to *all* people, more specifically to the BIPOC (Black, Indigenous, and People of Color) population. Interestingly it has also been lauded for its consideration of the same. Although both feminist and race movements share a common goal of promoting fairness and parity, examining the inclusive and exclusive facets of their interconnectedness, and recognizing their merits and critiques is essential.

The feminist movements have often failed to include racial and class identities and, in fact, often marginalized Black and Brown voices, as pronounced by BIPOC scholars (hooks, 2000/2015; Jackson, et al., 2021). The racial segregation in the early part of the feminist movement may have contributed to perpetuating White supremacy at the expense of BIPOC (Hardy, 2023). As the feminist movement emerged, White feminists disregarded the intersectionality of women of color. They focused only on sexist behaviors, valuing sex and gender over race, "suggesting a hierarchy of oppression exists, with sexism in the first place, evokes a sense of competing concerns that is unnecessary" (hooks, 2015, p. 36). This lack of oppressive intersectional acknowledgment demonstrates the lack of inclusivity and sensitivity of early White feminists to BIPOC. Collins (2000) suggested, "This historical suppression of Black women's ideas has had a pronounced influence on feminist theory" (p. 8). It has also been suggested that BIPOC were only called upon when needed to help further feminist goals (hooks, 2000/2015). Throughout the early evolution and development of the feminist movements, the agenda was set by and in the best interests of White, heterosexual, and cisgender women (Mena, 2022; Springer, 2002).

During the third and fourth wave of feminist theory, the acknowledgment of the intersectionality of BIPOC individuals emerged and began to foster inclusivity by recognizing the unique experiences and challenges faced by marginalized women of color (Brown, 2018; Crenshaw, 1989). Racism, sexism, and classism, which all intersect to shape unique oppressed experiences, came to be better understood. Feminist intersectional therapy became more relevant to the lived realities of diverse people: men and women, White and BIPOC.

The strength of feminist intersectionality is that it challenges the reductionist notion of a singular feminist narrative based on simply sex/gender. It allows for the notion of unique lived experiences that are difficult to norm to a Eurocentric, heteronormative, Christian-dominant, patriarchal society (Collins, 1990/2000; Crenshaw, 1989; hooks, 2000/2015). Because of oppressive social, cultural, and political "norms," BIPOC populations are susceptible to internalized sexism and racism (Hardy, 2023). It is for this reason that acceptance of their unique experiences becomes imperative.

Third- and fourth-wave feminist therapy acknowledges and honors the diverse experiences of all people while exposing the limitations of a myopic homogeneous movement of the early feminist foundations (Brown, 2018). Feminist intersectional therapy recognizes, for example, that the struggles faced by White women likely differ from those faced by BIPOC women. Therefore, their experiences and clinical needs should be addressed with the appropriate focus on multiple oppressions that each person must navigate. This recognition paves the way for a more nuanced and clinically practical approach to achieving intersectional parity in therapy. Moreover, it allows for an understanding of the multiple oppressions of each person, and perhaps a curative experience whereby the therapist can truly "see" the person before them.

Despite its strengths and uniqueness, intersectionality within feminist theory has faced criticism from the BIPOC population. Some believe mainstream feminism has co-opted the concept, reducing its transformational potential (Nash, 2019). Critics say intersectionality has been reduced to a mere buzzword without meaningful action (Davis, 2008).

Third- and fourth-wave feminism has embraced multiculturalism and multiple oppressions as an integral part of its theoretical and therapeutic perspective (see e.g., Brown, 2018; Enns & Williams, 2013). Occasionally, there have been voices who have asserted that feminism and multiculturalism are in conflict with each other (see, e.g., Kukathas, 2001; Okin, 2005). Concerns raised by these authors suggest a binary between the goals of feminism and the goals of multiculturalism, and posited that one movement would "win out" over the other (Weinbaum, 2001), either through an emphasis on women's equality in patriarchal cultures worldwide (imposing feminist values / women's rights on all cultures; Okin, 2005), or on cultural relativism (allowing cultures to retain traditions, even ones that kept women disempowered; Kukathas, 2001).

## Feminist Multicultural and Social Justice Therapy

As stated, feminist therapy was founded on the White women's feminist movement focused on oppression due to sexism and advocating for gender equality. Multicultural therapy has primarily focused on oppression due to race and ethnicity. Traditionally, "both of these philosophies have focused on single domains of diversity" (Horne & Arora, 2013, p. 246). Feminist intersectional therapy aims to integrate all clinical theories of oppression to create a healing, empowering, and authentic experience for the BIPOC population.

Across mental health disciplines, multicultural and social justice competencies must be considered for their alignment with feminist therapeutic competencies. *Standards and Indicators for Cultural Competence in Social Work Practice* (NASW, 2015); the *Multicultural Guidelines: An Ecological Approach to Context, Identity, and Intersectionality* from the American Psychological Association (APA, 2017); and the *Multicultural and Social Justice Counseling Competencies: Guidelines for the Counseling Profession* (MSJCC; Ratts et al., 2016) all provide a framework for therapists to integrate culture and social justice into clinical practice, teaching, scholarship, and supervision.

The MSJCC model (Ratts et al., 2016) will be the foundation for layering additional feminist intersectional conceptualizations for competencies. There are four areas that feminist therapists must consider to be competent in working with BIPOC. These include counselor self-awareness, client worldview, the counseling relationship, and counseling and advocacy interventions.

## Self-Awareness

Feminist therapists must become aware of their own social, cultural, and political identity and their own social, cultural, and political biases, internalized and externalized, that may hinder them from building a solid therapeutic relationship. They must consciously be aware of their attitudes and beliefs, develop a deep understanding of their intersectional, social, cultural, and political identities, and act to improve their self-awareness. One tool that might assist the therapist in enriching their self-awareness is completing a feminist cultural autobiography to explore personal cultural heritage and identities, embedded biases and assumptions, and recognize their privileges and oppressions. Understanding the self allows the therapist to understand how their culture impacts the therapeutic relationship.

## Client Worldview

Feminist therapists honor clients' narratives and must believe clients' experiences and perceptions of interactions with the oppressive constructs and systems in the Eurocentric, heteronormative, Christian-dominant patriarchal society that oppressed and created psychic injuries to non-majority people and thoughts. Feminist therapists must never invalidate the client's worldview, especially if that worldview is discrepant to the feminist therapists' worldview.

## Feminist Therapeutic Relationship

Feminist therapists must be transparent about their own knowledge, skills, and awareness related to the therapeutic process. All therapist encounters with clients are unique intersectional social, cultural, and political experiences, even when race/ethnicity matches. Feminist therapists, through egalitarian discussions with their clients, must be aware of how client and therapist cultural identities, beliefs, assumptions, and positionality influence the therapeutic relationship. Power should be acknowledged and discussed, with the goal of the client ultimately becoming empowered within the therapeutic relationship and out of it. Transparency will allow for cross-cultural communication and can aid in building a solid therapeutic alliance. Therapists must honor the client by pronouncing their name correctly, using nicknames if desired, and ensuring their pronouns are congruent with their identities. Likewise, the feminist therapist wants to flatten hierarchies by becoming equal in name usage (both first names or surnames) and, if therapeutically appropriate, sharing apparent intersectional identities.

## Counseling and Advocacy Interventions

One way to enhance intersectional multicultural understanding around how client and therapist worldview influences the therapeutic relationship is the discussion of identity development. When working with Black / African American clients, the Cross Racial Identity Scale (CRIS) (Vandiver et al., 2000) can assess Black racial identity development. Other racial identity development models include (but are not limited to) Ferdman and Gallegos's (2001) model of Latino identity development, Poston's (1990) biracial identity development model, and Kim's (1981) Asian American identity development model.

## Critical Race Theory and White Supremacy Culture

Critical race theory (CRT) was conceived as a legal theory traditionally taught in law school and research-based doctoral programs (Fair Fight Initiative, n.d.). It is not taught in the traditional preschool to high school curricula and is rarely taught in most majors in higher education (Fair Fight Initiative, n.d.). Three legal scholars of color provided the foundation for CRT: Derrick Bell (Bell, 1992), Kimberlé Crenshaw (Crenshaw,1988), and Richard Delgado (Delgado, & Stefancic, 2012). According to Crenshaw et al. (1995), CRT examines how legal systems have historically enabled racial oppression through practices like slavery, genocide, and colonialism, and how these influences persist in modern society. CRT posits that American culture incorporated racism from its beginning and is still meant to marginalize and oppress Black and Brown members while privileging White members. As a result, White supremacy is interwoven into all the social and cultural systems, including, but not limited to, the legal/criminal justice system, housing/financial markets, the health system, the job market, and the education system. CRT aims to explain racism's structural nature and eliminate all race-based and other unjust hierarchies, thus making society more equitable (Crenshaw et al., 1995; Fair Fight Initiative, n.d.).

According to Jones and Okun (n.d.) White supremacy refers to

> the ways in which these ruling class elite or the power elite in the colonies of what was to become the United States used the pseudo-scientific concept of race to create whiteness and a hierarchy of racialized value in order to disconnect and divide white people from Black, Indigenous, and People of Color (BIPOC); disconnect and divide Black, Indigenous, and People of Color from each other; and disconnect and divide white people from other white people. (Jones & Okun, n.d., p. 1)

Therefore, White supremacy culture is the

> widespread ideology baked into the beliefs, values, norms, and standards of our groups (many if not most of them), our communities, our towns, our states, our nation, teaching us both overtly and covertly that whiteness holds value, whiteness is the value. (Jones & Okun, n.d, p. 1)

No one is exempt from the impact of White supremacy culture; there are clearly disproportionate impacts on some people with specific intersectional identities (Grishow-Schade, 2024).

Widespread discrimination is evident for all non-white non-male persons. Because of the unique history of colonialism and race-based oppression, a great deal of research has focused on race, and in particular the Black experience. While this is so, it is also well established that the experiences of Indigenous and other persons of color (for example, Hispanic/Latinx, Asian, etc.) are impacted by White supremacy culture (Grishow-Schade, 2024).

In the legal/criminal justice system, Black men receive harsher sentences than White men who commit the same or similar crimes (United States Sentencing Commission, 2023). According to Konish (2022), Black homebuyers were denied mortgages twice as much as the overall population of borrowers in the nation's largest 50 metropolitan areas. Racism is embedded into the education system. The "school to prison pipeline" refers to a nationwide system of policies that disadvantages students of color and pushes them out of school into the criminal justice system (New York Civil Liberties Union, 2007). Higher suspension rates for Black and Brown students, and higher suspension rates for Black students with learning disabilities appear to lead to Black and Brown students being more likely to be involved with the criminal justice system (American Civil Liberties Union, 2023).

In the healthcare system, White supremacy impacts medical practice; for example, there may be a perception that men and women and Black and White persons have different pain tolerances resulting in discriminatory withholding of pain management or even life-saving treatment (New England Journal of Medicine, 2020; Schoenthaler & Williams, 2022). Black patients, especially Black women, have more negative health outcomes than White patients. Black women have a maternal mortality rate that is 2.6 times higher than that of White women (Hoyart, 2023). According to McDowell (2022), Black women have a 40% higher breast cancer death rate than White women. In the United States, White doctors make up 56% of the physician workforce, whereas only 5% are Black (Huertas, 2020). Racist admission policies and hiring policies appear to account for a lack of representation in colleges/universities, graduate and doctoral programs, medical and law schools, and in teaching.

The legacy of these examples of oppression exists today in different forms including poverty rates, learned helplessness, and internalized racism. The practice of *redlining* in the 1950s (when city governments drew red lines around specific neighborhoods based on race) is an example of intentional oppression (Faster Capital, 2024). Banks refused to give mortgages to Black residents of those redlined neighborhoods, and the government did not provide any resources to those neighborhoods. This deliberate racist practice allowed White people to come into those neighborhoods and buy/build property. The property owners priced Black residents out of the neighborhoods and paved the way for gentrification. This contributes to poverty today since Black and Brown people have not been able to build inheritances and pass on generational money the way that many White people have gained wealth (De los Santos et al., 2021; Faster Capital, 2024).

In the 2020–2021 school year, 6.1% of public-school teachers were Black, a non-representative number compared to student population (USAFacts, 2023). Williams (2010) found that school counselors were more apt to guide White students into college preparatory tracks than Black students and were more apt to see college as an option for White students than for Black students. According to the United Negro College Fund (UNCF, n.d.), Black students, whose behaviors may be the result of their home life rather than defiance, or who may have intellectual disorders, are overly tracked into special education programs at disproportionate rates.

Although CRT was born in the legal system, there are clinical implications that may help a feminist intersectional therapist examine and contextualize the suffering, pain, and behaviors of clients. Feminists have, since the third wave, touted the notion of multiple oppressions (Collins, 1990/2000; Spelman, 1988). CRT may be viewed as the next logical way of examining and putting into context the suffering, pain, and behaviors of clients. Helping clients understand how their intersectional identities are privileged or oppressed within Eurocentric, heteronormative, Christian-dominant, patriarchal constructs and systems gives context to their life experiences. Additionally, understanding how these patriarchal constructs create and promote oppressive legacies to prevent the success of the BIPOC population in this country may help to alleviate racial trauma. Hardy (2023) discusses how the gaslighting of society makes oppressed people believe that if they work hard enough, they can achieve, so there must be something wrong with them, which leads to internalized messages of inherent inferiority. The feminist therapist can use a CRT lens to help clients deconstruct racist systems, challenge these systems, become aware of the plight of the BIPOC population and their experience with oppression, and advocate at microsystemic and macrosystemic levels.

## Becoming Antiracist

Helms's (1995) theory of White racial identity development (WRID) presents a developmental process where individuals move from a lack of awareness of racism toward increased racial consciousness to becoming nonracist. Malott et al. (2015) extend one's development from nonracist to antiracist. To be an antiracist is to possess a heightened understanding of racism and White supremacy that manifests in action (Kendi, 2019). Kendi (2019) argues that in the fight against racism, there is no middle ground; people are either promoting racial equality or sustaining racial inequality through their actions or inactions. For the feminist therapist, action can include a willingness to discuss how one's intersectional identity impacts therapy, advocacy, and dismantling systems (Shand-Lubbers, & Baden, 2023).

## Feminist Intersectionality Therapy: Working with the BIPOC Population

When it comes to adequately serving the mental health needs of BIPOC individuals in the United States, traditional therapeutic models appear to be less than ideal (Abrams et al., 2019). Interventions must be culturally tailored as they are almost four times more effective than non-tailored interventions (Ward & Brown, 2015). Research also suggests that it is important for practitioners who serve this population to work toward utilizing a framework that does not focus on symptoms but instead on the factors that may have contributed to these symptoms, such as culture, society, and historical influences (Abrams et al., 2019). The utilization of feminist intersectional therapy stands as a paramount approach for fostering comprehensive and inclusive care.

An assumption in mainstream feminism was that race and class could be separated from gender (hooks, 1984). Collins and Bilge (2016) suggested that the lives of individuals are influenced and shaped by multiple axes rather than singular ones. A feminist intersectional framework can provide more nuanced and empathetic support tailored to the individual's unique experiences. Feminist intersectional therapy goes beyond a one-size-fits-all approach, delving into the complex intersections that shape one's worldview in order to promote a deeper understanding of the client's lived experiences. It also facilitates a more inclusive and empowering therapeutic environment with the goal of having a better ability to navigate and advocate in oppressive systems. In essence, embracing feminist intersectional therapy in a mental health clinical setting reflects a commitment to affirming diverse identities and deconstructing and dismantling systemic barriers, ultimately contributing to more effective and equitable mental health outcomes for individuals.

BIPOC populations have faced gross generalizations that make it difficult to adequately understand the unique needs and strengths of these populations (Armour-Burton & Etland, 2020). This feminist intersectional therapy model is a culturally sensitive, nonlinear clinical therapy model for working with BIPOC populations. It prioritizes intersectionality and acknowledges multiple oppressions and their impact on the client's well-being. When working with a BIPOC client—individual, relationship, or family therapy—feminist intersectional theory emphasizes areas such as communal healing, recognizes historical traumas, fosters empowerment through collaborative egalitarian therapeutic relationships, addresses systemic influences, promoting cultural validation and ensures holistic and equitable mental health support.

# Feminist Intersectional Therapy Model for BIPOC Populations

## Step 0.5: Doing Your Ongoing Self-Analysis

Feminist therapists must ensure that they are competent to work with BIPOC clients. They must have knowledge, skills, and self-awareness. Knowledge refers to one's ability to have sufficient information about BIPOC persons. One should be mindful that no one can be fully knowledgeable because the social, cultural, and political landscape are ever-changing. Likewise, keeping current with new environmental events, ecosystem changes, and new oppressive stressors is imperative for the feminist therapist. Skills refers to the ways in which therapy interacts differently with a BIPOC client from a White client (e.g., using the interventions listed here). Self-awareness refers to the requirement that a therapist be engaged in constant introspection. It can be helpful to understand their own intersectional identity, biases, and transferences.

## Step 1: The Feminist Intersectional Therapy Relationship

Feminist intersectional therapists value therapeutic transparency. They acknowledge any obvious differences between the client and themselves and discuss any concerns around those differences. Broaching might help provide feminist therapists with a framework to initiate difficult conversations. Additionally, a goal is not to be seen as an expert in the client's life. This is accomplished by flattening the hierarchy between client and therapist. That might be done with appropriate therapeutic self-disclosure, posturing as a fellow traveler (Yalom, 1980), demystifying the therapeutic process, power monitoring, and relinquishing power by taking a less directive stance.

## Step 2: Feminist Intersectional Exploration

In egalitarian collaboration with the client, feminist therapists examine the many facets of the client's intersectionality. This may go beyond race, sex, socioeconomics, gender, and sexuality to more nuanced areas such as skin tone, abilities, disabilities, geography and neighborhoods, histories of interaction with oppressive systems, education, talents, spiritual beliefs, and so forth. The purpose of this step is assessment. The therapist must garner a clear understanding of who the client is and what has impacted them.

## Step 3: Identity and Cultural Validation

It is important to validate the client's experiences. Psychoeducation around CRT and White supremacy culture aid in an understanding of the origins of the client's current distress. The feminist clinician may want to explore any possible internalized racism (examine self-talk, self-esteem, private beliefs about success, etc.) and possible areas of learned helplessness. The goal of this stage is to empower clients by allowing them to see the contexts of all that they endured.

## Step 4: Empowerment and Realities

In this stage, the feminist therapist helps the client strategize how to become more empowered and navigate the oppressive systems with as much advantage as possible. The feminist therapist and client can use the power analysis to review one person or system at a time to learn strategies for navigating with more power. However, *caution must be noted*: (1) the client needs to understand safety concerns and consequences associated with each empowerment; (2) although the goal is empowerment, not all systems can be navigated successfully. Clients should not internalize failures; in this case, aiming for personal power can be useful. In the case of the BIPOC population, clients may not be able to obtain the same opportunities as their White counterparts. In shifting perspective away from internal locus (e.g., "I couldn't make this happen") to an externalized one (e.g., "the system won't allow for this yet"), clients can maintain personal power in the face of oppressive systems.

## Step 5: Feminist Advocacy and Community Engagement

This is an action stage whereby the feminist therapist models self-empowered advocacy behaviors. Additionally, the client may desire to put their power into action. This can mean personal power (e.g., asserting their voice as desired, rethinking ways of feeling about themselves, changing a dynamic with one person, etc.). It can also mean community power (e.g., serving the community to help others' suffering), advocating for change toward equality, or protesting. Serving the community is known to be curative (Adler, 1956/1964).

## Step 6: Know More, Do More

The client is encouraged to share what they have learned with others, continue to educate themselves on oppressive systems, not internalize social, cultural, and political norms, and find communities that support their empowerment. They should be able to leave therapy with an increased consciousness that is generalizable to the next challenging life event.

# Feminist Intersectional Clinical Applications with the BIPOC Population

Feminist therapists aim to create a safe and affirming space where BIPOC individuals can freely discuss the multiple complexities of their lived experiences, consider the impact of various social structures on their mental health, and find empowerment to navigate oppression in the future better. Helping clients find empowerment to navigate societal expectations, challenge oppressive norms, and build a more authentic self-concept becomes central to the therapeutic journey, fostering personal growth and well-being for BIPOC.

## Feminist Intersectional Broaching

Broaching behavior is a consistent, open attitude where the therapist genuinely commits to inviting the clients to explore culture. It is initiated by the feminist therapist at the onset of the therapeutic relationship and is integrated throughout the relationship. Of note is the premise that White therapists-in-training may find cultural broaching more difficult than Black or Brown therapists-in-training because of their discomfort with talking about race/ethnicity. As they progress, they may become more comfortable addressing issues of race/ethnicity. The cultural broaching model (Day-Vines et al., 2007) may be useful.

## Feminist Ecological Exploration

Therapists can expand on Bronfenbrenner's ecological systems model (Bronfenbrenner, 1979; Guy-Evans, 2024) to explore how social, cultural, and political systems (education, legal, religious, etc.) may impact the client. When using an ecological model as a feminist therapist, you must consider the oppressive/privileged nature of each of those systems and expand on their impact. For example, you might indicate legal involvement for a client but will also need to note how being a member of a BIPOC population has interplayed with their involvement in that legal system.

## Feminist Identity Mapping Exercise (Social Atom Adaptation)

Clients create visual identity maps, incorporating aspects of their race, gender, sexuality, and many other intersecting identities. The client can place the identities as close to them or further away based on how much they embrace that identity. Each identity can be discussed as a continuum of privilege or oppression. Additionally, the clinician can help the client review if they have control over that identity or not. For example, they do not have control over race but might have some control over education. The goal is to aid the client in having a clear picture of their identities and how that has impacted their thoughts, behaviors, and oppressions from society.

## Feminist Intersectional Genogram

The therapist assists the client in identifying social, cultural, and political injuries as well as strengths in each generation. Using the feminist genogram can highlight how various oppressed intersectional identities allow for the passing down (through generations) of messages and experiences that influence a client's current identity.

## Feminist Intersectional Media Analysis

Using bibliotherapy, video therapy, or social media, the client can explore how oppressive social, cultural, and political norms influence us all. A goal is to help the client understand how marginalization and oppression are keeping White supremacy concepts in place and discuss how to navigate and/or protest and/or advocate these oppressive systems. Consciousness raising can be initiated without direct conversation. Additionally, clients may view representations of their intersecting identities. This may allow for the discussion of self-perception, family dynamics, and societal pressures to conform to societal norms that a client might not otherwise be aware of or comfortable speaking about. Taking the notion of bibliotherapy a step further, one might consider the use of a feminist intersectional book/movie club as a means of additional support. The feminist therapist might want to consider establishing an intersectional book/movie club where clients can gather that explores literature/film that delves into diverse perspectives on race, gender, and other intersecting identities. The therapist might discuss insights both in group and during individual therapy sessions. These activities aim to enhance consciousness around intersectionality, fostering a deeper understanding of how various identities intersect and influence individual and familial experiences and to make people feel not so isolated.

## Feminist Intersectional Story Circles

A feminist therapist can create a support space for clients who have analyzed their intersectional identities to share personal stories related to how their identities have limited, suppressed, or promoted their wellness. Additionally, BIPOC people can tell stories of their families and their endurance within the oppressive society. The goal of this activity is to remove isolation and thoughts around internalized oppression while promoting empathy and a supportive connection with others who have this higher consciousness. Ultimately, this can serve the purpose of empowerment.

## Feminist Intersectional Power Analysis

The feminist therapist helps the clients identify and list all people and systems in order to analyze each relationship and identify who has the power. The feminist therapist aids the client in determining who or what has the power through discussions: Are there any oppressive factors in the hierarchies within the relationship that may disempower the client? The therapist and client collaboratively look for patterns of who, what, and where the client can maintain empowerment in relationships and who, what, and where they may give it away. The goal of this activity is for the client to understand how they may maintain or give power away and decide if they would like to change that dynamic.

## Feminist Intersectional Timeline of Critical Incidents of Oppression

The clients construct a timeline chronicling key moments where oppression was experienced. For example, a client might note the first time they were called a slur or when they became aware of being part of a marginalized group (e.g., were diagnosed with an illness, etc.). Collaboratively, the feminist therapist and client can review their timeline and link previous incidents to any current challenges where appropriate. The feminist therapist can normalize reactions to oppression and aid the client in understanding the development of their current positioning.

## Cultural Ritual Participation

The feminist therapist can invite the client to share in cultural rituals and practices associated with the client's intersecting identities, fostering a deeper connection to cultural heritage. When a client is not familiar with rituals of their culture, and expresses an interest, the therapist might encourage investigation into such. A feminist therapist must always remain congruent and should not participate in anything disingenuous to themselves (i.e., the therapist should have a genuine interest in other cultural practices, or they should not engage in them). Proper therapeutic boundaries need to be maintained as well. Examples of cultural rituals might include culturally connected holidays, journeys to ancestral heritage sites, culturally connected acknowledgment ceremonies, healing or prayer circles, energy healing or cleansing, such as smudging, sweat lodge rituals, and reiki, breath work, chanting, and collective prayer.

## Attacking the Stigma

Clients might feel stigmas attached to their oppressed identities (Ford, 2021). This clinical application is a method whereby the feminist therapist collaboratively attempts to uncouple the patriarchal stigma from the client. The client defines their own meaning about what it is to be someone with a stigmatizing identity. There is an immense value in determining one's own meaning. In fact, this is at the crux of existential psychotherapy (Craig et al., 2016). The feminist therapist utilizes this concept to specifically explore what it means to be an oppressed person in society with the intention that the client can ultimately determine their own meaning, rejecting society's determination.

## Acceptance of Fictive Kin

Fictive kin are family members that are not related by blood (Chatters et al., 1994). People refer to fictive kin as "mom," "dad," "brother," "sister," "cousin," and so on. During the 1970s and 1980s, young queer and transgender people of color were kicked out of their homes because of their affectional orientation or gender identity/expression (Mena, 2022). In a similar fashion, it is not uncommon for BIPOC individuals to determine who they view as family. Feminist therapists will purposefully request that clients define their family outside of traditional constructs when relevant.

# Feminist Intersectional Model Example

Jason is a Black 18-year-old male. He explains to a school-based counselor that he has "severe anxiety" (in his words). He tells the counselor that his parents do not believe in therapy and that Jason, himself, is somewhat skeptical but is at a loss for what to do. He goes on to say that one night, while at the dinner table, his parents started discussing their pastor's sermon, repeating some of his anti-gay rhetoric. Jason expresses his hurt to his family and reveals that he is gay. His father calls the pastor and "outs" him. The church is a central part of Jason's community, which is predominantly Black. He lives in a redlined area of town where very few people ever "make it out." Everyone knows everyone, and soon Jason is ordered to the front of the church, where they pray over him in an attempt to "remove the demon." Jason is later reminded by his father that being a Black man in today's society is "difficult enough" and for that reason he "cannot also be gay." Since this incident Jason's anxiety has significantly increased.

*Step 0.5:* The feminist therapist challenges their own biases around race/ethnicity, affectional orientation, and religion/spirituality. Additionally, they conduct their own intersectional power analysis. The therapist is assured that they possess no bias that would interfere in working with this client.

*Step 1:* The feminist therapist engages in ongoing power monitoring and broaches the subjects of race/ethnicity, affectional orientation, and religion/spirituality differences in the relationship. The therapist may say, "Jason, as we build our relationship, I notice that we have some cultural differences regarding race/ethnicity, age, sex/gender, and affectional orientation and those differences could impact our relationship. How are you sitting with me as your therapist?"

*Step 2:* The therapist uses an ecological model to assess the people and systems in Jason's life and where he has experienced privilege and oppression. The therapist utilizes a timeline to determine any critical incidents or traumas of a social, cultural, or political nature to garner an understanding of their interaction with his current intersectional identity. Together they conclude that Jason's multiple oppressions are related to his socioeconomic status, the educational system he attends that does not provide enough opportunity, the neighborhood that he lives in, his pastor and church and its mainstream Christian beliefs, his mother and father, his Blackness, and his gayness.

*Step 3:* Using psychoeducation, including bibliotherapy, the therapist addresses how systems and structures based in racism/White supremacy, patriarchy, and heteronormativity have impacted Jason. The therapist begins the process of consciousness raising and validates Jason's experiences. For example, the therapist begins to understand that Jason's anxiety is a culmination of many incidents of bias beginning at a very young age. Jason has internalized the idea that "Black folk" never leave his community. This has been reinforced by messages from his family, the educational system, the media that he watches, and more. Being a gay male confounds his feeling that he "isn't good enough" and his church appears to have confirmed that. Jason's anxiety is not the result of something within him but instead a result of something outside of him; an oppressive society that has told him his whole life that he does not belong and that he is not good enough.

*Step 4:* The therapist helps Jason to identify those structures that are supportive and oppressive in his life. The therapist suggests Clay Cane's 2015 documentary "Holler if You Hear Me: Black and Gay in The Church" for Jason to watch, with the intention that it will assist Jason, first, in seeing his intersectional identity represented in an empowered way; and then, second, assist him in gaining a sense of personal power.

*Step 5:* The therapist may attack the stigma. The goal is for Jason to restructure his beliefs about being a Black gay male and replace negative messages with positive or neutral ones. Even though Jason wishes to continue active engagement in Christianity, he may grow to see the illegitimacy of the messenger (his pastor). He can put the fault in his pastor's interpretation of religious messages while allowing for his own interpretation of his religion/spirituality. In other words, Jason can define his own meaning. He also sheds the internalized feelings that he is not good enough, which have developed because of the many ways that society sees Black men. He comes to see those messages as illegitimate.

*Step 6:* Jason and his therapist collaborate on ways for him to share what he has learned from his therapeutic process. He creates a prayer circle that includes other marginalized persons. Jason views this as a curative experience. Advocacy for others becomes a central part of his life and his severe anxiety does not return.

# Feminist Intersectional Strengths, Criticisms, and Cautions

Feminist intersectional theory (FIT) addresses the social, cultural, and political constructs as primary to the therapy instead of other theories that may focus on assimilating clients to broken systems (Warner & Shields, 2018). FIT can offer a context and voice to those in society who have been marginalized and overlooked.

One potential criticism of this theory is that therapists may impose feminist agendas, without alignment from the client, and this can undermine the therapeutic relationship. Another critique is the potential overemphasis on environmental factors in the theory, which may neglect the role of biological influences on social development. The theory's strength lies in its ability to see the whole person in their entirety with all their intersectional identities. FIT does not ignore biology or other factors; what it does is introduce commonly ignored factors into a therapeutic setting. For the BIPOC population, relief can be garnered when they are not only fully seen by their therapist but also when they can fully see themselves as a product of their environment, an environment that has historically served to disempower and oppress them.

Lastly, feminist therapists need to be aware of "anti-woke" legislation (Florida's 2022 Stop WOKE Act HB 7/SB 148; West Virginia's 2024 Anti-Woke Act SB 870). It is illegal in some places (e.g., some schools) to espouse that "individuals are inherently racist, sexist, or oppressive, whether consciously or unconsciously" (Reilly, 2022, p. 1). Conversely, this awareness and consciousness raising is essential to the therapeutic process when working with the BIPOC population. Feminist therapists may find it challenging to work within the law's oppressive parameters while honoring the theory's spirit. They may be confronted by the law and will need to take care to protect the client from any potential assault from the legal system. This may be an area where consultation and advocacy are called for.

# What If?

What if everyone recognized that people are influenced by their environments including Eurocentric White supremacy culture?

What if people were immune to the messages of society?

What if things had gone differently historically (e.g., Indigenous people ruled, Whites were enslaved, etc.)?

What if religious figures were (correctly) depicted as persons of color throughout the West?

What if critical race theory was largely embraced by all as true?

What if there was an equalized playing field for persons of color? How would it happen? Who would resist? What would change?

What if all lives mattered equally, and there was no need to assert that Black lives matter?

What if society eventually all became the same color?

# References

Abrams, J. A., Hill, A., & Maxwell, M. (2019). Underneath the mask: Racially traumatic experiences and mental health issues among African American women in therapy. *Journal of Counseling Psychology, 66*(5), 576–589. https://doi.org/10.1037/cou0000342

Adler, A. (1964). *The individual psychology of Alfred Adler*. Harper Perennial. (Original work published 1956)

American Civil Liberties Union (2023). Why access to education is key to systemic equality. *American Civil Liberties Union*. https://www.aclu.org/news/racial-justice/why-access-to-education-is-key-to-systemic-equality

American Psychological Association. 2017. *Multicultural guidelines: An ecological approach to context, identity, and intersectionality*. http://www.apa.org/about/policy/multicultural-guidelines.pdf

Armour-Burton, T., & Etland, C. (2020). Black feminist thought: A paradigm to examine breast cancer disparities. *Nursing Research, 69*(4), 272–279. https://doi.org/10.1097/nnr.0000000000000426

Bell, Derrick A. (1992). *Faces at the bottom of the well: The permanence of racism*. Basic Books.

Bronfenbrenner, U. (1979). *The ecology of human development: Experiments by nature and design*. Harvard University Press.

Brown, L. (2018). *Feminist therapy* (2nd ed.). American Psychological Association.

Cane, C. (2015). *Holler if you hear me: Black and gay in the church* [Documentary]. BET.com.

Chatters, L. M., Taylor, R. J., & Jayakody, R. (1994). Fictive kinship relations in black extended families. *Journal of Comparative Family Studies, 25*(3), 297–312.

Cohen, J., Howard, M., & Nussbaum, M. C. (1999). *Is multiculturalism bad for women?* Princeton University Press.

Collins P. H. (2000). *Black feminist thought: Knowledge, consciousness, and the politics of empowerment*. Routledge. (Original work published 1990)

Collins, P. H., & Bilge, S. (2016). *Intersectionality*. Polity Press.

Craig, M., Vos, J., Cooper, M., & Correia, E. A. (2016). Existential psychotherapies. In D. J. Cain, K. Keenan, & S. Rubin (Eds.), *Humanistic psychotherapies: Handbook of research and practice* (2nd ed., pp. 283–317). American Psychological Association.

Crenshaw, K. W. (1988). Race, reform, and retrenchment: Transformation and legitimation in antidiscrimination law. *Harvard Law Review, 101*(7), 1331–1387.

Crenshaw, K. (1989). Demarginalizing the intersection of race and sex: A Black feminist critique of antidiscrimination doctrine, feminist theory, and antiracist politics. In K. Bartlett (Ed.), *Feminist legal theory* (pp. 57–80). Routledge.

Crenshaw, K., Gotanda, N., Peller, G., & Kendell, T. (1995). *Critical race theory: The key writings that formed the movement*. The New Press.

Davis, K. (2008). Intersectionality as buzzword: A sociology of science perspective on what makes a feminist theory successful. *Feminist Theory, 9*(1), 67–85. https://doi.org/10.1177/1464700108086364

Day-Vines, N. L., Wood, S. M., Grothaus, T., Craigen, L., Holman, A., Dotson-Blake, K. D., & Douglass, M. J. (2007). Broaching the subjects of race, ethnicity, and culture during the counseling process. *Journal of Counseling and Development, 85*(4), 401–409.

Delgado, R., & Stefancic, J. (2012). *Critical race theory: An introduction*. New York University Press.

De los Santos, H., Jiang, K., Bernardi, J., & Okechukwu, C. (2021). *From redlining to gentrification: The policy of the past that affects health outcomes today*. https://info.primarycare.hms.harvard.edu/perspectives/articles/redlining-gentrification-health-outcomes

Enns, C. Z., & Williams, E. N. (Eds.). (2013). *The Oxford handbook of feminist multicultural counseling psychology*. Oxford University Press.

Fair Fight Initiative (n.d.). *Critical race theory: What is critical race theory?* https://www.fairfightinitiative.org/critical-race-theory/?gad_source=1&gclid=CjwKCAjwxNW2BhAkEiwA24Cm9GLxdu3pkURgbBLjZBor2YD5kc0rPj5h660I2VkolNx9nUVS_OsnhBoCoXAQAvD_BwE

Faster Capital (2024). *Gentrification: Redlining's influence on gentrification: A closer look*. https://fastercapital.com/content/Gentrification--Redlining-s-Influence-on-Gentrification--A-Closer-Look.html

Ferdman, B. M., & Gallegos, P. I. (2001). Latinos and racial identity development. In C. L. Wijeyesinghe & B. W. Jackson III (Eds.), *New perspectives on racial identity development: A theoretical and practical anthology* (pp. 32–66). NYU Press.

Ford, D. J. (2021). The salve and the sting of religion/spirituality in queer and transgender BIPOC. In K. L. Nadal & M. R. Scharron-del Rio (Eds.), *Queer psychology: Intersectional perspectives* (pp. 275–290). Springer.

Grady, C. (2018). "The waves of feminism, and why people keep fighting over them, explained." Vox, July 20, 2018, Vox Media, LLC., Washington, DC.

Grishow-Schade, L. (2024) Preventing white supremacy: An applied conceptualization for the helping professions. *Discover Global Society, 2*, 52. https://doi.org/10.1007/s44282-024-00084-2

Guy-Evans, O. (2024). Bronfenbrenner's ecological systems theory. *SimplyPsychology*. https://www.simplypsychology.org/bronfenbrenner.html

Hardy, K. V. (2023). *Racial trauma: Clinical strategies and techniques for healing invisible wounds*. W. W. Norton.

Helms, J. E. (1995). An update of Helm's white and people of color racial identity models. In J. G. Ponterotto, J. M. Cassas, L. A. Suzuki, & C. M. Alexander (Eds.), *Handbook of multicultural counseling* (pp. 181–198). SAGE Publications.

hooks, B. (1984). *Feminist theory: From margin to center*. South End Press.

hooks, B. (2015). *Feminism is for everybody: Passionate politics*. South End Press. (Original work published 2000)

Horne, S. G. & Arora, K. S. (2013). Feminist multicultural counseling psychology in transnational contexts. In C. Enns & E. N. Williams (Eds.), *Oxford handbook of feminist multicultural counseling psychology* (pp. 240–254). Oxford University Press.

Hoyart, D. L. (2023). *Maternal mortality rates in the United States, 2021*. https://www.cdc.gov/nchs/data/hestat/maternal-mortality/2021/maternal-mortality-rates-2021.htm#:~:text=In%202021%2C%20the%20maternal%20mortality,(Figure%201%20and%20Table)

Huertas, R. (2020). *Minority patients benefit from having minority doctors, but that's a hard match to make*. https://www.michiganmedicine.org/health-lab/minority-patients-benefit-having-minority-doctors-thats-hard-match-make

Jackson S., Bailey M., & Welles B. (2021). *#HashtagActivism: Networks of race and gender justice*. MIT Press.

Jones, T., & Okun, T. (n.d.). What is white supremacy culture? *Simply*. https://www.whitesupremacyculture.info/what-is-it.html

Jones, C. T., & Welfare, L. E. (2017). Broaching behaviors of licensed professional counselors: A qualitative inquiry. *Journal of Addictions & Offender Counseling, 38*, 48–64. https://doi.org/10.1002/jaoc.12028

Jonsson T. (2014). White feminist stories: Locating race in representations of feminism in *The Guardian. Feminist Media Studies, 14*(6), 1012–1027.

Kendi, I. X. (2019). *How to be an antiracist*. Bodley Head.

Kim, J. (1981). Processes of Asian American identity development: A study of Japanese American women's perceptions of their struggle to achieve positive identities as Americans of Asian ancestry. *Dissertation Abstracts International, 42*(3), 1058B.

Konish, L. (2022). *Mortgage denial rate for Black borrowers is twice that of overall population, report finds*. CNBC. https://www.cnbc.com/2022/08/27/black-borrowers-mortgage-denial-rate-twice-that-of-overall-population.html

Kukathas, C. (2001). Is feminism bad for multiculturalism? *Public Affairs Quarterly 15*(2), 83–98.

Malott, K. M., Paone, T. R., Schaefle, S., Cates, J., & Haizlip, B. (2015). Expanding white racial identity theory: A qualitative investigation of whites engaged in antiracist action. *Journal of Counseling & Development, 93*(3), 333–343. https://doi.org/10.1002/jcad.12031

McDowell, S. (2022). *Breast cancer death rates are highest for black women—again*. https://www. cancer.org/research/acs-research-news/breast-cancer-death-rates-are-highest-for-black-women-again.html#:~:text=Breast%20cancer%20is%20the%20second,in%20Black%20and%20 Hispanic%20women

Mena, A. J. (2022) Special issue on BIPOC and LGBTQ feminist radical visionaries: Special issue dedicated to the memory of Jean Lau Chin. *Women & Therapy, 45*(4), 269–273.

Nash J. C. (2019) *Black feminism reimagined: After intersectionality*. Duke University Press.

National Association of Social Workers. (2015). *Standards and indicators for cultural competence in social work practice*. NASW Press.

New England Journal of Medicine. (2020). Taking black pain seriously [A 2016 study details the differences in pain perception between men and women]. *New England Journal of Medicine*. https://www.nejm.org/doi/full/10.1056/NEJMpv2024759#:~:text=A%202016%20study%20 details%20the,endings%2C%20and%20hence%20less%20sensitive

New York Civil Liberties Union. (2007). *The student safety act*. https://www.nyclu.org/migrated-page/ student-safety-act

Okin, S. M. (2005). Multiculturalism and feminism: No simple questions, no simple answers. In A. Eisenberg & J. Spinner-Halev (Eds.), *Minorities within minorities: Equality, rights and diversity* (pp. 67–89). Cambridge University Press.

Poston, W. C. (1990). The Biracial Identity Development Model: A needed addition. *Journal of Counseling & Development, 69*(2), 152–155. https://doi.org/10.1002/j.1556-6676.1990. tb01477.x

Ratts, M. J., Singh, A. A., Nassar-McMillan, S., Butler, S. K., & McCullough, J. R. (2016). Multicultural and social justice counseling competencies: Guidelines for the counseling profession. *Journal of Multicultural Counseling and Development, 44*(1), 28–48. https://doi. org/10.1002/jmcd.12035

Reilly, K. (2022). Florida's governor just signed the "Stop Woke Act": Here's what it means for schools and businesses. *TIME*. https://time.com/6168753/florida-stop-woke-law

Schoenthaler, A., & Williams, N. (2022). Looking beneath the surface: Racial bias in the treatment and management of pain. *JAMA Network Open, 5*(6), 1–3.

Shand-Lubbers, R. M., & Baden, A. L. (2023). Becoming a white antiracist counselor: A framework of identity development. *Counselor Education and Supervision, 62*(3), 276–294. https://doi. org/10.1002/ceas.12272

Song, S. (2007). *Justice, gender, and the politics of multiculturalism: Part I*. Cambridge University Press.

Spelman, E. V. (1988). *Inessential woman: Problems of exclusion in feminist thought*. Beacon Press.

Springer, K. (2002). Third wave Black feminism? *Signs: Journal of Women in Culture and Society, 27*(4), 1059–1082.

United Negro College Fund. (n.d.). *Education inequality: K–12 disparity facts*. https://uncf.org/pages/ k-12-disparity-facts-and-stats

USAFacts. (2023). *How many Black male teachers are there in the US?* https://usafacts.org/articles/ how-many-black-male-teachers-are-there-in-the-us/

United States Sentencing Commission. (2023). *2023 guidelines manual annotated*. https://www.ussc. gov/guidelines/2023-guidelines-manual-annotated

Vandiver, B. J., Cross, W. E., Jr., Fhagen-Smith, P. E., Worrell, F. C., Swim, J., & Caldwell, L. (2000). *Cross Racial Identity Scale (CRIS)* [Database record]. PsycTESTS. https://doi.org/10.1037/ t01825-000

Ward, E. C., & Brown, R. L. (2015). A culturally adapted depression intervention for African American adults experiencing depression: Oh happy day. *American Journal of Orthopsychiatry, 85*(1), 11–22. https://doi.org/10.1037/ort0000027

Warner, L. R., & Shields, S. A. (2018). Intersectionality as a framework for theory and research in feminist psychology. In N. K. Dess, J. Marecek, & L. C. Bell (Eds.), *Gender, sex, and sexualities: Psychological perspectives* (pp. 29–52). Oxford University Press.

Watts, S., & Stenner, P. (2005). Doing Q methodology: Theory, method, and interpretation. *Qualitative Research in Psychology*, 2(1), 67–91. https://doi.org/10.1191/1478088705qp022oa

Weinbaum, A. E. (2001). Book review: *Is multiculturalism bad for women?* Susan Moller Okin with respondents. *Signs*, 27(1), 294–299.

Williams, T. M. (2010). *Black students perceptions of their access to precollege counseling practices* (Publication No. 40) [Doctoral dissertation, St. John Fisher University]. Fisher Digital Publications.

Yalom, I. D. (1980). *Existential psychotherapy*. Basic Books.

Zakaria R. (2021). *Against white feminism: Notes on disruption*. W. W. Norton.

# 15

# Feminist Intersectional Therapy: Nondominant Gender and Affectional Identities

## Chase Morgan-Swaney, David Julius Ford Jr., Liz Curtis, and Amy Nourie

*The Eurocentric, Christian-dominant, heteronormative, patriarchal norms of society marginalize and oppress people's intersectional affectional orientations, causing great suffering that needs to be honored in therapy.*

## Feminist Perspectives with Nondominant Gender and Affectional Identities

Feminist theory is a crucial framework for mental health professionals navigating the contemporary expanded consciousness. Fourth-wave feminist theory provides a unique multisystemic lens through which to examine and raise consciousness of the lived intersectional experiences of diverse clients in their healing processes. Central to contemporary feminist theory is the concept of intersectionality, a term coined by Kimberlé Crenshaw (1989). It emphasizes the interconnected nature of social categories such as gender identity and expression, affectional identity (otherwise referred to as sexual orientation), race, and disability, recognizing that these intersecting identities create unique and complex experiences of power and oppression. Working with lesbian, gay, bisexual, transgender, gender-expansive, queer, intersex, asexual, pansexual, and polysexual (LGBTGEQIAP+) identities, a feminist lens necessitates a nuanced understanding of how these identities intersect and influence mental health, wellness, and the broader human experience.

When clinically applied to LGBTGEQIAP+ identities, feminist intersectional theoretical perspectives can play a pivotal role in acknowledging and deconstructing the impact that systems of oppression have on an individual's personal growth, self-efficacy, and overall mental health. For the purposes of this chapter, we will hereby refer to LGBTGEQIAP+ identities as nondominant gender and affectional identities.

## The Sociopolitical and Historical Case for Feminist Intersectional Theory with Nondominant Gender and Affectional Identities

The United States has a long history of laws discriminating against and punishing nondominant gender and affectional identities. Although many Indigenous populations respected and embraced *two-spirit* individuals, a contemporary umbrella term often used to denote gender variance beyond the traditional binary, colonizers forced the suppression of these identities (Balsam et al., 2004). In the American colonies, nondominant affectional relationships were usually not mentioned. Instead, there were laws against sodomy or "lewd behavior," which were considered abhorrent sexual offenses along with rape and incest (Woods, 2017). Illinois became the first state to decriminalize sexual behavior among same-gender sexual partners in 1962, with most other states following suit by the 1980s. However, it was not until 2003 that these laws were deemed unconstitutional by the U.S. Supreme Court in *Lawrence v. Texas*, overturning legislation in the remaining 14 states (Leslie, 2000). Despite the invalidation of sodomy laws and the inability to enforce these rules, 12 states still have legislation criminalizing consensual, non-procreative sexual intercourse (Peterson, 2021). While these laws were usually not enforced, in the mental health professions, homosexuality was still pathologized in one form or another (e.g., sociopathic personality disturbance, sexual deviation, etc.) in the *Diagnostic and Statistical Manual of Mental Disorders* (DSM) until 2013 (Drescher, 2015).

Despite high levels of public support for the rights of nondominant gender and affectional identities in the United States, states continue to propose and pass discriminatory and dangerous laws that ban access to gender-affirming care for minors and use of gender identity–congruent bathrooms, subject young athletes participating in sports to forced genital examinations, ban access to affirming literature in school and public libraries, and subject students to forced outing of their nondominant gender and affectional identities by school officials to their parents or legal guardians. According to the Human Rights Campaign (HRC), 2023 was a record-breaking year for discriminatory legislation, including over 500 bills proposed in state legislatures, with more than 70 passed into law (Peele, 2023).

## Navigating the Intersection of Feminist Intersectional Theory, Queer Theory, and Nondominant Gender and Affectional Identities

In 1980, author and poet Adrienne Rich suggested that compulsory heterosexuality was a systemic issue even within feminist theory and scholarship. In fact, when addressing several influential and educational feminist books of the time, Rich noted that none of these texts acknowledged "the institution of heterosexuality itself as a beachhead of male dominance" (Rich, 1980, p. 633). Rich's compulsory heterosexuality may have served as an introduction to heteronormativity, a concept universalized by Warner in 1991, which includes an assumption of the gender binary, and that the prescriptive heterosexual identity equates to marriage between two people of the opposite sex and reproduction. Many individuals could be highlighted for bringing queer theory closer to the mainstream, including Michel Foucault (*The History of Sexuality*), Eve Kosofsky Sedwick (*Epistemology of the Closet*), and Judith Butler (*Gender Trouble*). The history of queer theory would not be complete, however, without mentioning queer theorists of color, including Audre Lorde, Gloria Anzaldúa, and Cathy Cohen. While these are only a few of the many influential queer theorists, mental health professionals need to understand the deep connection between queer and feminist intersectional theories, especially when working with and advocating for nondominant gender and affectional clients.

## Addressing Systemic Oppression in Mental Health

Feminist intersectional theory encourages a critical examination of the Eurocentric patriarchal, heteronormative, Christian-dominant systemic structures that oppress nondominant gender and affectional clients. This historical systemic legacy of oppression is ever present, and it continues to impact norms, conceptualizations, and implicit and explicit biases within the mental health professions. Examining how systemic oppression has influenced mental health theories, modalities, and approaches involves exploring the impact of discriminatory policies, social attitudes, and institutionalized barriers related to seeking, accessing, and receiving safe, quality, and affirming mental health care (Morgan-Swaney, 2023). For example, "conversion therapy" (i.e., nondominant gender and affectional identity change efforts) continues to be permitted in the majority of U.S. states despite prohibitions by the leading mental health professional associations and well-documented instances of harm resulting from its use (Ausloos et al., 2024). In feminist therapy, clinicians collaborate with clients to develop strategies for navigating these systemic challenges, fostering resilience, and, as appropriate, advocating for social change throughout the clinical process.

Fourth-wave feminist clinicians also actively engage in intersectional advocacy for equity, recognizing that the fight for nondominant gender and affectional liberation intersects with broader social justice issues related to other diverse identities, backgrounds, and human experiences. This involves actively challenging discriminatory practices, promoting justice, equity, inclusion, and belonging, and advocating for policies that address the specific needs of nondominant gender and affectional populations. Through a feminist intersectional lens, clinicians are accomplices in deconstructing the broader systems of oppression that create and exacerbate mental health disparities (Cor & Chan, 2017).

## De-norming Heteronormativity and Cisnormativity

Feminist intersectional therapy challenges heteronormativity and cisnormativity, which presume that all individuals are heterosexual and cisgender and that heterosexual and cisgender identities are the preferred or correct way of being (Hudson, 2019; Oswald et al., 2009). For nondominant gender and affectional clients, existing within these patriarchal frameworks of erasure can lead to disempowering feelings and experiences of invisibility, marginalization, internalized stigma, and overt prejudice and hostility, known as homomisia and transmisia (Simmons University, 2019). Feminist clinicians strive to create a safe and affirming space that empowers clients and normalizes, equitizes, and legitimizes nondominant gender and affectional identities, behaviors, and forms of expression (Ginicola et al., 2017). The feminist clinician's goal is to help the client to be resilient in response to living in heteronormative and cisnormative systems. In some cases, the clinician can use social justice advocacy as an intentionally applied therapeutic technique that can move toward dismantling these oppressive and damaging systems if the client is so inclined.

Feminist intersectional therapy also strongly emphasizes empowering clients to name and claim their intersectional lived narratives and experiences. Working with nondominant gender and affectional clients means examining the unique strengths and marginalized oppressive challenges to move them toward personal empowerment. Clinicians employing feminist intersectional theory actively listen for power and oppression themes, validate marginalization experiences, amplify voices that feel like imposters, and empower people to assert themselves toward their truths, internally and externally. Feminist clinicians recognize the importance of client-led power sharing in exploring the influence of oppressive societal forces on their mental health and wellness (Brown, 2018; Evans et al., 2011).

# Therapeutic Relationship with Nondominant Gender and Affectional Clients

Traditional therapeutic relationships typically consist of a hierarchy-enhanced power dynamic in which clinicians organically possess greater power than clients due to their expertise. From a feminist perspective, this is problematic because clinicians in a hierarchy-enhanced power dynamic may be operating as experts regarding clients' concerns without giving necessary weight and deference to clients' lived expertise (i.e., centering their identities and experiences). Additionally, it is difficult to empower clients within the therapeutic relationship when the clinician holds the majority of the actual or perceived power. As a result, these clinicians may unwittingly serve as agents of oppression when serving nondominant gender and affectional clients, making cis- and heteronormative assumptions or encouraging adaptation to disaffirming environments. A feminist therapeutic relationship requires hierarchy-attenuated power dynamics rooted in mutuality and equity, where power is shared, and the client is the expert (i.e., egalitarian relationships). Relationships informed by the tenets of feminist intersectional theory aim to avoid replicating the power imbalances that nondominant gender and affectional populations experience in society (Evans et al., 2011).

For nondominant gender and affectional clients, the therapeutic relationship may be one of the few places where they feel fully seen and heard. Therefore, establishing trust and safety through transparency is paramount. Clinicians should demonstrate cultural humility, which involves a flexible understanding of nondominant gender and affectional identities, including affirming and up-to-date language and terminology. Clinicians should continuously learn to stay informed about these identities' evolving language and forms of expression. Additionally, feminist clinicians challenge binary thinking, such as the rigid categorizations of gender and affectional identities. As such, feminist clinicians should create a physical, intellectual, and emotional space where nonbinary, gender-expansive, and queer identities are honored and celebrated instead of erased and condemned. Similarly, nondominant gender and affectional clients have natural desires, wants, needs, and dreams that are often othered or pathologized. Feminist clinicians should actively normalize, equitize, and legitimize these experiences, acknowledging the adverse impact of centering cisgenderism and heterosexuality in society (Ginicola et al., 2017).

Additionally, the feminist clinician creates an environment that facilitates openness and trust in the therapeutic relationship (i.e., brave spaces). Unlike safe spaces that can uphold dominant traits and oppressive forces (e.g., whiteness and cis/heteronormativity) where someone can (and does) retreat when they feel uncomfortable or challenged, *brave* spaces (Arao & Clemens, 2013) require the courage to be authentic, the courage to sit with discomfort, and the courage to grow and be challenged. Not everyone has the privilege to retreat. Brave spaces allow for courageous conversations, and the clinician shoulders the responsibility for creating those spaces. Brave spaces enable clients to discuss difficult experiences and diagnoses with their clinicians without being judged or blamed. For example, when clients have been diagnosed with human immunodeficiency virus (HIV), they may be afraid to tell anyone, especially their clinician, due to societal stigma and shame surrounding the condition. Because the risk of contracting HIV is disproportionately higher among certain multiply marginalized nondominant gender and affectional populations, it is of particular importance that feminist clinicians establish brave spaces to broach HIV status with young Black men with nondominant affectional identities and Black transgender women, among others (Quinn et al., 2023).

# Feminist Therapeutic Relationship Praxis: Multicultural and Social Justice Frame

Each mental health discipline embraces diversity, multicultural competencies, and social justice. One example is the *Multicultural and Social Justice Counseling Competencies* (MSJCC; Ratts et al., 2016), which provides a framework that feminist clinicians can use to establish brave spaces and help address nondominant gender and affectional clients' experiences with their diagnoses. First, the feminist clinician assesses their own positionality and that of the client based on their levels of marginalization and privilege. By virtue of the client's intersectional identity as a nondominant gender and affectional person living in a cishet-dominant society, they face marginalization via anti-queer or anti-trans prejudice, discrimination, and oppression. The clinician recognizes that the client possesses that marginalized identity, recognizes what privileged and marginalized identities each have, and gives the clinician the tools to build an egalitarian relationship.

Next, the MSJCC prompts the clinician to assess their level of self-awareness regarding their intersectional cultural identities, their prejudices and biases, and their degree of cultural knowledge. Feminist clinicians must be open to exploring their own affectional and gender identities and any shame attached to them. Clinicians, too, must address any lack of knowledge they possess concerning nondominant gender and affectional identities. Actions the feminist clinician can take may include immersing themselves in nondominant gender and affectional communities, volunteering with organizations like the Trevor Project, obtaining professional development sponsored by the American Counseling Association's (ACA) Society for Sexual, Affectional, Intersex, and Gender Expansive Identities (SAIGE), the National Association of Social Workers (NASW) National Committee on Lesbian, Gay, Bisexual, Transgender, and Queer+ Issues (NCLGBTQ+), and the American Psychological Association's (APA) Society for the Psychology of Sexual Orientation and Gender Diversity (SPSOGD), and learning contemporary terminology in use by and for nondominant gender and affectional populations. Lastly, because some nondominant gender and affectional populations have an elevated risk of contracting HIV, feminist clinicians should also learn about HIV, including homomisic misinformation and myths surrounding the condition, how HIV can affect client health, how it is transmitted, and how it is safely and effectively prevented and managed.

The feminist clinician must be attuned to and validate the client's lived experiences and worldview. Nondominant gender and affectional clients experience discrimination across their ecological systems and often experience microaggressions from unknowing mental health professionals or, worse, mental health professionals consciously engaging in harmful "conversion therapy" practices. Nondominant gender and affectional clients are also subject to destructive and oppressive "anti-woke" laws and policies directed toward their human existence and their communities (e.g., "don't say gay" legislation and other religious or conscience exemptions permitting clinicians to opt out of serving nondominant gender and affectional clients). The feminist clinician must consider these oppressive underpinnings to lived experiences and how they may impact the client, even if the presenting concern does not concern their affectional or gender identity.

Due to multiple oppressions that influence the client's worldview, many people may not trust clinicians. As such, the feminist clinician must build trust with the client through transparency and collaboration. Cultural broaching (Day-Vines et al., 2007) prompts the clinician to initiate courageous conversations around race, ethnicity, HIV status, nondominant gender and affectional identities, and other aspects of cultural identity at the beginning and throughout the egalitarian therapeutic relationship. Cultural broaching requires appropriate therapeutic self-disclosure and cultural humility on the part of the feminist clinician, which often helps build trust and levy the power differential inherent in the therapeutic relationship. The feminist clinician acknowledges that they do not have the same intersectional experiences as the client but hopes to understand their lived experience and worldview.

Using therapeutic competencies, such as the MSJCC, as a framework, feminist clinicians advocate for and with nondominant gender and affectional clients at the intrapersonal, interpersonal, institutional, community, public policy, and international levels. At the institutional and community levels, feminist clinicians could help to ensure that there are social supports and spaces for community building for nondominant gender and affectional clients (e.g., community centers, affinity spaces, specialized clinics), as well as to make sure that those in the community are aware of such resources. At the public policy level, feminist clinicians can advocate for the repeal of laws that criminalize, marginalize, oppress, and discriminate against nondominant gender and affectional identities (e.g., ban conversion therapy in all states for minors and adults, repeal laws that criminalize HIV diagnosis or mandate HIV status disclosure in all instances). At the international level, feminist clinicians may be involved in global efforts to stop the murder and genocide of nondominant gender and affectional populations and provide destigmatizing education about nondominant gender and affectional identities.

# A Feminist Intersectional Model with Nondominant Gender and Affectional Clients

Feminist intersectional therapy provides a comprehensive framework for working collaboratively with nondominant gender and affectional clients. It emphasizes the importance of intersectionality, challenges oppressive presuppositions, amplifies and centers nondominant voices, and advocates for change at various levels. By incorporating feminist intersectional theoretical perspectives into a therapeutic model, clinicians can establish affirming, empowering, and liberating therapeutic spaces for nondominant gender and affectional clients. Each of the four intentions of the following proposed model has a corresponding aim and common features.

## Primary Intention: Establish a Healing Relationship with Transparency and Affirmation

The corresponding aim of the primary intention is to create an informed, affirming, and brave space. A common feature of this intention is to be aware of and generally knowledgeable about nondominant gender and affectional identities and related sociocultural experiences (e.g., homomisic and transmisic microaggressions, chosen families, etc.), with a particular emphasis on disaffirming and harmful experiences in the healthcare system (e.g., nondominant gender and affectional identity change efforts). Another common feature is ensuring that environmental aspects reflect the belonging of nondominant gender and affectional identities and experiences in the therapeutic space (e.g., inclusive intake documentation, representative office decor, etc.). Lastly, feminist clinicians build rapport through actively listening to understand nondominant gender and affectional clients' lived experiences embedded in their distinct sociocultural contexts, naming both sources of strength and challenge.

## Secondary Intention: Explore Intersectional Identities and Raise Critical Consciousness

The corresponding aim of the secondary intention is to facilitate self-discovery and externalize nondominant gender and affectional clients' concerns by connecting them to identity-based systems of oppression in society. A common feature of this intention is to invite nondominant gender and affectional clients to stand in their additional identities (e.g., age, ability, race, ethnicity, class, religion, etc.) and share their lived experiences therein. Another common feature is collaboratively identifying and exploring cultural sources of resilience and oppression at the various intersections of nondominant gender and affectional clients' unique privileged and minoritized identities. Lastly, feminist clinicians raise nondominant gender and affectional clients' critical consciousness by connecting their concerns to their experience of identity-based systemic oppression (e.g., cisheteronormativity, homo- and transmisia, etc.) to reduce internalized prejudice and self-blame.

## Tertiary Intention: Collaboratively Address Concerns with Empowerment and Advocacy

The corresponding aim of the tertiary intention is to foster identity empowerment and engage various forms of multi-level advocacy, as determined and led by nondominant gender and affectional clients. A common feature of this intention is to collaborate with nondominant gender and affectional clients to identify and pursue desired means of facilitating identity empowerment in and out of the therapeutic space (e.g., engaging queer media content in therapy, connecting with other nondominant gender and affectional individuals in the community, etc.), accounting for clients' degree of safety and outness in their life spaces. Another common feature is to collaborate with nondominant gender and affectional clients to identify and pursue desired means of advocating for themselves or their communities to address their unique concerns, developing any necessary skill sets and increasing clients' advocacy self-efficacy.

## Quaternary Intention: Close the Relationship with Reflection and a Spirit of Celebration

The corresponding aim of the quaternary intention is to collaboratively review and celebrate nondominant gender and affectional clients' journeys, acknowledging their growth and reinforcing their strengths. A common feature of this intention is to collaboratively review the clients' journey toward addressing their concerns, highlighting the areas where they grew (e.g., identity empowerment, self-advocacy, social activism, etc.). Another common feature is to reinforce and celebrate clients' various sources of strength and resilience at the intrapersonal (e.g., identity pride), interpersonal (e.g., chosen families), and suprapersonal levels (e.g., community activism). Finally, feminist clinicians engage in intentional self-disclosure about their experience working alongside their nondominant gender and affectional clients and how the process has moved them, expressing gratitude for clients' willingness to allow us to join them on their healing journey.

This is one possible conceptualization of a feminist intersectional model that may serve as a general guide to working alongside nondominant gender and affectional clients, and the intentions do not necessarily follow a linear progression in practice. Feminist clinicians and nondominant gender and affectional clients may revisit or cycle through intentions as needed. It is essential to tailor the therapeutic process to everyone's unique experiences and remain cognizant that honoring the relationship is the underpinning of the entire process. Additionally, ongoing power monitoring, self-reflection, and education for the clinician are crucial to providing culturally humble and affirming support in feminist therapy (Brown, 2018; Evans et al., 2011).

# Feminist Intersectional Applications with Nondominant Gender and Affectional Clients

When working with nondominant gender and affectional clients, the methods utilized should maintain an intersectional core and consistently seek to empower them. Collaborative, client-led therapeutic goals might include gaining intrapersonal insight, fostering social connection, encouraging assertiveness and self-advocacy, increasing boundary-setting skills, reclaiming power, and offering various avenues for social justice advocacy work. It is imperative that maintaining a transparent, egalitarian therapeutic relationship remains at the top of the priority list when considering feminist intersectional application.

## Intersectional Label Analysis

Feminist therapists inherently reject labels, but clinicians must recognize that labels can be meaningful for some nondominant gender and affectional clients. Identity labels can foster a sense of in-group safety and belonging that cisgender and heterosexual groups may not immediately provide. Identity labels can also contribute to a deep understanding of one's sense of self when this self may have been marginalized, suppressed, oppressed, or even rejected. Therapeutic intersectional label analysis takes this further by recognizing how a person might be viewed, judged, and therefore mistreated by the oppressive, biased systems around them. An intersectional label analysis is a method that may help clients look critically at their Eurocentric, cisheteronormative, Christian-dominant, patriarchal injuries. Nondominant gender and affectional clients are keenly aware of their intersectional identities and subsequently associated oppressions, even if they do not put a voice to them.

It may be helpful for the feminist clinician to create the safety of the therapeutic relationship to explore how clients' multiple identities interplay with their nondominant gender and affectional identities. For example, what does it mean in this society to be a gay, Black, cisgender man who identifies as a Christian? What identities would this client feel they may have to hide in certain social settings, and if not, how would they be treated or even harmed? Does living in nondominant gender and affectional identities make any other aspect of a client's identity more difficult? Feminist clinicians emphasize the client's strengths throughout this collaborative exploration technique, as empowerment is always an overarching goal with a feminist approach. For instance, has living in a nondominant gender and affectional identity made any other aspect of a client's identity more joyful or provided more growth opportunities? In what social settings, if any, does this client feel every aspect of their identity is safe? Does the client think that living in nondominant gender and affectional identities affords them any protections when considering their additional intersecting identities? In the broader context, intersectional label analysis is an opportunity for consciousness-raising when healing with nondominant gender and affectional clients.

## Assertiveness and Self-Advocacy

Assertiveness and self-advocacy are essential for empowering nondominant gender and affectional clients in a world that seeks to disempower them. An example could be collaboratively equipping clients with a set of responses for when they are misgendered or called by their dead names. Role-playing examples of these responses before the next incident might help elicit new thoughts and responses. Another example could be preparing the client with exit plans for emotionally difficult scenarios, like a holiday gathering with extended family. Feminist clinicians work with the client to decide in advance when a boundary is crossed, how long to sustain the situation and when they should leave the setting, what words they can say to leave or not, and decide how they might choose to feel empowered (as opposed to emotionally isolated) ahead of their exit. A self-advocacy method could be as simple as asking the client, "What do your body and mind need to experience calm right now?" and encouraging their ability to attune and listen to the needs of their mind and body.

Assertiveness and self-advocacy opportunities will present themselves in myriad ways for nondominant gender and affectional clients in healthcare settings, from encountering disaffirming and non-inclusive intake forms to navigating gatekeeping experiences when accessing gender-affirming medical and surgical procedures. Feminist therapists should help empower clients in self-advocacy when traversing the healthcare system and any other oppressive systems, remembering they have the autonomy to wield that empowerment or not. There is no judgment from the clinician if the client decides to remain nonassertive. Self-advocacy can range from speaking up for oneself to political action. It is important to note that self-advocacy is solely client-led, and a feminist therapist should never impose their values on nondominant gender and affectional clients or force them to engage in advocacy consciously or unconsciously.

## Feminist Intersectional Power Analysis

A feminist intersectional power analysis is an opportunity to examine how the social, cultural, and political patriarchy has taken power away from nondominant gender and affectional clients and how they can create strategies for empowerment going forward. A power analysis consists of collaboratively analyzing all the people and systems clients interact with. This can be done by listing names of people in different facets of the client's life and then using a Likert scale to determine who has the power in each situation. Power exists in various capacities (e.g., somatic, interpersonal, political, etc.), and it can often be determined by who needs whom more, real or perceived hierarchies of power, and who cares more about the relationship. Once this is completed, collaboratively look for themes of gender positions, type of relationship, and so on., when the client tends not to maintain a position of power. Likewise, the same analysis can be completed with systems. For example, an ecological systems frame (Bronfenbrenner, 1992) could be applied, or the client can list and examine every system they need to interact with or depend on in their community. Discussing the sources of disempowerment can help the client understand that these beliefs can be contextualized and challenged. This is also an opportunity to help clients discover ways to reclaim their power.

## Psychoeducation for Nondominant Gender and Affectional Clients

Research demonstrates that bibliotherapy and cinematherapy can be quite effective in promoting insight, growth, and healing through the use of popular media (Berg-Cross et al., 1990; Sacilotto et al., 2022). Nondominant gender and affectional clients often do not see themselves represented in media, and if they do, it may be in a disparaging, stigmatizing, or stereotypical manner. This can lead to feelings of individual and collective dismissal and erasure from the social, cultural, and political milieu. A feminist psychoeducation technique might ask nondominant gender and affectional clients to share a book, movie, television show, song, or other media where they felt their identity was well represented. Feminist clinicians who recommend a particular form of media must be familiar with its contents, which can be discussed and applied to the client's individualized worldview and context. As such, feminist therapists using this method should remain current in the latest queer media and have examples ready to share with clients. This traditional feminist therapy application could work well in individual or group settings.

## Community and Peer Education and Advocacy

Feminist therapists may advocate by offering education on topics that improve the mental health profession and aid in promoting beneficence and nonmaleficence when working with minoritized populations, such as nondominant gender and affectional identities. As advocates, mental health professionals can offer training or workshops on the contemporary nondominant gender and affectional lexicon, learning to create brave spaces, and other best practices when working clinically with this population. Community education could include offering support groups for families of nondominant gender and affectional youth or training materials for working with nondominant gender and affectional students at local schools. Such efforts can also include becoming involved and organizing others to advocate against oppressive, discriminatory policies that often infiltrate communities and schools.

# Feminist Intersectional Example: Ramiz (They/Them)

Ramiz, a 27-year-old nonbinary person (they/them), seeks counseling to explore their experiences of anxiety, depression, and difficulty establishing boundaries in relationships. In addition to their nonbinary gender identity, Ramiz's affectional identity is queer, and they have recently come out to their religiously conservative family, who have been unsupportive of their gender and affectional expansiveness. They work in a predominantly male industry, where they often feel marginalized and isolated due to their nondominant gender and affectional identities.

## Creating an Informed, Affirming, and Brave Space

In the initial sessions, the counselor takes time to establish a healing relationship built on trust, affirmation, and transparency. The counselor holds space for Ramiz's identities and experiences, ensuring they feel seen, heard, and valued. As appropriate, the counselor shares their knowledge of contemporary nondominant gender and affectional experiences and demystifies the feminist approach, explaining how this framework will guide the counseling process. Ramiz is explicitly encouraged to express themselves freely without fear of judgment, and the counselor emphasizes that this is a space where Ramiz's identities and experiences will be honored as they are explored.

## Facilitating Self-Discovery and Externalizing Concerns

The counselor guides Ramiz through a process of self-discovery, helping them understand how their internalized negativity and self-blame are linked to external systems of oppression. By externalizing these concerns, Ramiz begins to see their struggles not as personal shortcomings but as reactions to societal prejudices and discrimination, namely homomisia, transmisia, and Islamomisia. For example, Ramiz initially blames themselves for their inability to assert boundaries with their family. Through discussions, they come to realize that their difficulty stems from their family's adoption of traditional Islamic patriarchal norms and expectations. This realization helps Ramiz reduce self-blame and fosters a sense of compassion toward themselves.

## Intersectional Label Analysis and Power Analysis

The counselor uses intersectional label analysis to explore how Ramiz's many identities—nonbinary, queer, and Muslim—intersect and impact their lived experience. Together, they discuss how identity labels contribute to Ramiz's empowerment and disempowerment within their family, workplace, and mosque. In a power analysis, the counselor helps Ramiz explore and assess the power dynamics at play in their life, particularly in their family and professional environment. They explore how these dynamics have contributed to Ramiz's feelings of anxiety and depression, as well as their struggles with assertiveness and boundary-setting. The counselor highlights the systemic nature of these issues, connecting them to broader societal patterns of oppression based on Ramiz's minoritized identities.

## Fostering Identity Empowerment and Engaging in Advocacy

As Ramiz becomes more aware of the external factors contributing to their struggles, the counselor shifts the focus to fostering empowerment. Ramiz expresses a desire to be more assertive in their interactions with their family and colleagues. The counselor supports Ramiz in developing self-advocacy skills, such as assertiveness, where they practice setting boundaries and expressing their needs safely and clearly. Ramiz also expresses interest in advocating for greater inclusivity and fostering a sense of belonging within their workplace.

Together with the counselor, they explore ways to engage in advocacy that feels safe and manageable, such as joining an employee resource group or affinity space dedicated to nondominant gender and affectional identities. The counselor encourages Ramiz in these efforts, reinforcing that they innately deserve a space in which they belong. As part of their advocacy efforts, Ramiz decides to host a community education session at a local affirming mosque on the importance of using correct pronouns and understanding gender-expansive identities. This experience is particularly healing for Ramiz as they can stand in their nonbinary, queer, and Muslim identities in a noncompromising manner with pride.

## Reflecting on and Celebrating Ramiz's Journey

As the counseling process ends, the counselor collaboratively reviews and celebrates Ramiz's journey. They acknowledge the growth Ramiz has made in terms of self-discovery, empowerment, and advocacy. Additionally, Ramiz and the counselor highlight the sources of strength and resilience they have fostered at the intrapersonal, interpersonal, and suprapersonal levels, namely their new affinity space with fellow nondominant gender and affectional colleagues at work and their burgeoning relationships with congregants at the local affirming mosque. Lastly, they celebrate Ramiz's courage, and the counselor expresses gratitude for Ramiz's willingness to invite them into their life to come alongside them on this journey.

# Strengths and Criticisms

Feminist intersectional therapy could be ideal for marginalized communities like nondominant gender and affectional folks because it aims to afford what the client may not be provided in daily life, which are opportunities for empowerment, collaboration, asserting wants and needs, and genuine respect. Feminist methods aid nondominant gender and affectional clients in navigating a world not conducive to belonging and equip them with assertiveness skills and tools to find and establish community. Feminist therapy promotes reclaiming personal power and teaches the client how to wield it effectively, which is imperative for oppressed folks with power taken from them at virtually all systemic levels. Another strength is the social justice and advocacy framework, which encourages clients and clinicians alike, if desired and as appropriate, to take an active role in the change they wish to see socially, politically, and culturally.

Real-world client feedback provides insight into the criticisms of applying feminist intersectional therapy with nondominant gender and affectional identities. Anecdotally, some clients have reported that strongly identifying with their nondominant gender or affectional identity labels only serves to heighten their sense of otherness and exclusion from society. Clients may feel that they do not want to focus so much on their differences but rather on what likens them to cisgender and heterosexual identities, as this may serve to enhance feelings of safety or belonging. Additionally, some multiply minoritized clients may experience a more pressing need to "pass" or be perceived as cisgender and heterosexual by others in their communities due to elevated rates of homo- and transmisia.

Another criticism of feminist intersectional therapy is its emphasis on social activism, which is not well understood as many mental health professionals believe it to be a necessary component of every feminist therapeutic process. Quite the contrary, feminist clinicians who promote or encourage engagement in social activism as a goal of the healing process without collaborating with nondominant gender and affectional clients are violating the core feminist tenet of honoring clients' autonomy and right to engage in self-direction. As such, feminist therapists must be careful not to push their values, beliefs, or agenda, consciously or unconsciously, onto their clients.

# Final Thoughts

In applying fourth-wave feminist theory to healing work with nondominant gender and affectional clients, it is crucial to recognize the intersectional nature of identities and the complex power dynamics that shape these individuals' lived experiences. Feminist intersectional theory, with its emphasis on challenging oppressive power structures and advocating for equity, provides a valuable framework for understanding and addressing the unique challenges faced by nondominant gender and affectional clients. Feminist clinicians can create a more welcoming and affirming healing environment by centering nondominant gender and affectional clients' diverse and intersecting identities and experiences. This involves not only understanding sociocultural, political, and historical issues related to inhabiting nondominant gender and affectional identities in society but also considering how these lived experiences intersect with other aspects of identity, such as race, class, and ability, in empowering and disempowering ways.

Feminist clinicians must exercise cultural humility to continually recognize and address their own biases and assumptions, which may, if unattended, inadvertently replicate systemic oppression in the healing space. Furthermore, feminist intersectional theory encourages clinicians to adopt a collaborative approach, empowering clients to take a directive role in healing work. This empowerment can extend beyond the clinical space, as nondominant gender and affectional clients are encouraged to advocate for themselves and their communities if it aligns with their goals.

Incorporating feminist intersectional principles into clinical practice requires a commitment to ongoing self-reflection, education, and advocacy among clinicians. Feminist clinicians must remain attuned to the evolving discourse on gender and affectional identity. They must ensure that the latest research and best practices inform their approach, emphasizing particularly the work of nondominant gender and affectional scholars and clinicians who engage in healing work alongside similarly situated clients. By doing so, feminist clinicians can better support their nondominant gender and affectional clients in navigating the nuances of their identities and lived experiences in their unique societal contexts, ultimately fostering self-acceptance, empowerment, and client-directed change.

# What If?

What if nondominant gender and affectional identities and experiences were honored as superior instead of inferior?

What if the total population numbers were equally representative of nondominant gender and affectional identities and cisgender and heterosexual identities?

What if the landmark U.S. Supreme Court decisions regarding marriage equality, same-sex intimate relations, and protections against employment discrimination for nondominant gender and affectional identities were overturned?

What if gender-expansive youth and their parents, guardians, or caregivers were able to make healthcare decisions with their providers without government involvement?

# References

Arao, B., & Clemens, K. (2013). From safe spaces to brave spaces: A new way to frame dialogue around diversity and social justice. In L. Landreman (Ed.), *The art of effective facilitation: Reflections from social justice educators* (pp. 135–150). Stylus.

Ausloos, C. D., Pinto, S. A., & Morgan-Swaney, C. T. T. (2024). Romantic and affectional identity and queer oppression. In J. Cook & M. Clark (Eds.), *Multicultural and social justice counseling: A systemic, person-centered, and ethical approach.* Cognella.

Balsam, K. F., Huang, B., Fieland, K. C., Simoni, J. M., & Walters, K. L. (2004). Culture, trauma, and wellness: A comparison of heterosexual and lesbian, gay, bisexual, and two-spirit Native Americans. *Cultural Diversity and Ethnic Minority Psychology, 10*(3), 287–301. https://doi.org/10.1037/1099-9809.10.3.287

Berg-Cross, L., Jennings, P., & Baruch, R. (1990). Cinematherapy: Theory and application. *Psychotherapy in Private Practice, 8,* 135–156. https://doi.org/10.1300/j294v08n01_15

Bronfenbrenner, U. (1992). Ecological systems theory. In R. Vasta (Ed.), *Six theories of child development: Revised formulations and current issues* (pp. 187–249). Jessica Kingsley Publishers.

Brown, L. S. (2018). *Feminist therapy.* American Psychological Association.

Butler, J. (2006). *Gender trouble.* Routledge.

Cor, D. N., & Chan, C. D. (2017). Intersectional feminism and LGBTIQQA+ psychology: Understanding our present by exploring our past. In R. Ruth & E. Santacruz (Eds.), *LGBT psychology and mental health: Emerging research and advances* (pp. 109–132). Praeger.

Crenshaw, K. (1989). Demarginalizing the intersection of race and sex: A Black feminist critique of antidiscrimination doctrine, feminist theory, and antiracist politics. In K. Bartlett (Ed.), *Feminist legal theory* (pp. 57–80). Routledge.

Day-Vines, N. L., Wood, S. M., Grothaus, T., Craigen, L., Holman, A., Dotson-Blake, K., & Douglass, M. J. (2007). Broaching the subjects of race, ethnicity, and culture during the counseling process. *Journal of Counseling & Development, 85*(4), 401–409.

Drescher, J. (2015). Out of DSM: Depathologizing homosexuality. *Behavioral Science, 4*(5), 565–575. https://doi.org/10.3390%2Fbs5040565

Evans, K. M., Kincade, E. A., & Seem, S. R. (2011). *Introduction to feminist therapy: Strategies for social and individual change.* SAGE.

Foucault, M. (1926–1984). *The history of sexuality.* Pantheon Books.

Ginicola, M. M., Smith, C., & Filmore, J. M. (Eds.). (2017). *Affirmative counseling with LGBTQI+ people.* American Counseling Association.

Hudson, K. D. (2019). (Un)doing transmisogynist stigma in health care settings: Experiences of ten transgender women of color. *Journal of Progressive Human Services*, *30*(1), 69–87. https://doi.org/10.1080/10428232.2017.1412768

Leslie, C. R. (2000). Creating criminals: The injuries inflicted by "unenforced" sodomy laws. *Harvard Civil Rights – Civil Liberties Law Review*, *35*(1), 103–182. https://heinonline.org/HOL/P?h=hein.journals/hcrcl35&i=109

Merriam-Webster. (n.d.). Microaggression. In *Merriam-Webster.com dictionary*. Retrieved December 12, 2023, from https://www.merriam-webster.com/dictionary/microaggression

Morgan-Swaney, C. T. T. (2023). *The contribution of affirmative training and implicit bias on new professionals' affectional identity counselor competencies* (Publication No. 30980008) [Doctoral dissertation, The University of Akron]. ProQuest Dissertations Publishing.

Oswald, R., Kuvalanka, K., Blume, L., & Berkowitz, D. (2009). Queering the family. In S. A. Lloyd, A. L. Few, & K. R. Allen (Eds.), *Handbook of feminist family studies* (pp. 43–55). SAGE.

Peele, C. (May 23, 2023). *Roundup of anti-LGBTQ+ legislation advancing in states across the country*. Human Rights Campaign. https://www.hrc.org/press-releases/roundup-of-anti-lgbtq-legislation-advancing-in-states-across-the-country

Peterson, J. C. (2021). The walking dead: How the criminal regulation of sodomy survived *Lawrence v. Texas*. *Missouri Law Review*, *86*(3), 857–902. https://heinonline.org/HOL/P?h=hein.journals/molr86&i=875

Quinn, K. G., Dickson-Gomez, J., Craig, A., John, S. A., & Walsh, J. L. (2023). Intersectional discrimination and PrEP use among young black sexual minority individuals: The importance of black LGBTQ communities and social support. *AIDS and Behavior*, *27*(1), 290–302. https://doi.org/10.1007/s10461-022-03763-w

Ratts, M. J., Singh, A. A., Nassar-McMillan, S., Butler, S. K., & McCullough, J. R. (2016). Multicultural and social justice counseling competencies: Guidelines for the counseling profession. *Journal of Multicultural Counseling and Development*, *44*(1), 28–48. https://doi.org/10.1002/jmcd.12035

Rich, A. (1980). Compulsory heterosexuality and lesbian existence. *Signs*, *5*(4), 631–660. https://www.jstor.org/stable/3173834

Sacilotto, E., Salvato, G., Villa, F., Salvi, F., & Bottini, G. (2022). Through the looking glass: A scoping review of cinema and video therapy. *Front. Psychol.*, 12:732246. https://doi.org/10.3389/fpsyg.2021.732246

Sedgwick, E. K. (1990). *Epistemology of the closet*. University of California Press.

Simmons University Library. *Anti-oppression: Anti-transmisia*. (2019). https://simmons.libguides.com/anti-oppression/anti-transmisia

Warner, M. (1991). Introduction: Fear of a queer planet. *Social Text*, *29*, 3–17. https://www.jstor.org/stable/466295

Woods, J. B. (2017). LGBT identity and crime. *California Law Review*, *105*(3), 667–733. https://www.jstor.org/stable/44630758

# 16

# Feminist Intersectional Therapy with Children and Adolescents

## *Joelle Zabotka, Dominique Maywald, Amy Nourie, and Sedaria LaNora Williams*

*Children and adolescents are uniquely disempowered in a patriarchal system.*

## Feminist Intersectional Theory and Children/Adolescents: No Power

An overarching feminist theory goal of empowerment may be no more poignantly utilized than in a child and adolescent therapy discussion. Clearly, "The fundamental condition of childhood is powerlessness" (Smiley, 1991). As individuals without social, cultural, or political power, it is imperative to recognize that children and adolescents do not typically present themselves or initiate the therapeutic process. Cox (1997) stated, "What is unique in the child treatment situation is that children are not autonomous individuals" (p. 90). In fact, in most settings, they do not even have personal power and cannot seek therapy without guardian consent. Anderson (1997) refers to "adults, agencies or governments who have power over and responsibility for children and adolescents" (p. 1) as "powerholders." Thus, the power in the therapy process for children and adolescents is inherently even more unbalanced than the therapeutic power dynamics an adult may encounter from the beginning of the process. Additionally, feminist clinicians are often called upon to intervene with children and adolescents experiencing mental illness, behavioral and academic-related issues, as well as situational/family issues that the child or adolescent has no power to control.

Societal, cultural, and political structures/systems do not empower children nor adolescents. For example, the United States child welfare system, though varied state to state, is structured to protect the safety of children and adolescents, without necessarily providing input or choice in decision-making. Schools are structured around hierarchy, in which the students possess the least amount of power in the system. Children often possess the greatest vulnerability is school shootings yet have little power or voice in addressing these tragedies. The devastation is addressed by adults—educators, policymakers, law enforcement personnel—who may not fully seek or understand the children's perspectives.

Given the lack of power to make decisions for themselves within families and societies, children and adolescents must be considered a marginalized and even oppressed population when it relates to empowerment. While some may not view children and adolescents as a marginalized group, research suggests that any population that has encountered financial, social, political, and cultural marginalization due to circumstances beyond their control—such as poverty, discrimination, violence, trauma, dislocation, and disenfranchisement—should be considered as such (Murthy, 2022). It is, therefore, essential for the feminist therapist to treat children and adolescents who have experienced these challenges with equal care and respect, including providing a voice that is heard and valued.

# Feminist Theory and Oppressive, Socially Learned Limitations

Feminism, as a social and political movement, plays an integral part in addressing the unique challenges faced by children and adolescents within societal, cultural, and political structures. For example, societal expectations around body image impact children and adolescents. Second-wave feminism drew attention to the ways young girls were socialized to equate self-worth with physical attributes, resulting in damage, including low self-esteem and eating disorders (Bearman et al., 2006).

As early as the 1980s, Hill and Lynch (1983) stated that girls and boys encounter societal expectations that may push them to adhere to traditional gender roles and face increased pressure to conform to culturally sanctioned gender roles. Gender roles refer to the social expectations and norms, established by the Eurocentric, heteronormative, Christian-dominant, patriarchal legacy that dictate distinctive behaviors, activities, and characteristics assigned to individuals based on gender. These roles often continue to promote and reinforce traditional stereotypes, which perpetuate an oppressive binary view of gender, limit the potential of children and adolescents, and do not provide a nuanced, intersectional perspective on gender. Feminism challenges these gender roles by advocating for gender equality, examining the restrictive nature of societal expectations, and including intersectionality in exploring identities.

Children's first point of reference for forming and socializing gender role attitudes is the family. However, a family receives their view of gender roles from the restrictive patriarchal society (Ullrich et al., 2022). Eagly and Wood (2012) suggested that through societal observations, children and adolescents develop attitudes toward their roles based on what they see in the home and outside world. In other words, unknowingly (and often unconsciously), families and social norms shape children and adolescents as they continue to be raised with embedded patriarchal ideals of "norms" that oppress people who do not fit these molds. This is where feminist intersectional therapy with children and adolescents may be helpful.

# Feminist Intersectional Therapy

Feminist intersectional therapy examines the impact of gender and other intersecting identities on young individuals and questions existing power dynamics. Feminist therapists aim to develop a more unbiased atmosphere for their growth and development. Society imposes rigid Eurocentric, heteronormative, Christian-dominant, patriarchal-driven identities on children and adolescents through myriad means, including socialization processes, media representations, and institutional practices. Feminist therapists can help children and adolescents by focusing on the effects of social identities and their broader implications for societal structures.

Feminist therapy has moved beyond gender as its main focus with the third and fourth waves of evolution to a more inclusive understanding of oppression. Gender can no longer be viewed without an intersectional lens to help children and adolescents better understand their lived experiences; acknowledging that multiple oppressions may have as much impact as gender. For example, it is difficult to argue that a 10-year-old White, cisgender male child, from an intact family and an expensive neighborhood has a different life experience than a 10-year-old transgender Hispanic child who is from a low socioeconomic neighborhood with few resources. The feminist therapist must consider the vast intersectional privileges and oppressions that each child, adolescent, parent, and family have in order to understand their experiences properly. Conceptualizing and attempting to fit children and adolescents into the rigid patriarchal systems, as has traditionally been done, can serve to harm. Feminist therapists attempt to help children, adolescents, parents, and families navigate these oppressive systems while advocating for equality for all.

# Feminist Intersectional Parenting

Since children have no power in society or the health care system, the feminist intersectional therapy must involve the parent/guardian or other "powerholders" at some level in the therapeutic process. Fortunately, children and adolescents can often benefit from involved parents and/or caregivers to promote a holistic approach to intervention. This parental/caregiver involvement often allows clinicians to gain insights into the dynamics and parenting styles within the family. The feminist clinician then has the potential to offer parenting support and psychoeducation, in addition to assisting the parent(s)/caregiver(s) in reinforcing therapeutic strategies beyond the counseling session. As a result, it may be beneficial to offer an examination of parenting from a feminist intersectional perspective for parents as well as the client.

There are many theories surrounding parenting and mothering. Matricentric feminism, for instance, suggests that the category of mother is independent of the category of woman and, therefore, "mothers are oppressed under patriarchy as women and as mothers" (O'Reilly, 2019, p. 15). Similar to intersectionality, maternal theories often embrace identity politics and include motherhood as an institution in the political, patriarchal system (Rich, 1995). While mothering is often seen as gendered, the act of mothering includes traits such as nurturing, protecting, and raising children, which is the duty of all parents and extended families of all genders, not just biological mothers.

Many parenting models and, in fact, the entire child welfare system, are based on the concepts of "good" and "bad" parenting. Various intersecting identities affect whether parents are considered good or bad; and, of course, good children come from good parents. This widespread goal of "good parenting" is often supported by "evidence" driven by the norm of patriarchal superiority that points to best parents being contained in White, middle-class, two-parent (cis/het) families. Families, especially mothers, that do not fit into this mold are othered and pathologized, "lending support to notions that the mothering of Black women and working-class women is necessarily problematic" (Unger, 2001, p. 178). Collins (1994) argues that women of color may feel powerless and invisible not only due to patriarchy but also due to American social institutions derived from the patriarchy. "Shifting the center to accommodate this diversity promises to recontextualize motherhood and point us toward feminist theorizing that embraces difference as an essential part of commonality" (Collins, 1994, p. 62). This feminist intersectional model intends to help in that shift.

What, then, is feminist parenting? It is not necessarily the act of parenting while also ascribing to feminist ideology. In fact, many parents would not define themselves as feminists or even be interested in feminist ideology. Instead, feminist intersectional parenting is a model of raising children that includes shared values by most people: advocacy for equality, empathy for others, dignity for the self and others, and inclusivity for all. Although feminist therapy and its value system may not yet be a part of the mainstream in parenting frameworks, it is important to offer a guide for parents who wish to eschew power dynamics and instead learn to focus on a shared power based on equity and social justice. A feminist therapeutic perspective on balancing power dynamics in parent-child relationships requires a shift from traditional parenting norms and may cause anxiety for parents and even evoke criticism from the ecosystems. Parents and caregivers can consider creating an affirming environment that empowers their children through open communication, shared decision-making, challenging gendered expectations and fostering empathy.

Feminist clinicians working with children and adolescents may maintain a dual focus, addressing both the presenting issue(s) brought forth by the youth and family, while at the same time working toward empowerment of the child/adolescent and challenging the hierarchical structure. Additionally, feminist clinicians can focus on power dynamics, gender norms, and intersectionality.

# Unique Challenges for Feminist Therapists with Children and Adolescents

There exist many challenges to working with children from a fourth-wave feminist intersectional perspective. One of those challenges is the balance of attempting to flatten the hierarchies and decrease the power differential between clinicians and youth/families while at the same time holding the responsibilities of mandated reporting, which is tied to maintaining licensure, following the law, malpractice, and so on. Mandated reporting is an essential component of clinical work, including feminist clinical practice. Clinicians are legally obligated to report suspicions of abuse or neglect to appropriate authorities, a mandate intended to safeguard vulnerable populations. The mandated reporting process should align with feminist clinical values, emphasizing the importance of ethical and empathic practice.

Mandated reporting laws in the United States were first developed in the 1960s after Kempe et al. published a journal article identifying the "battered child syndrome" (1962). Within a few years, all 50 states passed mandatory reporting laws in this new, modern era of child protection (Brown & Gallagher, 2014; Myers, 2008). Feminist clinicians understand that these laws are meant to help prevent the abuse and neglect of children. However, it is important to also understand the limitations of these laws and the harm they may produce, whether this is intentional or not. Mandatory reporting policies might lead to over-surveillance of marginalized communities, especially single mothers in communities of color. Unintended repercussions of mandatory reporting laws include an increase in unfounded reports, a broad distrust among neighbors, and many clinicians unwilling to report suspected abuse because of the consequences to the family as well as general lack of help by child welfare entities (Myers, 2008).

In cases where a report is filed, feminist clinicians should advocate for outcomes that are minimally intrusive and maximally beneficial for the family system, prioritizing their well-being and welfare. Feminist clinicians are encouraged to involve clients in the reporting process whenever feasible. This involvement can include discussing potential implications and providing support through the process, aiming to alleviate feelings of powerlessness and betrayal. Recognizing the potential trauma of the mandated reporting process for children and their families, feminist clinicians are urged to offer emotional support and culturally affirming resources. These resources may assist clients in navigating the complexities of life post-mandated reports.

Additional challenges are centered on issues of power. There may be instances when the child or adolescent is well-engaged with the clinician and would like to continue therapy but is not able to make that decision. Similarly, if an agency or supervisor does not support this perspective, for example, the presenting issue is met, but the farther-reaching efforts around empowerment, intersectional identities, advocacy, and self-awareness are still being advanced, the process may be terminated. Finally, although the focus of this chapter is on children and adolescent work, the importance of the inclusion of the parent/caregiver in the process has been discussed. Should the parent/caregiver not support feminist intersectional conceptualizations, the process may also halt.

# Feminist Intersectional Child and Adolescent Model: Youth Empowerment

Important areas to consider in this model include clinician attention toward self in practice, position to and within the work, establishing a safe and culturally affirming therapeutic relationship, enhancing communication and negotiation skills, and addressing power dynamics and advocacy.

## Stage One: The Self of the Feminist Clinician

This stage prompts the clinician to assess the impact of their "service/work" with clients. The feminist practitioner becomes the focal point for critical reflection, directing attention to the complex dimensions with clinical practice. In essence, critical self-reflection and an understanding of positionality move beyond theoretical concepts and become applicable and practical tools for practitioners to engage in transformative and ethical practices (Collins, 2019). A feminist approach requires clinicians to be conscious of how their positionality may shape their perspectives and responses to clients (Brown, 2018). This awareness fosters a commitment to adapting therapeutic strategies to meet the unique needs and experiences of each individual client. Practitioners delve into an honest and critical evaluation of their own positionality, exploring the extent to which the client felt genuinely "heard" or potentially "led." Was the practitioner able to remain vigilant to feminist principles throughout the intervention process?

A key facet of this stage involves analysis of the clinician's adeptness at managing and balancing myriad expectations of both parents/caregivers and the child or adolescent client. This demands a distinct understanding of feminist principles, culture, power dynamics within familial relationships, and the ability to navigate these intricacies without perpetuating oppression (Jordan, 2010). Being able to successfully navigate this stage requires the clinician to survey their values, principles, biases, and assumptions related to parenting. Recognizing and addressing these biases is crucial for maintaining an unbiased and feminist intersectional approach. Are the feminist practitioner's interventions influenced by personal and societal expectations or prejudices?

Lastly, the feminist clinician's needs come into view. Advancing social justice, in any capacity, is arduous. Burnout may not be avoidable. Feminist practitioners must be encouraged to sustain the good fight and persevere as individuals while never projecting this same passion onto clients consciously or unconsciously. Societal inequities impacting young folks and their families are plentiful and are not quickly or quietly remedied. Feminist practitioners are expected to advocate to dismantle all forms of violence, gender-based oppression, intersectional marginalization, oppression, exploitation, and injustice. To nurture advocacy endurance, feminist practitioners can be encouraged to prioritize their emotional, spiritual, physical, communal, and mental well-being needs (see, e.g., Norcross & VandenBos, 2018).

Self-awareness and self-compassion are essential for maintaining the emotional well-being of the feminist practitioner. Conscientious efforts are made to assess and advocate for these needs. This includes creating a support system, both within and outside the clinical practice realm, and establishing mechanisms for ongoing self-assessment, self-compassion, and self-care. In doing so, the feminist clinician ensures their capacity to provide effective, ethical, and empathic feminist intersectional interventions while remaining attuned to the evolving landscape of clinical feminist-informed practice. Some thoughts and reminders follow.

## Continued Professional Development/Training

Feminist clinicians seek training grounded in feminist theory to assist in exploring bias. Training events serve as an opportunity to build a supportive network of like-minded clinicians. Engaging in professional groups, forums, or associations dedicated to feminist therapy creates a community where clinicians can share experiences, seek advice, and find mentorship. This network becomes a valuable resource for clinical consultation, offering diverse perspectives and support in challenging cases. Additionally, this strategy opens avenues for creating a referral network that aligns with feminist values.

## Reflective Journaling and Positionality Analysis

Clinicians engage in reflective journaling as a key technique for self-assessment and critical reflection. This involves writing about their experiences with clients, and focusing on how their own identities, beliefs, and biases might influence their practice. For instance, a clinician might write about how their cultural background influenced their interpretation of a family's dynamics or how their personal experiences with gender roles impacted their response to a client's situation. This reflective practice helps the clinician to recognize and mitigate any potential biases, ensuring that their interventions are client-centered and not clouded by personal perspectives. Additionally, this technique prompts practitioners to ponder if their interventions inadvertently led clients or if they remained true to feminist principles of empowering and hearing clients.

## *Balancing Multiple Perspectives*

This effort involves clinicians consciously navigating and balancing the diverse expectations of parents/caregivers and child or adolescent clients. Role-playing exercises, supervision, and peer consultations can be used to enhance this skill. For example, in a case where a clinician is working with a family, they might role-play both the child's and the parent's perspectives with a colleague to gain deeper insight into the family dynamics. This practice aids in understanding the complex interplay of feminist principles, cultural contexts, and power dynamics within families. It ensures that the clinician's interventions do not perpetuate oppression and are sensitive to the nuances of each family's unique cultural makeup and presenting situation. The clinician continuously evaluates if their interventions are influenced by personal or societal biases, especially concerning parenting roles, norms, and expectations.

## *Practitioner Self-Care, Self-Compassion, and Advocacy Endurance*

To address burnout and sustain the long-term commitment required for advancing social justice, clinicians are encouraged to prioritize their holistic well-being. This includes regular self-assessment of emotional, spiritual, physical, and mental health needs. Clinicians might engage in activities such as mindfulness meditation, attending self-care workshops, or participating in support groups that focus on the challenges of feminist clinical practice.

Establishing a robust support system within and outside the clinical setting is vital. This support could come from colleagues, professional mentors, or external networks that provide a space for sharing experiences and strategies for self-care. This ensures that clinicians maintain their emotional well-being, enabling them to continue providing effective, ethical, and empathic interventions. The focus here is not just on self-care as a routine but as an integral part of feminist practice that acknowledges the emotional labor involved in dismantling systemic oppression. It also involves creating mechanisms for ongoing self-assessment, such as regular check-ins with a mentor or supervisor, and self-care plans that are revisited and revised as needed.

# Stage Two: Establishing a Safe and Culturally Affirming Therapeutic Relationship

No matter the age of the child, adolescent or adult, establishing a safe and culturally affirming therapeutic relationship is imperative, beginning with the very first client contact. As stated, it is most common for children and adolescents to present for therapy by a parent or caregiver and not through their own undertaking. Therefore, the issue of a hierarchical power differential is immediately present and serves to reinforce patriarchal norms. For this reason, it is important for the clinician to empower the child or adolescent, as well as the parent(s) or caregiver(s) to define the issues that brought them to the counseling setting. Active listening with use of empathy, validation of the child or adolescent's unique strengths and experiences can build a safe and judgment-free environment that transcends traditional power imbalances (Rogers, 1961).

Most importantly, the narratives that the client and family express must be believed. The feminist therapist is in a unique position because, often, hearing two conflicting stories organically positions the therapist as a judge of "normal." Feminist therapists reject the concept of "normal." Conversely, as an adult often raised in a patriarchal society, it is almost natural for the therapist to understand the adult perspective of desiring the child or adolescent to fit into the patriarchal norm and systems. The successful feminist therapist remains out of the judging role, no matter how much it is provoked.

Utilizing the feminist therapeutic underpinning of transparency and demystifying the therapeutic process while building a therapeutic relationship will also assist in promoting equality and empowerment. With the goal of establishing egalitarian therapeutic relationships all around, the feminist clinician must recognize and acknowledge the power dynamics between the client and themselves, as well as the parent/caregivers and themselves, and work toward shifting the power to the client and the parents/caregivers. Although these therapeutic establishments of safety may seem unrelated to the presenting problem, these feminist relationship qualities will serve for an egalitarian, collaborative exploration of the problem.

## Stage Three: Enhancing Communication and Negotiation/ Navigation Skills

Cultivating a higher awareness of the Eurocentric, heteronormative, Christian-dominant, patriarchal social, cultural, and political landscape is an integral step in increasing critical consciousness. Oppressive social structures have a pivotal role in shaping both individual and collective identities. Feminist clinicians strive to explore with clients to gain a deeper understanding of the world around them. When children and adolescents recognize the interconnectedness of various social identities, feminist clinicians can encourage the exploration of intersectionality, which may be very different from their existing life scripts.

Understanding intersectionality may assist in a recognition of how unique, privileged, and oppressive identities shape them and their peers with different access to resources and experiences of discrimination. When children and adolescents achieve this level of understanding, it could promote cultural affirmation, foster empathy for self and others, and emphasize the solidarity among oppressive and marginalized populations. When feminist practitioners encourage critical thinking about societal expectations and stereotypes, this can help young people view themselves as free from restrictive norms. It can also embolden children and adolescents to question systemic injustices, challenge patriarchal structures, and participate in dismantling oppressive norms.

Equipping children and adolescents with developmentally appropriate feminist communication skills to navigate bureaucratic and institutional landscapes (schools, child welfare, hospitals, etc.) is empowering. Feminist practitioners place emphasis on strengths-based affirming language that validates their lived experiences and reinforces self-worth. Feminist therapists also seek to monitor the power within the therapeutic relationship through open, transparent two-way conversations with the goal of promoting more power for the client. Feminist communication skills are crucial elements for encouraging the agency and voice of children and adolescents because, as stated, many of the systems they will interact with have a history of being rigid, oppressive, and systemically unjust. Feminist clinicians encourage autonomy in communication, allowing children and adolescents to articulate and voice their needs, preferences, and opinions. Children and adolescents who have developed effective communication strategies to navigate oppressive, unjust systems will learn to demonstrate and hopefully generalize agency, autonomy, self-efficacy and resilience.

An aspect of developmentally appropriate feminist communication skills includes helping children and adolescents understand relational reciprocity from an empowered perspective. Relational reciprocity focuses on the reciprocal or "give and take" dynamic within communication and relationships (Gilligan, 1982). A young person's ability to demonstrate empathy toward others will have a positive impact on their overall social functioning (Yoo et al., 2013). Reciprocity, by nature, suggests equality within communication; however, with children and adolescents, there is a consistent hierarchy between adults and authority figures that often interferes with equality. Exploring empowered relational reciprocity might encourage children and adolescents to engage in productive assertive and empowering interactions, listen and hear diverse perspectives and appreciate unique intersectional individuality.

Navigation and negotiation skills are necessary for self-advocacy and boundary setting. Clinical feminist negotiation extends beyond the traditional definitions to include the ability to navigate complex oppressive systems, socially normed peer pressures, societal definitions of success and "good," and conflicts with caregivers who often have assimilated and share the embedded patriarchal values of society. Negotiation/navigation skills may contribute to individual growth through learning assertiveness and how to present opinions, as well as advocating within the overall landscape of equitable social dynamics.

How can a feminist therapist explore critical thinking, negotiation, and negotiation skills with children who cannot think critically and have no real social power? How do they help children be assertive with their teacher, parents, and other adults, without them being seen as "disrespectful"? The answer is, of course, that everything needs to be in a developmentally appropriate context, and it may best serve the child/adolescent if the feminist therapist can bring the people who have the power (parents, school, doctors, etc.) to collaborate and support the empowerment goals. Lastly, feminist therapists are committed to advocating for their clients as well as the greater society to support the clients in their goals.

## Stage Four: Addressing Power Dynamics, Assertiveness and Advocacy

If clinicians are truly working from the feminist perspective, they must create an egalitarian relationship that promotes equality in which the child or adolescent feels heard and valued. Creating a balanced egalitarian relationship with children and adolescents is particularly challenging. It might require the work of examining oppressive social, cultural, and political norms that promote the hierarchies and oppressive structures within gender roles, age roles, cultural roles, and so on, that maintain an imbalance of power for children and adolescents. Transparently addressing the power dynamics also involves children's lived intersectional experiences and supporting their participation in developmentally empowered decision-making.

### *Assertiveness and Advocacy*

Infusing assertiveness and advocacy skills into feminist clinical work with children and adolescents may strengthen their ability to assert themselves and contribute to positive social change across their lifespan. Advocacy-oriented interventions can positively impact mental health outcomes (Kottman & Meany-Walen, 2016). Teaching self-advocacy can serve to empower children and adolescents with the language to communicate their needs assertively. Feminist clinicians can help young clients understand their rights and articulate what they need to feel supported within various contexts (educational systems, juvenile justice systems, child welfare systems, healthcare systems, and interpersonal relationships). Feminist clinicians' modeling advocacy can contribute to holistic approaches that address both individual and systemic challenges.

When considering power dynamics, the parent/caregiver-child relationship must also be addressed. Fostering open and safe communication encourages children to express their thoughts and feelings without fear of reprisal. However, parents must be open to these new communications and not interpret them as disrespect or as a loss of their parental control. Feminist therapists must help parents/caregivers understand that if their child is empowered, the parents do not lose power. Clinicians can teach parents to listen and hear their children, without aligning with their decisions. As the clinician works to equalize power within the therapeutic relationship, they will encourage the same from parent/caregiver. Positive parenting outcomes have been linked to developmentally appropriate shared decision-making, responsiveness, and encouraging open dialogue between parents and children (Baumrind, 1967; Baumrind et al., 2010). Therapeutic interventions should include a parenting approach, when possible, with both the parent/caregiver and young person as this approach can build a foundation toward parenting from an empowerment feminist perspective.

# Feminist Intersectional Therapeutic Applications

## Applications with Parents/Caregivers

### Validate Experience of Parenting and Psychoeducation Growth

Parents often learn how to parent from their own experiences of being parented, even when they do not agree with the way they were parented. Many parents desire to change these patterns that can be taught through psychoeducation. Feminist principles encourage parents to challenge their patterns and promote equality and empowerment within their parenting.

### Understanding Intersectional Identities of Their Family

The feminist therapist can help the parents explore the unique characteristics of each member of the family and assess each child's needs based on intersecting identities. Traditional parenting may strive to apply the same expectations to all children, but how each child experiences intersecting identities may vary. The feminist therapist might guide parents to value each child's individuality and understand that each child may interact with and be affected by the family system in a unique way.

### Power Discussions

Working with parents around shared power includes understanding how validating children to have a voice does not mean they get their way; it means they are heard. The feminist therapist may discuss areas where children can get their way. An example of this technique may focus on helping parents to recognize when to give more autonomy to the child—for example, allowing the child to pick food for dinner or what to wear—this helps highlight when the parent can allow the child more control.

### Systems Reviews

The feminist therapist may discuss with parents all the systems that they are working within for their children or themselves and help them understand the Eurocentric, heteronormative, Christian-dominant patriarchal influences of the systems. They may also discuss with them how they may want to navigate these systems with assertiveness and/or advocacy.

## *Understanding Decision-Making*

How do parents make decisions? Is there decision anxiety, automatic thoughts from their childhood, not making decisions at all and waiting for someone else to make them, and so forth? Feminist therapists can help parents become aware of their process to help them make more empowered, intentional decisions. Decision-making can connect to many other areas of parenting.

# Applications Working with Parents/Caregivers and Children/Adolescents

*Note:* Each of these activities must be developmentally adjusted.

## *Play Together*

In session, the feminist intersectional clinician provides the child and their parent/caregiver with art supplies and asks them to create a piece of art that represents "strength" as they see it. Each person creates their own piece, and afterward, they share their creations. The feminist therapist can discuss how each person's concept of strength may differ and how societal norms, gender expectations, and personal experiences shape these ideas. The discussion can lead to a conversation about redefining strength in a way that is inclusive and empowering for everyone.

## *Assessing Power*

The clinician introduces the concept of "Power Mapping," a creative exercise where the child and their family visually map out the sources of power and influence in their lives. The clinician provides a large sheet of paper and colored markers. Ask each person to draw a central circle representing their home, then draw lines outward to other circles representing school, friends, community, media, and other significant influences. Together, they discuss how each of these influences impacts their thoughts, behaviors, and roles within the family. This technique allows the child and their parent/caregiver to explore and understand how external societal pressures, including patriarchal norms and expectations, shape their interactions and self-perceptions. This technique can begin a conversation about how to balance these influences and create a home environment where everyone feels empowered, equally valued and heard, and safe to explore diversity of thought.

## *Autonomy, Navigating, and Negotiating Exercises*

Feminist therapists can help children and adolescents negotiate with parent(s) or caregiver(s) for desired items or privileges, supporting a sense of empowerment and autonomy. It is important to remain mindful around the developmental capability of the child/adolescent and awareness of their level of ability. The practice of communicating, negotiating, and being heard is an important one for adolescents and supports the developmental shift toward greater autonomy. The process may also enhance communication and reduce conflicts (Steinberg, 2014). Likewise, the feminist therapist can teach parents the best responses for when they would like to grant the child/adolescent request and when they do not. Communication about power involves being heard and truly considered regarding reasoning for choices or suggestions and plans to fulfill those. Any significant parental challenges with communication should be handled privately and not in front of the child.

## Power Reversal

The clinician may suggest a role reversal exercise where the child and a parent/caregiver or sibling switch roles. This role reversal disrupts traditional power dynamics and fosters mutual respect (Jordan, 2010). Empowering the child or adolescent to lead may promote the development of an autonomous, self-defined identity (Anderson & Hill, 1997; Brown, 2018). Moreover, this intervention bolsters relational skills like active listening, empathy, and collaboration. When caregivers learn from their children, it deepens their understanding and appreciation of the young individual's capabilities and viewpoint. This can advance not only personal and familial relationships but also exemplify egalitarian, respectful connections applicable in wider societal interactions (Worell & Remer, 2003). This technique encourages empathy and understanding by allowing each family member to experience life from the other's perspective. As they act out common scenarios (e.g., getting ready for school, discussing a disagreement), the clinician pauses the exercise to discuss what they notice about power dynamics, communication patterns, and emotional responses. This can be an opportunity to challenge and reframe traditional expectations within the family system.

# Working with Child/Adolescent Individually

## Role-Play Assertiveness

The child/adolescent can identify a need or desire and practice role-play with the feminist clinician to express this need assertively and confidently. This exercise can help build skills that encourage assertiveness in everyday interactions.

## Creative Empowerment

The feminist therapist invites the child or adolescent to create a story. Begin with a simple prompt like "Once upon a time, in a world where everyone's voice mattered, there was a young hero/heroine." As the child/adolescent adds to the story, they weave in their perspectives, feelings, and experiences. The clinician guides the process by gently integrating feminist concepts such as equality, empowerment, and challenging traditional intersectional identities and social roles, encouraging the child/adolescent to explore how these themes can be reflected in their real-life interactions.

## Digital Advocacy for Children and Adolescents

This approach may serve to empower younger clients by amplifying their voices as allies in supporting social causes; it also provides an invaluable opportunity to rebalance the power dynamics that exist within the client-clinician relationship. Child and adolescent clients are better positioned to contribute/teach/speak to the sharing and usage of technology applications with clinicians who may not be as well versed in current social platforms. When youth are motivated to teach someone from another generation a skill, the therapeutic relationship becomes a collaborative space, promoting authentic, open, and transparent discussions. This egalitarian approach may not only enrich the therapeutic process but also signify a paradigm shift toward an affirmative and empowering model of feminist intervention.

**Responsible Use.** Gain parental consent and assent from the child and adolescent client. Explore and evaluate how children and adolescents use technology and social media. Educate young people on the safe use of technology and social media. Discuss the potential impact of virtual content.

**Educate.** Teach children and adolescents about social issues that may be impacting their layers of intersectionality. Feminist clinicians can use developmentally appropriate resources and discussion to help youth understand the broad context of systemic inequalities.

**Identify.** Feminist clinicians may facilitate discussions to identify the social causes that resonate with clients, encouraging them to explore, question, and express their passions, without imposing their own values on the clients.

**Digital Content Creation.** Using AI or user-friendly platforms (Canva, Instagram, etc.), allow children and adolescents, with appropriate consent and permissions, to create virtual vision boards or journals.

**Storytelling.** Feminist clinicians might emphasize the power of storytelling to cultivate empathy within their peers and adults. Children and adolescents can be guided in crafting powerful narratives, humanizing and highlighting the intersectional aspects of social issues.

**Advocacy.** Assist children and adolescents, with parental permission, in creating and curating content for sharing on social media platforms. Teach clients how to use hashtags effectively and engage with communities addressing similar social causes to amplify their messages. Practitioners can encourage constructive conversation with like-minded peers and reinforce the strength that lies within peer collaboration.

# Feminist Intersectional Therapy Example

Billy is a 12-year-old bi-racial, cisgender boy who was raised Protestant and comes from a working-class family. He is attending sixth grade in one of the local private schools. He receives a merit scholarship based on his high scores. The school counselor contacted his mother, June, with some concerns several months into the school year. Teachers have reported that Billy is behind academically despite having been an A student in past grades. Most days, Billy does not come to school with his homework complete. Teachers have noted that Billy is inattentive and appears tired. During lunchtime, Billy mostly prefers to sit alone. He has participated on the school soccer team but did not go out for the team during recent try outs.

June is 32 years old and works full time as a paralegal. She does not receive consistent child support payments from or consistent contact with Billy's father. She and Billy do not have family in the area, but June has a supportive circle of friends she can rely upon. The only life change that June can identify is Pedro, her boyfriend, joining their household. Pedro moved in with her and Billy after a few months of dating.

## Stage One: Practice and Position

The clinician is engaged in critical self-reflection to engage in transformative and ethical clinical practice as described in the model.

## Stage Two: The Therapeutic Relationship

Throughout the establishment of the therapeutic relationship, the clinician remains attuned to the feminist perspective, focusing on dismantling traditional power hierarchies and promoting empowerment. This not only addresses the immediate concerns brought to therapy but also supports Billy's overall growth and development within the context of his family and social environment. The clinician begins with a warm, welcoming approach, and a physical environment that feels safe and nonthreatening to Billy and June. The clinician openly addresses the inherent power differentials present in the therapy room, especially considering Billy's age and the referral circumstances. This is done to validate Billy's experience and make it clear that his perspective is valuable and respected. The clinician actively listens to both Billy and June, demonstrating empathy and understanding.

Focusing on Billy, the clinician encourages him to share about himself, his interests, and his feelings regarding the changes in his life, including the recent academic challenges and the introduction of Pedro into his household. The clinician honors Billy's choices about what to share or not share. This practice reinforces the notion that Billy has control over his experience, encouraging a sense of safety and power and putting Billy in a position of authority over his narrative. The clinician is aware of and sensitive to any cultural dynamics that may be relevant to Billy's situation, including the intersectionality of his race, gender, socioeconomic status (while attending a private school) in addition to his family structure and the dynamics of having a nonbiological parental figure in the home.

The clinician works to establish an egalitarian relationship with Billy. This involves acknowledging and openly discussing the inherent power dynamics in the therapeutic relationship, especially given Billy's age. The clinician challenges traditional social, cultural, patriarchal models and structures within gender roles, age roles, and cultural roles. This might involve discussions about how these roles influence Billy's life and encouraging him to question and explore these dynamics in school, at home, with friends, and so on.

In working with June, the clinician asks about her experiences as a single parent, acknowledging the challenges she faces. This involves exploring June's own perceptions of parenting, including how her experiences and values shape her approach to raising Billy. The clinician validates June's efforts and experiences as a parent while also exploring any biases or assumptions she may hold about parenting. This helps normalize her experience and provides a supportive space for her to express any concerns or challenges. She acknowledges that Pedro moved in quickly with her and Billy. He is trying to help take some parenting stress off her by stepping up to parent Billy.

## Stage Three: Enhancing Communication Skills

Throughout this process, the clinician emphasizes shared power and dismantling oppressive norms. This approach is designed to address Billy's immediate needs and equip him with the skills necessary for healthy interpersonal relationships and self-advocacy. In a supportive environment where Billy feels heard and validated, the clinician works with Billy to develop his communication skills, emphasizing the importance of expressing his thoughts and feelings clearly. This involves role-playing exercises where Billy practices articulating his needs and preferences in various scenarios, such as conversations with teachers or interactions with peers. The clinician also encourages Billy to explore his thoughts and feelings about the changes in his life, including the shift in his academic performance and his adjustment to Pedro joining the household.

Billy is encouraged to engage in discussions about relational reciprocity and learn about the importance of mutual respect and understanding in relationships. The clinician uses examples relevant to Billy's age, such as balancing listening and speaking in conversations with friends or family members. Teaching Billy about empathy and hearing others' perspectives is crucial. This involves discussing how to respond empathetically to peers or family members and understanding the impact of his actions on others.

Billy learns negotiation skills as a form of self-advocacy and boundary setting. The clinician introduces scenarios where Billy practices negotiating skills with June around topics such as curfew times or his preferences regarding household routines. The clinician also helps Billy understand how to navigate complex systems, like school dynamics, and how to deal effectively with peer pressure.

### Joint Sessions with June and Billy

In joint sessions, both June and Billy are invited to create a nonverbal piece of art expressing their views about the word "family." This activity helps both understand each other's perspectives and foster a collaborative family dynamic. The clinician facilitates discussions between Billy and June, highlighting differences in how they see Pedro. Billy likes Pedro but does not want to see him as a father; he worries he would betray his own father if he did that. June recognizes that Pedro is a new addition to the family, and they are all still trying to learn how to be a family together. She does really enjoy her relationship with Pedro and how much Pedro likes Billy.

### Empowering Billy

Since Billy is 12 years old, strategies for empowering younger children can be introduced, giving Billy more control over certain aspects of his life, such as choosing extracurricular activities or managing his homework schedule. Because of the family evolution, it may be possible for Billy to have a greater voice in how this new configuration will work.

## Stage Four: Addressing Power Dynamics and Assertiveness

Throughout stage 3, the clinician's focus is on empowering Billy to understand and navigate the power dynamics in his life, while also equipping him with the skills and confidence to be an advocate for himself and others. This intervention stage is designed to foster Billy's personal growth and identity as an individual who can effectively communicate, advocate, and contribute positively to his social environment.

### Infusing Advocacy Skills

The clinician introduces advocacy-oriented interventions, teaching Billy how to assert himself to tell June and Pedro what he is feeling and what he needs from them to feel less worried. This involves giving Billy the language and tools to communicate his needs assertively with June and Pedro as well as in other contexts.

### Empowering Billy as an Ally

Billy is encouraged to see himself as an ally, amplifying his voice in supporting social causes he connects to—in his case, perhaps this includes connecting with other children in blended families. The feminist clinician encourages Billy to share his knowledge or skills, particularly in areas where he feels confident, such as technology or social media, to have the opportunity to teach his therapist something.

### Digital Advocacy with Billy

The clinician explores responsible use of technology and social media with Billy, gaining consent from June and assent from Billy. Discussions include the safe use of technology and the potential impact of virtual content. Educating Billy about social issues impacting his intersecting identities is a key component. This is a way for him to connect with other children in blended families, with permission and oversight by June. The clinician also uses developmentally appropriate resources to help Billy understand systemic inequalities he connects with or is interested in. The clinician facilitates digital content creation, like virtual vision boards or journals, using AI or user-friendly platforms, with appropriate consents. Emphasizing the power of storytelling, the clinician guides Billy in crafting narratives highlighting social issues of interest and cultivating empathy and understanding among his peers and adults. Billy is assisted in creating and curating content for sharing on social media platforms, teaching him to use hashtags effectively and engage with communities addressing similar social causes.

### Working with June

In tandem with Billy's individual work, the clinician also engages June in cultivating and maintaining open and safe communication. This involves encouraging June to listen to Billy's thoughts and feelings and validate his perspective, especially as it relates to the evolution of their family. The clinician also works on strategies with June to empower Billy, such as a power reversal where Billy teaches June and Pedro soccer drills, thereby reinforcing a balanced parent-child dynamic.

# What If?

What if children had more autonomy in education systems surrounding what they wanted to learn?

What if all education systems taught autonomy, agency, assertiveness, and empowerment?

What if society supported people who do not fit into the "norms" and rewarded diversity rather than tolerating it?

What if society did not have definitions of success always leading toward capitalism?

What if creativity and thinking/ behaving differently were rewarded?

# References

Anderson, G. (1997). Introduction: Children, adolescents, and their powerholders in therapy settings. In G. Anderson & M. Hill (Eds), *Children's rights, therapists' responsibilities*. Haworth Press.

Anderson, G., & Hill, M. (1997). *Children's rights: Therapist responsibilities*. Haworth Press.

Baumrind, D. (1967). Child-care practices anteceding three patterns of preschool behavior. *Genetic Psychology Monographs*, 75, 43–88.

Baumrind, D., Larzelere, R. E., & Owens, E. B. (2010). Effects of preschool parents' power assertive patterns and practices on adolescent development. *Parenting*, 10(3), 157–201. https://doi.org/10.1080/15295190903290790

Bearman, S. K., Presnell, K., Martinez, E., & Stice, E. (2006). The skinny on body dissatisfaction: A longitudinal study of adolescent girls and boys. *Journal of Youth & Adolescence, 35*(2), 217–229.

Brown, L. (2018). *Feminist therapy* (2nd ed., pp. 217–229). American Psychological Association.

Brown, L. G., & Gallagher, K. (2014). Mandatory reporting of abuse: A historical perspective of the evolution of the state's current mandatory laws with a review of the laws in the Commonwealth of Pennsylvania. *Villanova Law Review, 59*(6), 37.

Collins. P. H. (1994). Shifting the center: Race, class, and feminist theorizing about motherhood. In E. N. Glenn, L. Grace Chang, & L. R. Forcey (Eds.), *Mothering: Ideology, experience, and agency* (pp. 45–66). Routledge.

Cox, N. (1997). Treating parents and children together: A feminist look at exclusionary practices in family therapy and child psychotherapy. In G. Anderson & M. Hill (Eds), *Children's rights, therapists' responsibilities.* Haworth Press.

Eagly, A. H., & Wood, W. (2012). Social role theory. In P. A. M. Van Lange, A. W. Kruglanski, & E. T. Higgins (Eds.), *Handbook of theories of social psychology* (pp. 458–476). SAGE. https://doi.org/10.4135/9781446249222.n49

Gilligan, C. (1982). *In a different voice: Psychological theory and women's development.* Harvard University Press.

Hill, J. P., & Lynch, M. E. (1983). The intensification of gender-related role expectations during early adolescence. In J. Brooks-Gunn & A. C. Petersen. (Eds.), *Girls at puberty* (pp. 201–228). Springer. https://doi.org/10.1007/978-1-4899-0354-9_10

Hill Collins, P. (2019). *Intersectionality as critical social theory.* Duke University Press

Kempe, C. H., Silverman, F. N., Steele, B. F., Droegemueller, W., & Silver, H. K. (1962). The battered-child syndrome. *JAMA, 181*(1), 17–24.

Jordan, J. V. (2010). *Relational-cultural therapy.* American Psychological Association.

Kottman, T., & Meany-Walen, K. (2016). *Partners in play: An Adlerian approach to play therapy* (3rd ed.). American Counseling Association.

Murthy, V. H. (2022). The mental health of minority and marginalized young people: An opportunity for action. *Public Health Reports, 137*(4), 613–616. https://doi.org/10.1177/00333549221102390

Myers, J. E. B. (2008). A short history of child protection in America. *Family Law Quarterly 42*(3), 449–463. http://www.jstor.org/stable/25740668

Norcross, J. C., & VandenBos, G. R. (2018). *Leaving it at the office: A guide to psychotherapist self-care.* Guilford Press.

O'Reilly, A. (2019). Matricentric feminism: A feminism for mothers. In L. O'Brien Hallstein, A. O'Reilly, & M. Giles (Eds.), *The Routledge companion to motherhood* (pp. 51–60). Routledge.

Rich, A. (1995). *Of woman born: Motherhood as experience and institution.* W. W. Norton.

Rogers, C. (1961). *On becoming a person: A therapist's view of psychotherapy.* Houghton Mifflin.

Smiley, J. (1991). *A thousand acres.* Alfred A. Knopf.

Steinberg, L. (2014). *Age of opportunity: Lessons from the new science of adolescence.* Houghton Mifflin Harcourt.

Ullrich, R., Becker, M., & Scharf, J. (2022). The development of gender role attitudes during adolescence: Effects of sex, socioeconomic background, and cognitive abilities. *Journal of Youth and Adolescence, 51*(11), 2114–2129. https://doi.org/10.1007/s10964-022-01651-z

Unger, R. K. (2001). *Handbook of the psychology of women and gender.* Wiley.

Worell, J., & Remer, P. (2003). *Feminist perspectives in therapy: Empowering diverse women* (2nd ed.). Wiley.

Yoo, H., Feng, X., & Day, R. (2013). Adolescents' empathy and prosocial behavior in the family context: A longitudinal study. *Journal of Youth Adolescence, 42*(12), 1858–1872. https://doi.org/10.1007/s10964-012-9900-6

# 17

# Feminist Intersectional Therapy and Disability

## *Kathleen McCleskey, Chase Morgan-Swaney, and Emily R. Miller*

*Patriarchal social and cultural norms honor people of ability. People with disabilities are often marginalized, oppressed, and even ignored by the greater society, creating undue intersectional suffering.*

## Feminist Intersectional Theory Perspectives on Counseling Disabled Populations

Feminist intersectional therapy with disabled populations involves honoring the strengths of the lived experiences of individuals with disabilities. Feminist clinicians aim to promote inclusive, accessible, and affirming support, dismantle societal barriers to belonging, and foster opportunities to thrive within anti-ableist economic, educational, and relational systems. Feminist theory emphasizes empowerment, social justice, and self-determination (Sprague & Hayes, 2000). As such, it is congruent for the feminist therapist to utilize identity-centered (e.g., disabled individuals) and person-centered language (e.g., individuals with disabilities) interchangeably, as this honors the terminology that most disabled folks prefer (Dunn & Andrews, 2015). While the nature of disability varies, and these variations are briefly explored in a subsequent section, this chapter focuses on working with disabled individuals more broadly.

Measuring prevalence rates of disability is complex and sources vary in their reports. Some sources report 13.4% of the U.S. population is disabled (U.S. Census Bureau, 2022) and others report over 30% of people have disabilities (Center for Disease Control and Prevention [CDC], 2024). These estimates can vary depending on the definition of disability; they can also vary despite using the same assessment questions due to differences in administration and response rates (CDC, 2024). Regardless of which prevalence statistics are used, many people are living with disabilities, and the chances are high that mental health clinicians will work with clients with disabilities (Olkin, 2017).

Modern feminist therapy acknowledges the primacy of intersectionality as it pertains to the influence of the convergence of disabled individuals' multiple identities and oppressive societal forces, such as patriarchy, ableism, and capitalism. For example, cisgender men who acquire disabilities following on-the-job injuries may experience internalized oppression and marginalization due to their perceived lack of self-worth or value to their families and communities, referred to as a "dilemma of disabled masculinity" (Barrett, 2014, p. 39). As a result, these men with disabilities can turn to substances to cope with their emotional and physical pains, which renders them vulnerable to exploitation by the pharmaceutical industry, as was seen during the opioid epidemic. Therapy from a feminist perspective explores the gradations of these intersections, understanding the interplay of disability, gender identity, gender socialization, patriarchy, ableism, and capitalism, among myriad others, in shaping the experiences of folks with disabilties.

## The Discourse of Disability

It is important to note that there have been different models explaining disability. Three of the most prevalent have been the moral model, the medical model, and the social model (Retief & Letšosa, 2018). Briefly, the moral model (also the oldest model), suggests that disability is a punishment for bad behavior or morals, or it is a test of faith to be endured. While this model may not be commonly used today, there are still people who ascribe to parts or all of it (Olkin, 2017).

The medical model is a deficit model that identifies what is "wrong" with the person and aims to try to "fix" them so that they are more "normal." This model gives great power to medical professionals as those who frame and diagnose the problem (Retief & Letšosa, 2018).

The social model suggests that disabilities are variations of human experiences, and that the disability ensues from the social construction of these variations as being undesirable and lesser (Retief & Letšosa, 2018). In this view, akin to feminist theory, people are disabled by oppressive social attitudes and restrictions.

Lastly, the World Health Organization (WHO) defines a disability as the "interaction between individuals with a health condition . . . with personal and environmental factors," which can include social, legal, and cultural attitudes and systems (WHO, 2024). Both the social model of disability and the WHO definitions take the construct of disability away from the individual and is congruent with the feminist view of disability as a social and environmental issue that privileges nondisabled people.

Serving individuals with disabilities using feminist intersectional theory, therefore, requires a nuanced understanding of the lexicon of disability and an awareness of the diverse intersectional experiences that folks with different variations of disability navigate. Other specific knowledge that can be helpful in understanding the distinctions between congenital (i.e., present from birth) and acquired disabilities (i.e., developed later in life) to the extent that it is important to those we serve. This distinction may or may not be significant depending on how it influences disabled individuals' self-perception, intersectional identity development, and degree of social marginalization or oppression. Folks with congenital disabilities may grapple with lifelong societal misperceptions, while those with acquired disabilities may be adapting to an evolving sense of identity. In sum, feminist clinicians must avoid overemphasizing this distinction if it is not meaningful to disabled clients, as this would represent an infringement on their autonomy to define their experience and what matters to them (Haegele & Hodge, 2016).

Feminist clinicians consider both salient (i.e., visible) and invisible disabilities. Salient disabilities, such as those affecting individuals' mobility, are typically apparent, while invisible disabilities, such as some chronic illnesses or iterations of neurodivergence, may not be easily discernible. Feminists possess a keen awareness of the oppressive societal forces associated with visible and invisible disabilities, recognizing that disabled folks' experiences can vary significantly based on the salience of the disability (McConnell & Minshew, 2023). For example, folks who are neurodiverse operate within an economic system that presupposes and privileges ableness and, as such, neurotypicality. As a result, neurodiverse individuals can often feel inadequate, unproductive, lazy, or broken in some fashion. In reality, feminist clinicians understand it is the ableist expectations of the economic system, not neurodiverse individuals, that are broken and in need of repair.

Social, legal, and educational definitions of disability vary in the Western world between systems, populations, cultures, and communities. The concept of disability studies aims to encapsulate a large and ever-changing definition of "disabled." Disability studies attempt to frame our worldview to one of inclusivity, as discussed earlier, where we can think of all types of people with all types of abilities (see, e.g., Olkin, 2017). By utilizing this change in worldview, the aim is to think of ways to foster a more inclusive, nuanced, and accessible world, whether that be social structures and legal works, or physical spaces and forms of accessibility. Feminist intersectional therapy is congruent with the conceptualization of disability as it interacts with other intersecting identities and how they are encountered and perceived within the therapeutic community.

## Systemic Impacts on People with Disability

There are many ways in which systems can be limiting and oppressive to disabled people. Healthcare, including mental health care, and medical benefits in the United States are inadequate to people with disabilities, which is something feminist counselors must consider when working with disabled individuals. Government healthcare benefits come with restricting limits for disabled individuals with heavy health expenses, often leaving no funding available for mental healthcare (Rowan et al., 2013). The overcomplication of healthcare in the United States for all individuals is made more difficult for those with disabilities who must often interact with oppressive marginalizing systems and who often have to fight for their rights to best practices in health. Marriage and employment bring complications to healthcare benefits in a different way than for nondisabled individuals. Some healthcare accounts and benefits have limits if an individual who is disabled is married, and many do not account for disabled individuals starting families, such as ABLE accounts (Social Security Administration, 2024). People with disabilities have been described as un "unrecognized health disparity population" (Krahn et al., 2015, p. S198).

Public education has challenges faced by students with disabilities. Disabled people have gained rights to public education due to the Individuals with Disabilities Education Act (IDEA); this has greatly increased the number of students recognized with disabilities and has been able to provide needed services (Williams, 2022). Systemically, however, there have been fewer special education teachers than are needed and more vacancies in special education than in other teaching specialties (Blad, 2024). While in school, students with disabilities may receive both the benefits of normalizing the disability population while simultaneously experiencing some educational and social segregation (Olkin, 2017). In higher education, marginalization for people with disabilities often persists. Those with visible disabilities may fare better than those with invisible disabilities, and those with mental health, emotional, or behavioral disorders have had problems connecting to support services, adjusting to college, and/or ultimately graduating (Safer et al., 2020).

Employment opportunities are another way that disabled people are systemically marginalized, oppressed, and even rejected. People with disabilities are much more likely to be unemployed or underemployed than are nondisabled people (Bureau of Labor Statistics, 2024; Smith et al., 2023). This underrepresentation in the workforce has social, cultural, and financial impact on both the disability community and the greater systemic culture. For example, many people with disabilities with fewer financial resources, despite potentially having higher healthcare-associated costs (Smith et al., 2023). It also reinforces patriarchal messages that people with disabilities are unable to work and are reliant on being cared for which serves to perpetuate systems that marginalize and oppress disabled people.

Disabled persons can also be marginalized related to dating and intimate relationships. Nondisabled females in the United States have been found to be more receptive to dating a disabled partner than were nondisabled males in the United States or nondisabled people of either gender in Taiwan or Singapore (Chen et al., 2002). People with some kinds of disabilities have been perceived as more attractive than those with other kinds of disabilities or more suited to dating rather than working with (see, e.g., Seo & Chen, 2009, for a review of this topic). Knowing someone with a disability also increases the likelihood of dating someone with a disability (Chen et al., 2002). One important aspect of romantic relationships and disability can be whether a relationship predates a disability or not (Olkin, 2017). Still, as a group, disabled people have often been viewed as asexual, not able to physically engage in sexual activities, or unable to understand sexuality (Mert Kastner, 2019).

For many years, the disability rights movement operated independently of the feminist movement, and vice versa, even though both share similar perspectives on systemic oppression, restricted possibilities, and a restricted view of "normal" (Garland-Thomson, 2003). Recent feminist intersectional perspectives have integrated disability and feminist studies and perspectives (see, e.g., Garland-Thomson, 2003; Nosek, 2010). In addition, Olkin (2017) developed disability-affirmative therapy (D-AT) to conceptualize disability within the therapeutic environment; Olkin (2017) identifies aspects of D-AT as having been influenced by feminist perspectives and as having elements that align with a feminist worldview.

# Feminist Intersectional Conceptualization with Clients with Disabilities

From a feminist intersectional perspective, it is imperative to contextualize the unique intersectional individual client within the oppressive systems they inhabit. Feminist conceptualizations must include the ecosystems surrounding the clients both directly (families, organizations, communities) and indirectly (norms, mores, culture) with the understanding of the oppressive influence of Eurocentric, heteronormative, Christian-dominant, patriarchal norms. The feminist therapist must also consider the clients intersectional identities that intersect with their experiences through gender binaries ableist expectations, available options, bias, and often stigmatized messaging. Cultural, social, and political messaging can be implicit, explicit, direct and/or indirect. A disabled person's agency, autonomy, and power opportunities must be considered when conceptualizing a client and their presenting issues within and among these oppressive interlocking marginalizing systems.

Because of the multiple ways in which people with disabilities can be marginalized, these dynamics must not become replicated in the therapeutic setting. One of the most healing factors of a feminist intersectional approach can be the egalitarian, power-sharing, truly collaborative therapeutic relationship. This flattened hierarchical relationship can be the vehicle to collaboratively explore the client's lived intersectional experiences, problem definition, and goals.

Through acknowledgment and monitoring of therapeutic power differentials, the feminist therapist hopes to aid clients to become more empowered. With disabled clients, many avenues of empowerment can be examined. Some empowerments can be internal, related to how a client defines a disability and its empowering or limiting impact on their life, whether or not they have an identity as a disabled person, and how any disability identity intersects with other social locations. Other potential areas for empowerment can include arenas already discussed—health care, education, employment, and relationships with others. The feminist clinician supports and empowers the client as much as possible in exercising autonomy and self-advocacy. This will include listening carefully (and asking the client) about language use and what language around disability empowers or disempowers them. It also might include exploring the client's stance on the prevalence of their disability related to the presenting issue. They made decide that their disability will not be very salient for every issue, or that disability can be the primary issue.

# A Feminist Intersectional Model for Working with Clients with Disabilities

## Creating an Affirming Environment

Before working with disabled clients, there is a great deal that a feminist clinician will do to prepare an affirming clinical environment. An essential first step is to become educated on disability history, disability culture, and disability rights. One way to do this is to become more fluent in the different models of disability. It is equally important to learn an overview of all the ways disability can impact a person, as well as the broad range of disabilities, including those that are visible and invisible. Some disabilities may have more predictable impacts on a person, and others (such as chronic illnesses) can have more fluid impacts (Brodt & Lewis, 2024). Miserandino (2003) created the spoon theory of disability; this theory has become popular with many people. It is the first theory developed by a nonacademic person based on lived experience and not research (Brodt & Lewis, 2024). Spoon theory describes how a person with a disability needs to manage their energy each day and how limited energy demands difficult choices (Miserandino, 2003). A person with a chronic illness has a limited number of "spoons" or units of energy per day, and they must carefully prioritize how those spoons are used.

Feminist therapists will benefit from learning from people with disabilities both in professional literature and personally and from approaching work with disabled persons with cultural humility, especially if they are not, themselves, part of the disability community. If the therapist is a member of the disability community, it is helpful to consider potential countertransference stemming from that, such as assuming similarities that may not be present, or assuming common experiences that may cause the therapist to not ask specific questions about those.

Another aspect of preparation involves practical matters. Feminist therapists need to assess physical and (if appropriate) virtual spaces for accessibility. Physical spaces include parking lots, entrances, waiting areas, bathrooms, hallways, and offices. A helpful perspective here is that of universal design (UD). UD contends that "products, environments, programmes, and services should be usable for different people" (Lid, 2014, p. 1345) and that "anything that makes an environment more accessible for someone, likely makes it more accessible for all" (Froehlich, 2024, personal communication).

Virtual spaces should also be assessed for accessibility. When counseling virtually, therapists should be familiar with assistive technologies and how to help clients access appropriate technology for virtual counseling. Technology-based platforms used by the therapist need to have accessibility features. Other accommodations should be available on an individual basis (e.g., sign language interpreters). Communication needs should be assessed in any modality with an understanding of how to access resources to assist clients who need them. Paperwork should use inclusive language, be available in alternative formats, and not contain any biased questions.

Three resources that may help gain an overview of therapeutic work with clients with disabilities are the American Psychological Association (APA) "Guidelines for Assessment and Intervention With Persons With Disabilities" (2022), the American Rehabilitation Counseling Association (ARCA) "Disability-Related Counseling Competencies" (2018) and the Commission on Rehabilitation Counselor Certification (CRCC) "Code of Professional Ethics for Certified Rehabilitation Counselors" (2023).

Another aspect of preparation for working with disabled clients is to use reflexive skills to examine potential countertransference or microaggressions with this population. Olkin (2017) describes how microaggressive comments and questions can signal to a client with disabilities that a therapist has bias and/or is uncomfortable with disability. Examples of microaggressions can include centering a disability as the only pertinent detail, asking extremely personal questions, infantilizing a person with a disability, or denying a disabled person their rights (Olkin et al., 2019). Using microaggressions may sometimes seem to a therapist to signify joining behavior ("I had a roommate who was disabled"). However, they often serve to signal bias to the client with a disability (Olkin, 2017). Not having an accessible office can also be a microaggression. Assuming a disabled person is asexual is a microaggression. Feminist therapists need to ensure that they examine personal beliefs and feelings about disability and do not recreate in the therapy room the same kind of devaluing and disaffirming experiences that clients likely experience outside of it.

## Meeting the Client

This stage is the beginning of the therapeutic journey with the client. When first meeting a client with a disability, a feminist clinician will provide a welcoming and affirming environment. This stage centers on learning and understanding who the client is holistically and how they identify themselves and their presenting issues. It is assumed at the beginning of this stage that informed consent, role induction, and so on will happen as they would for any client, and be done in an accessible, empowering, and affirming manner.

Collaboratively, the feminist therapist and the client discuss identity, issues, and goals. It is possible that in the first meeting, clients may begin to describe and discuss their intersecting identities, including disability-related identities. Feminist clinicians listen for marginalization in clients' stories, so being attuned to ableism as well as any other experiences of "isms" will be helpful while still centering the client's voice.

Also in this stage, the feminist clinician transparently discusses the therapeutic value for acknowledging and monitoring a power-sharing within therapeutic relationship. As part of power-sharing, and transparency, consistent with other multicultural values, a feminist clinician needs to appropriately take responsibility to learn more about any disability they do not understand, including any cultural, social, or political nuances associated with that particular disability. In this and subsequent stages, clients should not be expected to function as sole sources of education about their disabilities.

An important note to remember is that the presenting problem may be about any disabilities, may be connected to any disabilities, or may be unconnected to any disabilities. As an example, a blind cisgender male client may want to discuss being blind, may want to focus on job-related challenges that are connected to being blind, at least in part, or may want to talk about a relationship breakup that had nothing to do with his blindness but instead about their sexual incompatibility.

## Deeper Intersectional Exploration

In early sessions, deeper exploration of the client's life, intersecting identities, and presenting concerns can occur. In this stage, the feminist therapist and the client can collaboratively uncover if or how the presenting problems connect to any disability. After meeting the client, the feminist therapist will have researched knowledge about any of the client's disabilities to ask informed questions about the client's experiences. Again, this exploration needs to center the voice of the client and not to create a connection between the problem and disability if there is none.

This is also the stage where there can be more focus on intersectional identities, if the client is interested in that—as a person with a disability, but also in terms of gender, race, age, religion, affectional orientation, and so on—and how these identities intersect with the presenting problem and/or the disability. As part of this processing, the feminist therapist can note for the next stage and reflect on any ableism or other forms of bias or discrimination the client may have experienced or be experiencing currently.

## Situating the Problem and/or the Disability in Patriarchal Systems

A hallmark of feminist therapy is contextualizing clients and their problems within Eurocentric, heteronormative, cisgender, Christian-dominant, and ableist patriarchal systems. This contextualization includes probing into norms, expectations, values, and messages about differing social identities and how many systems are set up to reinforce those. Feminist therapists are transparent with clients about how this kind of context can be helpful. In this stage, and with the client's agreement, a feminist therapist can help the client to examine intersecting identities related to client presenting issues through this feminist intersectional lens.

For clients with disabilities, examining ableist culture would likely be helpful. This might include explorations of embedded family-of-origin messages and experiences, educational experiences, work experiences, dating experiences, health care experiences, previous therapy, microaggressions, and so on. Psychoeducation could be offered to frame all the "isms" of patriarchal culture and to explore the intersectionality of client identities within that frame as well as any connections to presenting problems. Additionally, the feminist therapist is helping the client determine the levels of privilege and oppression their identities have in society and how it may complicate the matters they are currently facing.

As part of these explorations, it might also be helpful to examine where clients identify as having power/autonomy and choices and where they do not, as well as where there are options to resist or reframe any patriarchal marginalization. Doing a power analysis could be helpful here, as could an intersectional gender analysis. Other possible exploration techniques could include an intersectional social atom or a feminist critical genogram.

## Collaboratively Exploring Impacts of Systemic Influences on the Problem

After identifying how patriarchal culture impacts clients, problem definition, and potential goals, a feminist clinician and a client can collaboratively reexamine whether any initial framing of problems or solutions now offers other frames. Does the client want to redefine problems with new context? Have any new problems emerged or been identified? Have any initial goals changed? How can the client use any new thoughts/information to navigate the oppressive systems with more power?

## Collaborative Goal-Setting with Empowerment

Discussion in the previous stage may, with some clients, reinforce initial ideas or understandings or expand or change them. For some clients, these kinds of consciousness-raising explorations may lead to "aha" moments around deeper issues such as identity definitions around being a person with a disability or around any other identities and identity intersections. If that occurs, the direction of the work may shift to spend time on these deeper issues before returning to initially defined problems or to new ones that may have emerged. The therapeutic goal is to raise consciousness to empower the client to make future decisions with more awareness.

Together, the feminist therapist and the client will form therapeutic goals, led by the client's empowered definition of desired goals and with the feminist therapist supporting, assisting, and collaborating. Feminist therapists ensure that collaborative work focuses on what clients choose as goals. It is possible that advocacy efforts and skills may be identified as part of the therapeutic work—either self-advocacy by the client or advocacy by the client for self and others. Advocacy must be included only if the client wants to include it, and any advocacy where the therapist collaborates with the client must be clearly endorsed by the client. Advocacy has always been a core value of feminist therapy but as feminist clinicians, we do not impose advocacy goals or requirements on clients. Therapists, as feminists, can take on advocacy goals themselves outside client goals.

## Collaborative Work toward Empowered Goals

After goals have been collaboratively decided, this stage is where further work is done consistent with reaching the client's specific goals formed from a higher consciousness. Often, an element of feminist therapeutic work involves the client becoming empowered to reject or resist patriarchal norms and expectations and instead to develop their affirming messages and expectations. However, feminist therapists *do not* impose these goals onto clients. A feminist therapist can regularly check with the client to ensure that the focus remains on goals the client has identified and endorsed.

In this work toward goals, feminist therapists might help clients continue to monitor patriarchal impacts of therapeutic work as well as their experiences of the therapy itself. Feminist therapists demystify the counseling process as part of the egalitarian relationship; this can be used in discussing reasoning for suggesting or considering particular interventions as well as in using immediacy to check in with how clients feel heard, valued, and helped (or not) in the therapeutic process. Creating and maintaining this power-sharing in therapy is one healing aspect of the work and can be especially powerful to clients who have been marginalized and disempowered. Overall, the feminist approach is concerned with increasing clients' autonomy and power and so continuing to notice and discuss how that is happening—or not—can be a guiding principle in the specific work with a particular client.

## Collaborative Agreement of When the Therapeutic Work Is Done

Also consistent with the power-sharing dynamic, feminist clinicians collaborate with clients to decide when to end the therapeutic relationship. When both agree to end the therapy, part of this stage of the clinical work can include reflecting together on the shared journey of the feminist therapist and client. Client growth can be highlighted through experiences of consciousness raising, empowerment, reframing, skill-building, relational assertiveness, and possibly advocacy. If there is disagreement between counselor and client about when to end the professional relationship, the client's autonomy is respected—clients are empowered to make their own decisions even if the feminist therapist does not agree with them.

# Feminist Intersectional Clinical Applications with Disabled Populations

We offer the following examples of how feminist intersectional theory might be implemented with disabled clients. We do not purport that these are the only, or the correct way, to do this, but only that they are some possibilities. In general, feminist techniques aim to raise consciousness in clients to help them situate themselves and their issues within the patriarchal systems discussed earlier.

## Power Analysis

Power analysis is a feminist therapy intervention that critically examines power dynamics within personal, interpersonal, and societal contexts (Evans et al., 2011). It aims to help clients with disabilities explore how power imbalances affect their relationships to self, others, and systems. Feminist clinicians may start by jointly identifying the clients' most influential intersections, examining how their relevant identities, experiences, and societal forces converge and, in so doing, enhance or attenuate power in different contexts. We want to invite clients to reflect on experiences with power, which may involve exploring relational dynamics and interactions with the systems they frequently navigate (e.g., healthcare).

One possible framework that may be helpful to use in a power analysis is from Nosek (2010). Nosek (2010) describes issues of concern to women with disabilities, but these can be used with people of all genders and provide specific, common experiences where disabled people may want to examine personal autonomy. These areas are "identity and self-worth, individual autonomy, connectedness and social support, control of one's body, sexuality, violence and abuse, discrimination, employment and income inequities, and health disparities" (Nosek, 2010, pp. 506–507). Having a client assess their levels of power in each of these domains could help uncover potential areas of therapeutic work and clarify domains where the client feels more and less empowered.

Feminist clinicians normalize disabled clients' reactions to disempowering experiences and provide a space for them to express the impact of power inequities on their well-being. Collaboratively, we identify sources of empowerment within clients and their spheres, including character strengths, personal values, religious or spiritual beliefs, supportive relationships, or involvement in meaningful activities. Feminist clinicians encourage clients with disabilities to wield these factors as they navigate and challenge oppressive power structures. Lastly, we want to facilitate the development of strategies clients can utilize to exert their power, such as assertiveness training, boundary setting, and self-advocacy in spaces where disabled clients desire a more egalitarian, hierarchy-attenuated experience of power.

## Self-Advocacy

Self-advocacy is a crucial aspect of feminist clinical application, empowering disabled individuals to assert their needs and rights (Evans et al., 2011). However, before clients with disabilities are encouraged to engage in self-advocacy, feminist clinicians must ensure that clients have cultivated an indomitable self-identity, power consciousness, and a sense of empowerment, as they are likely to face various forms of resistance to their attempts to meet their needs and exercise or advance their rights. Additionally, we want to work together to ensure that clients with disabilities understand the current legal and political landscape regarding their needs and rights, as possessing this information is critical for disabled clients to feel knowledgeable and efficacious in their abilities to engage in self-advocacy in various settings.

Once this foundation is established, feminist clinicians and disabled clients engage in skill-building and role-playing focused on communication, assertiveness, and negotiation, developing effective methods to use during self-advocacy. While possessing self-advocacy skills increases disabled clients' likelihood of success, working alongside clients to develop strategies to cope with disempowering results is also important. We encourage clients to engage their protective factors, including strengths, values, beliefs, supportive relationships, or meaningful activities, when their self-advocacy efforts do not result in the intended outcome. As clients with disabilities have experiences engaging in self-advocacy, feminist clinicians hold space for clients to reflect on the process, identifying strengths and areas for growth to prepare for future efforts. Lastly, we want to ensure that we celebrate with our disabled clients as they fulfill their needs and exercise their rights through self-advocacy, amplifying the power of their voice in shaping their experience.

## Feminist Genogram

Genograms can be used with individual clients as well as with partners or families. A feminist clinician can utilize the genogram format to help clients explore many aspects of their intersectional identities both in the past and in the present. One possible way to do this is through examining messages about the client's disability from members of the family. Were there family members who seemed to espouse different models of disability? Were there any who gave affirming messages and support? Were there any who gave disaffirming or disempowering messages about disability and/or other intersecting identities? How did messages, behaviors, and actions impact relationships or still impact them today?

Genograms can also be broadened to include other entities beyond family members. Social or community organizations, systems of care, education systems, and so on, could all be included on a genogram in creative ways to explore how those impacted family relationships and clients' development. As with the more traditional genogram, power in relation to systems and organizations could be mapped and assessed.

## Feminist Social Atom

Another way to use images to represent current relationships in a client's life is through a social atom. Social atoms were first developed and used by Moreno (1943) to give a graphic representation of the relational experiences of a person through manipulating symbols for different people, organizations, constructs, and so forth via size and proximity in relation to the individual. Social atoms are a snapshot in time and can be very helpful in assessing where a person is right now in terms of whichever relationships are explored.

When working with disabled clients, the client could select current relationships, entities, concerns, and the like, and graph their impact on the client at the moment. A client may put a mark, name, or symbol in the center of a piece of paper (or wherever they want to put it) to represent themselves. Then they may use symbols or words to depict, as an example, (1) a partner to whom they feel close, whose symbol would be next to/near the client's symbol, and would be the same size as the client's if the relationship was perceived as power-sharing and/or supportive; (2) a workplace or boss that may be looming overhead, large and close, if there are problems at work and the client feel less empowered there; (3) a symbol for a friend from whom the client gets great support but who lives far away—the symbol for the friend would represent both the level of support and the level of proximity, so possibly a large symbol far away; (4) an assistive device which the client is finding useful in reducing some kind of systemic barriers, which could be depicted by a large symbol near the client's symbol, and (5) an upcoming event for which the client has some anxiety and is thinking about but is not consumed with, which could be depicted by a medium sized symbol half the page away from the client's symbol.

Social atoms can be used by feminist therapist to help clients depict power in their lives today, worries they currently have, or even their intersectional identities in the moment in terms of which identities are at the forefront and which may be more in the background. If doing this latter example, it would be good to help the client generate all salient identities, perhaps both in terms of social locations (race, ethnicity, age, affectional orientation, religion, etc.) and also in terms of life roles (daughter, father, partner, student, worker, volunteer, leisure identities, etc.). Identities could then be graphically depicted in terms of current proximity, current impact, and current intersections. One of the advantages of using a social atom is that the client is able to choose what to focus on, to include, and to exclude. Having the client explore and explain the social atom can highlight potential areas with which to spend more time.

## Feminist Mask Exercise

The mask exercise is a creative technique used in art therapy (see, e.g., Barnum, 2022); it has also been used as a technique in other therapeutic disciplines. Clients are provided either an actual blank three-dimensional mask or a mask outline on paper (in which case there should be two, or one on each side of the paper); they are then asked to draw or to decorate the "outside" mask depicting aspects of themselves that they let the world see and also another version which is the "inside" mask, that is, aspects that they keep to themselves. It can be illuminating to explore with clients which aspects of themselves they share with the world and which they keep private or hidden.

A feminist therapist can offer the mask exercise with disabled clients as a way to explore several things. One possible exploration is that of intersectional identities, including any disability identity. Rather than only focus on what they share with the world, this can be reframed as depicting what the world expects or accepts from them. What parts of their intersecting identities are valued in patriarchal society (outer mask), and which are rejected (inner mask)? Or, in terms of their impairments or disabilities, what parts of themselves do they show or "lead with" in various venues (with family, at work/school, with friends, in medical settings, etc.), and which do they not show until later or not at all? How do various identities move into the foreground or into the background depending on the situation and people involved? Processing these with clients may clarify identity development, assertiveness, career, or relational opportunities for therapeutic work.

## The Feminist Egalitarian Therapeutic Relationship

A hallmark of a feminist approach is the egalitarian therapeutic relationship and it may be thought of as an (ongoing) technique, while also as a way of being with clients. As discussed before, one aim of feminist work is to not recreate inside the therapy relationship the same oppressions and marginalization that occur outside of it. Because of this, feminist clinicians need to monitor themselves and the relationship to ensure that they are sharing power wherever they can and not abusing the power they do have. With clients with disabilities, this also means that they view the client as the expert on their disability, that they seek input from the client about the therapeutic alliance, and that they work to ensure that they do not use microaggressions.

An egalitarian clinical relationship can, however, be challenging at times as therapists may work within systems that are rooted in patriarchal oppression, and both therapist and client live within the same patriarchal societal frameworks. As an example, training to be a clinician involves learning theories and techniques that may oppress clients, which were taught in a hierarchical system that may not have fostered empowerment. It could be a challenge to actually partner with clients and relinquish the role of being "in charge." Doing so requires that we trust our clients and their lived experiences to inform us about them; and we trust ourselves to be receptive to them. It also requires that we be aware enough to monitor power sharing and that we be invested enough to maintain collaborative discussion of power within the relationship. At times, we may also need to work within hierarchical systems and need to find collaborative ways to navigate those as much as possible.

When working with clients with disabilities, we know that there have been historical ways in which stigma and oppression have shaped the disability community. One way that has happened has been to see people with disabilities as being less capable and as needing more care. As therapists, we may find our own countertransference pulling us toward a more caretaking role. We must resist any such impulse. The healing nature of the egalitarian relationship springs from clients feeling our trust, our respect of their own voices and own wisdom, and knowing that we can combine their and our abilities to work together on their problems. With a person who feels empowered, such a relationship is affirming. With a person who feels disempowered, such a therapeutic relationship can be profoundly corrective. Wherever a disabled client already falls on the range of empowerment, the egalitarian therapeutic relationship can support them.

# Case Example: Applying a Feminist Model to Work with Disabled Clients

Alex, a 23-year-old nonbinary and autistic individual, is a recent college graduate freshly employed in the tech industry. While they enjoy the field immensely, they are experiencing challenges relating to their predominantly female colleagues and meeting their male supervisor's expectations. Fearful of losing their job, Alex presents to counseling to "figure out what's wrong" with them and learn how to "quickly correct the problems." Only formally identified as autistic during the latter half of college and newly exploring their nonbinary identity, Alex has not shared aspects of their lived experience with colleagues because no one at work has asked.

## Creating an Affirming Environment to Meet Alex where They Are

The clinician begins by establishing an environment for Alex that is both gender and neuro affirming. Before meeting with Alex, it is incumbent upon the therapist, who is a neurotypical cisgender woman, to establish a basic understanding of the contemporary cultural milieu surrounding neurodiversity and gender expansiveness, with a particular emphasis on familiarizing herself with the lived experiences of folks navigating the intersection of autistic and nonbinary identities. Likewise, the therapist must explore and appreciate how oppressive forces (e.g., ableism and neuronormativity, and transmisia and cisnormativity) influence the trajectory of autistic and nonbinary people's lives.

Additionally, the clinician must evaluate her intake paperwork to ensure that it can account for an inclusive range of neurodiverse and gender-expansive identities, expressions, and experiences. For example, she may include optional free-response questions about Alex's gender identity, lived name, and pronouns. She may ask how the physical space should be situated (e.g., visual, auditory, and tactile aspects of the environment). Common environmental considerations include offering options for dim lighting, noise reduction, and self-stimulating behaviors (or stimming).

The therapist must also maintain an awareness of heterogeneity. Alex's lived experience is unique and will not perfectly align with the therapist's more globalized understanding of the typical sociocultural experiences and needs of autistic and nonbinary folks. This is why she must regard Alex as the expert on their lived experience so that she can bracket any inapplicable knowledge of neurodiverse and gender-expansive culture and center Alex's experiences. Similarly, she defers to Alex to identify the nature of their presenting concerns, even as they situate their concerns intrapersonally ("figure out what's wrong [with me]"). The therapist devotes time during the initial appointment to generally orient Alex to the therapeutic process and invites them to ask questions, seek clarification, and offer feedback at any time throughout the process.

## Exploring and Situating Alex's Concerns in Patriarchal Systems

The therapist listens to Alex's experience of their presenting concerns and identifies how suprapersonal dynamics factor into Alex's experiences in their occupational environment. For instance, Alex shares that their male supervisor assumes they do not have any questions or concerns about their work tasks because they do not ask questions or express concerns during the daily staff meeting. As a result, Alex states they often find themselves with more work assignments than their colleagues, which increases their stress, rendering them less likely to engage with others and more likely to focus on meeting the increasingly inequitable demands of their workload.

Conceptualizing through a feminist lens, the therapist connects Alex's presenting concerns to ableism and neuronormativity, which relate to Alex's experience as an autistic person in the workforce. For example, Alex's supervisor assigns them more work than their colleagues because Alex does not ask questions or voice concerns about their work in daily staff meetings. This action is grounded in ableist misgivings that Alex must excel in their work because they do not say otherwise when they are afforded the opportunity to do so during the daily staff meetings. While most of Alex's colleagues actively participate in these meetings, it is a neuronormative assumption that this type of forum serves all employees well and, as such, the modality is a good fit for all employees.

Moreover, since Alex's male supervisor assumes their gender identity is also that of a cisgender man, sociocultural norms and expectations of masculinity likely lead Alex's supervisor to view them through the lens of the "strong and silent type" bias. In other words, unlike Alex's predominantly female colleagues, Alex's supervisor regards them as a "typical man" who "keeps his head down," does not "rock the boat," and focuses on excelling at their work. The clinician situates the presenting concerns as embedded in these systemic forces and Alex's occupational setting, focusing on how present workplace dynamics do not facilitate an affirming environment that meets Alex where they are.

## Mutual Identification of Systemic Influences on Alex's Concerns

The therapist and Alex mutually examine the impact of these systemic influences on Alex's workplace experiences. Through intersectional analysis, they discuss how the confluence of multiple factors—such as Alex's gender identity, neurodiversity, and workplace culture—influences how they experience their daily life. The therapist and Alex perform this intersectional analysis through the co-creation of a feminist genogram, which explores Alex's relationships with people and systems (e.g., family system, educational system, capitalist economic system, etc.) that proliferated and perpetuated ableism, neuronormativity, and cisnormativity throughout their life. This creative intervention helps Alex see their experiences through a multisystemic lens, reducing self-blame and pathologization of self through externalizing and contextualizing their presenting concerns. Furthermore, using a feminist genogram to conduct an intersectional analysis offers Alex a less verbal means of expression. However, the therapist does not want to assume that Alex would prefer to use or benefit from the use of more nonverbal interventions solely based on their neurodiversity.

## Setting Goals Collaboratively

The therapist and Alex collaboratively establish goals, which may include the following:

1  Learning to augment social skills in ways that feel authentic to Alex's communication style.
2  Building self-advocacy skills to increase Alex's sense of belonging in the workplace.
3  Engaging neurodiverse and gender-expansive culture to facilitate Alex's process of identity exploration.

## Jointly Working toward Goals: Self-Advocacy

The therapist presents Alex with a high-level overview of self-advocacy, including how various neurodiverse folks have described and engaged in it over time. The therapist is mindful of providing Alex with numerous accounts and definitions of self-advocacy so that Alex can establish a construct that is meaningful and resonant to them. Together, they jointly decide how Alex wants to engage in self-advocacy to meet their goal of increasing their sense of belonging in the workplace. Since it is workplace dynamics and not Alex that needs to change, Alex would like to schedule a one-on-one meeting with their human resources (HR) representative to ask for the necessary changes. Alex and the therapist collaboratively determine that Alex will ask for one-on-one meetings with their supervisor in addition to the daily staff meetings and access to one of the vacant private offices to use as needed.

Alex states they are not yet ready to disclose their minoritized identities to their HR representative. The therapist intentionally affirms Alex's in-session exercise of self-advocacy and honors their autonomy to decide whether and with whom they will share these aspects of themselves. Alex's requested changes are reasonable and flexible, and they deserve to experience a sense of belonging in their work environment without delay. As the work continues, the therapist devotes time during each session for Alex to share feedback about their experience of the therapeutic relationship, the process of working toward their goals, and their progress. In response to feedback, the clinician expresses gratitude and follows Alex's lead in co-constructing the path forward.

# Closing Thoughts

The intersection between feminism and disability as it pertains to counseling should focus on agency and autonomy. Autonomy looks different to different individuals. Bodily autonomy is a common overlap in the disability and feminist communities; reproductive rights including abortion, birth control, and other healthcare as well as wage gaps and theft and employment discrimination are intersections of identity for many disabled and nondisabled individuals, and as such they are important to be viewed in this context while counseling. The conditioned concept of "womanhood" often relies on "bodies that work as expected" (Webster, 2017). What happens when one doesn't fit that model? Feminism and feminist counseling must be able to shape itself to include the broad scope of disability as it pertains to differently abled people.

# What If?

What if bodies were not judged based on abilities but instead were all celebrated?

What if the concept of disability had never developed?

What if all public spaces were completely accessible?

What if all education took visible and invisible disabilities into account with all planning and implementation?

What if there were prominent leaders and role models in all societal areas who had disabilities?

# References

American Psychological Association. (2022). *APA guidelines for assessment and intervention with persons with disabilities.* https://www.apa.org/about/policy/guidelines-assessment-intervention-disabilities.pdf

APA Task Force on Guidelines for Assessment and Intervention with Persons With Disabilities. (2022). *APA guidelines for assessment and intervention with persons with disabilities.* American Psychological Association. https://www.apa.org/about/policy/guidelines-assessment-intervention-disabilities.pdf

Barrett, T. (2014). Disabled masculinities: A review and suggestions for further research. *Masculinities and Social Change, 3*(1), 36–61. http://doi.org/10.447/MCS.2014.41

Barnum, A. (2022, July 5). *The importance of mask making in art therapy.* https://barnumcounseling.com/2022/07/05/the-importance-of-mask-making-in-art-therapy

Blad, E. (2024, May 13). Retention is the missing ingredient in special education staffing. *Education Week.* https://www.edweek.org/leadership/retention-is-the-missing-ingredient-in-special-education-staffing/2024/05

Brodt, M., & Lewis, C. (2024). Beyond affirming: Expanding disability affirmative therapy using a case example. *Practice Innovations.* Advance online publication. https://doi.org/10.1037/pri0000249

Bureau of Labor Statistics. (2024). *Persons with a disability: Labor force characteristics—2023.* https://www.bls.gov/news.release/pdf/disabl.pdf

Centers for Disease Control and Prevention. (2024). *Disability datasets.* https://www.cdc.gov/ncbddd/disabilityandhealth/datasets.html

Chapin, M., McCarthy, H., Shaw, L., Bradham-Cousar, M., Chapman, R., Nosek, M., Peterson, S., Yilmaz, Z., & Ysasi, N. (2018). *Disability-related counseling competencies.* American Rehabilitation Counseling Association, a division of ACA. https://www.counseling.org/docs/default-source/competencies/arca-disability-related-counseling-competencies-v51519.pdf?sfvrsn=984f4bd0_1

Chen, R. K., Brodwin, M. G., Cardoso, E., & Chan, F. (2002). Attitudes toward people with disabilities in the social context of dating and marriage: A comparison of American, Taiwanese, and Singaporean college students. *Journal of Rehabilitation, 6*(4), 5–11.

Commission on Rehabilitation Counselor Certification. (2023). *Code of professional ethics for certified rehabilitation counselors.* Author. https://crccertification.com/wp-content/uploads/2023/04/2023-Code-of-Ethics.pdf

Dunn, D. S., & Andrews, E. E. (2015). Person-first and identity-first language: Developing psychologists' cultural competence using disability language. *American Psychologist, 70*(3), 255–264. https://doi.org/10.1037/a0038636

Evans, K. M., Kincade, E. A., & Seem, S. R. (2011). *Introduction to feminist therapy: Strategies for social and individual change.* SAGE.

Garland-Thomson, R. (2002). Integrating disability, transforming feminist theory. *NWSA Journal, 14*(3), 1–32. http://www.jstor.org/stable/4316922

Haegele, J. A., & Hodge, S. (2016). Disability discourse: Overview and critiques of the medical and social models. *Quest, 68*(2), 193–206. https://doi.org/10.1080/00336297.2016.1143849

Krahn, G. L., Walker, D. K., & Correa-De-Araujo, R. (2015). Persons with disabilities as an unrecognized health disparity population. *American Journal of Public Health, 105 Supplement 2,* S198-S206. https://doi.org/10.2105/AJPH.2014.302182

Lid, I. M. (2014). Universal design and disability: An interdisciplinary perspective. *Disability & Rehabilitation, 36*(16): 1344–1349. https://doi.org/10.3109/09638288.2014.931472

McConnell, E. A., & Minshew, R. (2023). Feminist therapy at the intersection of gender diversity and neurodiversity. *Women & Therapy, 46*(1), 36–57. https://doi.org/10.1080/02703149.2023.2189776

Mert Kastner, M. (2019). *Attitudes toward disabled people in the social context of dating, marriage, and work: Religiosity, religious orientation, conservatism and ambivalent sexism* [Unpublished master's thesis]. Middle East Technical University.

Miserandino, C. (2003). *The spoon theory*. https://butyoudontlooksick.com/articles/written-by-christine/the-spoon-theory

Moreno, J. L. (1943). Sociometry and the cultural order. *Sociometry, 6*(3), 299–344.

Nosek, M. A. (2010). Women's experience of disability. In R. G. Frank, M. Rosenthal, & B. Caplan (Eds.), *Handbook of rehabilitation psychology* (2nd ed., pp. 371–378). American Psychological Association. https://doi.org/10.1037/15972-025

Olkin, R. (2017). *Disability-affirmative therapy: A case formulation template for clients with disabilities*. Oxford University Press.

Olkin, R., Hayward, H. S., Abbene, M. S., & VanHeel, G. (2019). The experiences of microaggressions against women. *Journal of Social Issues, 75*(3), 757–785. https://doi.org/10.1111/josi.12342

Public Law 113–295 The Stephen Beck, Jr., Achieving a Better Life Experience Act (ABLE Act) – Enacted December 19, 2014

Retief, M., & Letšosa, R. (2018). Models of disability: A brief overview. *Theological Studies 74*(1), 1–8. https://doi.org/10.4102/hts.v74i1.4738

Rowan, K., McAlpine, D., & Blewett, L. (2013) Access and cost barriers to mental health care by insurance status, 1999 to 2010. *Health Affairs, 32*(10). https://doi.org/10.1377/hlthaff.2013.0133

Safer, A., Farmer, L., & Song, B. (2020). *Quantifying difficulties of university students with disabilities* (EJ1273641). ERIC. https://files.eric.ed.gov/fulltext/EJ1273641.pdf

Seo, W., & Chen, R. K. (2009). Attitudes of college students toward people with disabilities. *Journal of Applied Rehabilitation Counseling, 40*(4), 3–8.

Smith, T. J., Hugh, C., & Fontechia, S. (2023). Unemployment and underemployment of people with disabilities: An untapped resource within the global economy. *IntechOpen*. https://www.intechopen.com/online-first/1123171

Social Security Administration. (2024). *Spotlight on achieving a better life experience (ABLE) accounts*. https://www.ssa.gov/ssi/spotlights/spot-able.html

Sprague, J., & Hayes, J. (2000). Self-determination and empowerment: A feminist standpoint analysis of talk about disability. *American Journal of Community Psychology, 28*(5), 671–695. https://doi.org/10.1023/A:1005197704441

U. S. Census Bureau. (2022). *Disabled population in the United States*. https://www.census.gov/search-results.html?q=disability&page=1&stateGeo=none&searchtype=web&cssp=SERP&_charset_=UTF-8

Webster, L. (2017) The politics of being me. *Buzzfeed*. https://www.buzzfeed.com/lucywebster/how-feminism-informed-my-identity-as-a-disabled-woman

Williams, V. (2022). *47 years later, are we delivering on the promise of IDEA?* U.S. Department of Education. https://sites.ed.gov/osers/2022/11/47-years-later-are-we-delivering-on-the-promise-of-idea

World Health Organization. (Accessed 2024). *Disability*. https://www.who.int/health-topics/disability#tab=tab_1

# 18

# Feminist Intersectional Therapy: Empowered Aging for Older Adults

## Kathleen McCleskey, Mariah Moran, and Nicole Jackson Walker

*Patriarchal social, cultural, and political constructs value youth and often honor those who can earn money, are physically attractive, and can reproduce. Therefore, older adults can find themselves devalued, marginalized, and oppressed.*

Feminist therapy is foundationally concerned with examining issues of power and oppression and how those impact people's lives (Brown, 2018). Feminist therapists recognize that, in the United States, society is organized as a Eurocentric, heteronormative, Christian-dominant patriarchy where some social locations (White, cisgender male, heterosexual, Christian, young adult, able-bodied) are inherently privileged. In contrast, others (people of color, genders other than male, LGBTQ+, non-Christian, old, disabled) are marginalized. Therefore, a feminist therapist will take these patriarchal dynamics into account when thinking about a client's social location and cultural value of age.

Additionally, since the third wave of feminism, feminist therapy includes a focus on intersectionality, or the way that oppression of social identities is not simply additive but is rather exponential (Crenshaw, 1989). From this feminist intersectional framework, multiple social identities are not only considered singly; the nuanced way in which combinations of identities are experienced, perceived, and received must be examined and explored for privileges and marginalization that may impact the aging client. For example, a Chinese American, cisgender female elder, and a Caucasian, cisgender female elder are likely to have differing experiences of their racial, cultural, gender, and age-combined identities even though they may seem to share similar experiences of being older or of being female.

Being younger is prized in youth-oriented cultures like the United States (Berger, 2017). Being too old is not. Older adults may enjoy some privilege regarding financial stability, ability to retire, and breadth and depth of knowledge gained over their life thus far (Black & Stone, 2005). However, this is also a time when increasing disenfranchisement can begin.

In midlife and beyond, ageism can be seen in attitudes and behaviors toward older people (Berger, 2017; Brinkhof et al., 2022; Edström, 2018). This, coupled with the physical and systemic realities of aging means the latter half of life often includes multiple oppressions and marginalization. This chapter will explore how older age can be disempowering and how feminist therapists can work to help clients become more empowered as they age.

# Power/Lack of Power in Older Adults

## Middle Adulthood

Middle adulthood is the life stage before the final life stage of old age (Erikson, 1997). This stage of life is ambiguous as to when it begins and ends, though some consider it the span between ages 40 and 60 (Lachman et al., 2015). It has also become more varied in the last few decades related to opportunities, expectations, and media depictions (Chaudhuri, 2023). While historically, middle age adulthood used to be considered "old" by many, with a now longer overall life expectancy, this middle-aged adulthood stage of life is perceived as more productive. by comparison. This midlife period within the lifespan brings with it physical changes as well as social changes. Midlife is a time of rising gains in areas of happiness, knowledge, and emotional regulation; while at the same time, it is the start of declining physical and cognitive functioning (Lachman et al., 2015). During this time, people with uteruses will typically experience menopause, thereby losing the ability to have children, and people with penises will experience a decline in testosterone and a greater chance of problems with erections (Buehler, 2021). Socially, women may begin to feel invisible as their stereotypical attractiveness diminishes (Generation Menopause [GenM], 2021; Meagher, 2014), and heterosexual men may feel anxious about declining physical functioning. Intersectionally, appearance concerns for gay men (Lodge & Umberson, 2013) may have an even greater additional impact on a person Although there does not appear to be a common cause for all midlife crises, aging, itself, can be a cause (Lachman et al., 2015).

The lengthy period of midlife is also often a time of great role transition. Transitions that can occur during this time frame might include work transitions, parenting transitions as children are launched, caring for aging parents or relatives, and potentially looking toward retirement (Bateson, 2013; Chuang, 2019). Personal and social power in this stage can be both gained and lost. Financial stability may be attained, mastery can be gained in a job or career, successful parenting can be achieved, and recognition for these and other accomplishments may be acknowledged. At the same time, age-related health issues may begin to develop, and significant declines and losses may begin that continue into older adulthood, including deaths of significant persons and peers in an individual's life. Middle adulthood is a lengthy period in which people may peak in some life task areas and also begin to diminish in others. A feminist therapist helps a client understand their intersectional identities and transitioning social positioning to maximize their empowerment in navigating this middle adult stage.

## Older Adulthood

The transition from midlife into older adulthood can also be somewhat ambiguous. If one uses 60–65 years old as the beginning of older adulthood, then this last stage of aging may be the longest period of an individual's life. As of 2024, life expectancy in the United States is 80.2 years for females and 74.8 years for males (CDC, 2022), but many people live well beyond these ages, and the percentage of individuals who are 85 years or older is expected to be more than twice in 2040 than it was in 2022 (Administration on Aging, 2024). Additionally, projections indicate a swell of adults in U.S. society 65 years and older as baby boomers move into older adulthood, and this trend is predicted to continue for some time (Administration on Aging, 2024). Currently, no information on life expectancy is given by the CDC for transgender and nonbinary individuals.

A snapshot of current older adults can be gleaned from the Administration on Aging's 2023 annual report (published in 2024) on older Americans (where gender is reported as binary). In 2022, 17.3% of the U.S. population was 65 years of age or older; this number has increased 34% since 2012. Women outnumber men of all ages in this life stage, and the differences increase with age. Twenty-five percent of the elderly population identified as a racial minority, and that percentage is predicted to rise dramatically compared to White elders. More men in this life stage are married, and women are widowed at more than three times the rate of men. Many elders live with spouses, and many live alone (33% of women, and 22% of men), even when much older, when living alone becomes even more common; 1%–8% of elders live in nursing homes, with older people more likely to be in those settings.

Financially, older men have more resources than older women, with men having a median income of $37,430 compared to women's median of $24,630. Combined household incomes are higher if elders do not live alone. In 2022, just over 10% of older adults lived in poverty with another 4.7% at "near poor" levels. Poverty levels were lowest for non-Hispanic White elders (8.2%) and higher for Asian American elders (12.9%), Hispanic elders (16.9%), and African American elders (17.6%).

As can be seen, there are clear gender and racial disparities in income later in life, continuing earlier patterns throughout earning years. Older adults also spend more on health care costs than others; 13% of their spending is health care costs compared to 8% of spending for the total population. In terms of work, 19.2% of adults 65 years or older in 2023 were either currently employed or were actively trying to become employed.

In the last decades of life, many predictable losses occur. Typically, people will lose spouses, family members, and friends to death (Welzel et al., 2021). People are also more likely to lose aspects of their independence through physical aging, frailty, or health conditions (Administration on Aging, 2024). Many people need to give up driving as they age (Savoie et al., 2024), which greatly impacts independence and quality of life. Older adults typically retire during this stage or are no longer working full time (Administration on Aging, 2024). Additionally, some people may lose the ability to age in their homes. Separately, each of these losses can be profound—cumulatively, they can dissipate much of an individual's agency and autonomy.

There are also many gains in older adulthood. Even in very old age, older adults have been found to rate more gains than losses (Kaspar et al., 2023). In one study, only adults 90 years and older reported more developmental losses than gains, and even that seemed connected to institutional living (Kaspar et al., 2023). There can be growth found in relationships, in gaining knowledge, in understanding oneself, and in having a sense of personal freedom. As strategies, older adults may have adaptable goals (Kaspar et al., 2023) and/or use selective optimization with compensation (SOC) (Freund et al., 2017). In SOC, when resources (internal as well as external) are limited by aging, individuals select goals they are better able to achieve and use strategies to compensate in areas where goals are now harder to reach.

In older adulthood, Erikson (1950/1997) describes integrity as a sense of self-acceptance, contentment with life, and imminent death versus despair, or a lack of fulfillment or peace and the inability to come to terms with life, aging, and approaching death. Therefore, in embracing aging, people make meaning and find relief from suffering. Gerotranscendence describes a greater awareness of one's own life and connection to the universe, as well as a transcendent, perspective about life (Tornstam, 2005).

In gerotranscendence, a person may focus more on the abstract, such as spirituality or the passage of time; may experience a decrease in self-centeredness; and may focus more on connection with others. At the same time, the elder may also desire some withdrawal from the world, which is seen as natural even though societies and cultures may reject that notion. Gerotranscendence may be seen as enacting personal power to no longer center life around society and the world but instead to find a connection with greater and more meaningful things. Feminist therapists can help older adults discern how they make meaning of aging and empower them to examine and navigate how these gains and losses, new social positioning and gerotranscendence may or may not fit their current lived experiences.

## Stereotypes and Ageism

Stereotypes of older adulthood can include beliefs and attitudes of both younger people toward older people and also older people's beliefs toward aging. Stereotypes of elders can include both positive and negative attitudes and beliefs. North and Fiske (2013) studied differences between how older adults are viewed in terms of warmth and capability (descriptive), and how they are expected to behave (prescriptive). They found that older people were often rated as warm but incapable by younger raters, resulting in views of benevolent ageism. This changed in terms of elders who violated prescribed behaviors—they were rated negatively by younger raters resulting in views of hostile ageism. Younger raters had more negative reactions about these older individuals than any other age range (older, middle age, younger) did. The "violations" of expected behavior included not stepping aside from resources to make them available to younger people, taking up too many shared resources, including health-related resources, and trying to encroach on youth culture.

The "violation" of taking too many resources is perhaps illustrated in research about the COVID-19 pandemic. Flett and Heisel (2021) discuss the tensions during 2020 and 2021 between messages of protecting elders from COVID-19 and examples of elder neglect and abuse that were prevalent in news cycles. They concluded that, while purporting to want to protect elders and shield them from illness, actual actions to safeguard them fell short. Many needs of elders were not prioritized, even as they were dying at the highest rates, and this neglect conveyed to elders that they did not matter. Flett and Heisel (2021) report, "Indeed, some older people have wondered openly about exactly when they became disposable" (p. 2447). This divide between promoting positive messages about elders as a group (to the extent they are) and not immediately disrupting negative behaviors against that group illustrates how complex and deeply embedded oppressive norms can be, and how they impact people's lives.

Stereotypes of aging lead to ageist behaviors in different areas. Employment is one area where ageism has been documented and is connected to older adults' ideas of being less capable (Chasteen & Cary, 2015). Additionally, in a meta-review of global health outcomes research, Chang et al. (2020) found that ageism negatively impacted all four identified health structures which identified as not having access to health care, not being included in clinical trials, being devalued, and not having employment opportunities. Eleven specific health domains were identified within these structures where ageism was present and reported negative impacts on elders' mental health, quality of life, cognition, and longevity.

In addition, a stereotype threat occurs when an elder is exposed to a negative stereotype about elders and then confirms that stereotype behaviorally (see e.g., Brothers et al., 2021; Chasteen & Cary, 2015). For example, an elder who is told that older people tend to take too long to tell a story may become flustered and take longer than usual to tell a story, thereby confirming the stereotype. Stereotype threat has been found to have impacts on memory (Chasteen & Cary, 2015) and to be associated with worse physical health (Brothers et al., 2021).

Among other forms of marginalization, it is vital for feminist therapists to be versed in how isolation, neglect, and abuse of elders contribute to health outcomes (Teo et al., 2023). Incidences of abuse enacted upon the elderly are common and often overlooked (Yon et al., 2017). Elder abuse can be physical, psychological, financial, or sexual, and includes neglect and abandonment (U.S. Department of Justice, 2023). If working with elders, feminist therapists, along with all therapists should know the warning signs of elder abuse.

## Cultural Differences in Perspectives on Aging

There are cultural differences in how older adults are socially positioned and valued (Ackerman & Chopik, 2021; Fernandez-Ballesteros et al., 2020; Voss et al., 2018). This has resulted in dichotomous stereotypes that Western culture has negative views of old age and aging, while Asian or Indigenous cultures have more positive views. A negative stereotype might be that older adults are slow and that they create burdens as their health and mobility decline; the loss of their vitality and productivity is often viewed as embarrassing or a disappointment. On the other hand, a positive stereotype could be that older adults are more revered and valued for their wisdom gained over their lifespan.

Recent literature has confirmed differing cultural views of aging and older adults, but views are more intersectional and complex than these simple stereotypes suggest. In addition to intersectional identities, views on aging are also influenced by an interplay of multiple domains related to culture, such as family, friendships, autonomy, leisure, personality, finances, work, appearance, health, and fitness (De Paula Couto et al., 2022; Kornadt et al., 2020; Voss et al., 2018). For example, one culture may have positive views of older people related to finances and work and have negative views related to appearance and health. These cultural views on aging are partly developed due to socialization to family and broader cultural values (De Paula Couto et al., 2022). Furthermore, there is a suggestion of evidence that a rise in aging populations may be eroding traditionally positive views of elders in some Eastern countries, while some Western countries may hold more positive views of elders than previously assumed (North & Fiske, 2013).

Remembering that all these culturally and politically socialized views of older adults in the United States are also greatly influenced by the larger culture couched in Eurocentric, heteronormative, Christian-dominant, patriarchal norms, there is much grist for the feminist therapist. It is the examination of these often oppressive social values that creates an avenue to working with clients who may be grappling with aging or older adulthood. A feminist therapeutic perspective when working with clients who are aging is uniquely individualized through an intersectional lens, subjective in understanding the client's narrative and lived experiences, and honored with high esteem for the wisdom they possess in their own expertise about their lives.

For example, a 70-year-old Japanese American navigates the cultural values of American geopolitical and economic structures while also having a family cultural heritage of Japanese values. The American economic structures value autonomy, independence, self-sufficiency, financial success, upward social mobility, and dedication to work. The family cultural heritage may value collective responsibility, interdependency, cooperation, dedication to work, and financial success not to elevate one person, but to elevate the social standing and wealth of the entire family. It is the intersection and integration of these values for this older adult that must be further examined collaboratively with the feminist therapist in clinical practice.

A feminist therapeutic approach might examine the following topics: How do these personal cultural values shape their view of themselves? How might they clash with the traditional Eurocentric, heteronormative, Christian-dominant, and patriarchal social norms? What might empowerment and navigating with agency look like in older age?

### Transgender and Nonbinary Elders

There is a limited body of information about how the aging process impacts transgender/nonbinary (TNB) individuals. Two important aspects of aging for TNB individuals are that not all these elders may be "out" as TNB (Knochel & Seelman, 2020) and that TNB people have faced and continue to face discrimination (Witten, 2014). TNB elders of today have likely faced a lifetime of lack of marginalization, oppression, and even rejection. They may or may not have accessed gender-affirming care; if they did, they may have experienced discrimination from systems of care (Witten, 2014). Transgender individuals, specifically, have been shown to have a higher risk of mortality, and, as part of that, a higher rate of suicide and homicide (Jackson et al., 2023).

Knochel and Seelman (2020) discuss several issues that may be particularly salient for TNB elders. If individuals would like to receive gender-affirming surgery as older adults, there may be other health issues that complicate that process. If a person does transition, they may then identify to others as cisgender; in such a situation, the person could be "outed" as transgender if living in a care facility where physical care is given. Some elders may feel too old to try to receive gender-affirming care at all. In addition, health disparities that existed before older age continue in this stage, and TNB elders may anticipate receiving bias in care. End-of-life issues may be complicated by shifting legal identities, and there may be a lack of end-of-life planning for some. TNB older adults also report more mental health issues than other older adults. Feminist therapists should be aware of these unique potential intersectional biases that TNB adults may face as they age. Feminist therapists acknowledge and examine the possible complications and dangers that may exist for this population while empowering, navigating, and advocating within oppressive systems that often injure them.

## Feminist Intersectional Therapy Healing Factors for Aging and Older Adults

Feminist intersectional healing factors are explorations to raise consciousness, empower people, and advocate with/for clients for resisting social, cultural and political oppressions. Healing factors move people toward wellness. For those in midlife and beyond, specific oppressions must be taken into consideration such as stigma, stereotypes, and ageism. What does it mean to be empowered in aging? What are optimal ways to experience life as one continues to age? How do clients ultimately want to navigate from the latter part of their lives, including their deaths?

It is predictable that aging will often cause marginalization and oppression in some parts of life; therefore, the feminist therapist aims to help clients identify where they currently hold power and agency, where they may lose power and agency, and how to balance power so they retain as much autonomy as possible. Some of the work to help individuals age as they choose can begin decades earlier, in midlife. Feminist therapists can be proactive with younger clients by bringing up areas of life where power imbalances currently exist and how that may evolve in later years. For clients currently in midlife and older adulthood, examining all areas of power and autonomy may prove crucial for elder life satisfaction.

For a feminist therapist, one aspect of exploring autonomy and power in later life is to help clients recognize what they can control and what they cannot. Physical problems, illnesses, and losses may or may not be preventable or treatable. Clients' lives may be altered over time through loss of independence. Still, within each area of potentially lost autonomy, there are still choices. Feminist therapists can assist clients in discerning current choices and potential future decisions, can collaboratively explore options and make plans for the future, and can help empower them to advocate for autonomy in situations where their agency is threatened.

There is no situation where empowerment and agency are more important than in end-of-life issues and planning. Elders may seek input from medical providers, caregivers, family members, friends, and others, about serious health matters. Feminist therapists can assist people in midlife and beyond (or earlier) in considering end-of-life issues, wishes, and plans. These may include financial, spiritual, medical, moral, or cultural aspects of concerns; the feminist therapist should develop a good feminist network of providers in these areas that can be referral sources for clients. All referral sources should be vetted to provide unbiased, client-centered, culturally responsive, antiracist support.

In addition to issues of power and autonomy, the other area common in midlife and beyond is meaning-making (Erikson, 1950/1997). Feminist therapists can collaboratively, with older adults, examine life events through a feminist framework of societal, cultural, and patriarchal contexts around meaning-making. Meaning-making can occur in many areas of midlife and beyond—understanding life transitions, personal impacts, leaving a legacy, losses, and so on. As stated before, older adults often face multiple losses including loss of partners, siblings, peers, work life, independence, and health, as well as an anticipated loss associated with their own mortality. The experience of grief in older adulthood is almost guaranteed. Meaning-making can be a central concept in understanding the process of grief. With a feminist therapist, clients in midlife and older can examine meaning-making through a feminist intersectional lens of privilege and oppression to explore what an empowered future may entail.

# An Intersectional Feminist Model with Aging Older Adults

This is one conceptualization of a feminist intersectional model for feminist clinicians working with older adults. It is not intended to be utilized in steps or stages but left to the clinical creativity of the feminist therapist to use all or some parts of this feminist intersectional model.

## Transparency and Validation

Feminist therapists working with older adults maintain the same feminist underpinnings of transparency, egalitarianism, and power sharing. Feminist therapists may begin this process with therapeutic self-disclosure by using broaching to determine whether sharing their ages, intersectional identities, and stages of life might hold therapeutic value for the client. Although age is often apparent to one another, the transparency of stating this openly acknowledges the possible commonalities, yet unique intersectional differences between therapist and client may set the tone of egalitarianism and power sharing. Additionally, feminist therapists can also explain their approach regarding the egalitarian relationship, power sharing, and power monitoring that will be part of the therapy.

## Normalizing Aging without Marginalization

Clients may come to therapy to work on issues around aging, or they may come for other presenting problems and aging is in the background of the issue. Either way, feminist therapists can normalize the aging process and acknowledge any challenges or fears about aging. It is important to model (if age-appropriate) or discuss behavior of empowered aging and be mindful not to dismiss clients' concerns by pointing out that everyone experiences the same things. It may be useful to understand how this particular client and their intersectional identity view this aging process, and how it relates to the presenting problem. This normalization without marginalization can continue throughout the duration of the therapy.

## Reviewing Power in Previous Life Stages

Clients' presenting concerns can, as in any other feminist counseling, be primarily focused on current experiences. Yet, in the transitional stages of midlife and older adulthood, echoes of power from previous stages may also be present. It may be helpful to see if and how current issues are related to previous stages and if they follow or diverge from previous empowerment or disempowerment patterns. Family relationships, for example, can shift over these stages, and adult children can become caretakers or helpers for their parents. How relationships functioned in earlier stages may impact role shifts and power in the present. A power analysis may help to contextualize present issues not only related to power within societal, cultural, and patriarchal systems but also examining those systemic impacts of privilege and oppression over the life cycle.

## Examining Intersectional Identities

Whatever issues and concerns clients in midlife and older adulthood bring into therapy, it can be helpful to examine their current identities and beliefs through an intersectional lens. An intersectional power analysis might help the feminist therapist to examine how intersectional social locations of gender, race, ethnicity, ability, religion, affectional orientation, socioeconomc status (SES), and the like, are also intersecting with the social location of age. Understanding the historical and possibly personal legacy of privilege and oppression that the client has experienced may help raise their consciousness and empower the client with this awareness.

## Striving for Empowerment

As stated before, these mid and older stages in life will likely contain transitions and losses in addition to gains. As clients age, they are more likely to interact with systems such as Social Security and Medicare, as well as health care systems. Some of these systems may be or may feel disempowering for clients. Feminist therapists can work with to help empower clients to navigate these complicated and potentially oppressive systems they may encounter.

In addition, power may be shifting in many of their ecosystem relationships. For an adult in midlife who is caring for a parent, there may be ways in which each feels empowered and each feels disempowered. Likewise, within their employment or community, marginalization may begin to feel disempowering. A feminist therapist can work with clients to navigate power sharing in family and community relationships and help clients advocate for themselves.

## Advocacy

There are many opportunities for feminist and social justice advocacy with aging clients (with permission) and on behalf of clients. Together or separately, clients and therapists can advocate for increased services and treatments for older adults, including mental health care, transportation support, and social support. Feminist therapists can dispute negative stereotypes of aging now in professional arenas, and in personal arenas, should they choose. Feminist therapists can also be proactive about modeling and emphasizing positive aspects of aging by having posters, books, and/or films in their professional environment that portray positive older role models. Posters/artwork would be inclusive of all genders. Feminist therapists can also seek out "aging mentors" who could be available to connect with others who struggle with aspects of aging. Aging mentors could be elders who have successfully navigated some of the life changes previously discussed, and who have remained, or become, empowered in later life. Lastly, feminist therapists could find or help create events that promote positive aging, wisdom-sharing meetings, "owning the crone," and so on, perhaps partnering with senior service programs.

# Feminist Intersectional Applications for Empowered Aging

## Feminist Intersectional Consciousness Raising

With this technique, the goal of the therapist is to increase clients' awareness of how social, political, and cultural influences impact the client's current beliefs and behaviors. With this awareness, clients can be more empowered to review their current and former life stages in a patriarchal contextual manner with the hopes of understanding how they came to these beliefs or behaviors and whether they would like to maintain them. To implement this technique, the therapist can work with the client to generate all possible intersectional identities of the client, including (but not limited to) age, race, ethnicity, ability, affectional orientation, religion, spirituality, and so forth. The client can then identify the intersections of their identities, and can point to which intersecting identities are most important to them now, and which may have been important in the past. Raising consciousness about intersectional identities and the privileges, and oppressions that may be associated with each one not only raises consciousness and gives more knowledge and power to the client but can also set the stage to bring those intersections into other techniques or therapeutic work.

## Intersectional Power Analysis

A power analysis is a central technique from the early development of feminist therapy, and this addition of intersectional identities within power analysis serves as a more accurate understanding of the complications of social privilege and oppression. In this analysis, the client can identify people and organizations they interact with and rate on a Likert-type scale how much power they perceive they have in the relationship and how much the other person or systemic entity has, considering the intersectional identities they already identified. Do they perceive equal power, greater power, or less power with each person/system in their ecosystem? For example, does an older adult perceive having less power with their adult child caregiver because of being dependent on them? What is the power balance with doctors, managed care companies, spouses, children, the Social Security Administration, and so on?

When conducting an intersectional power analysis with an older adult, the feminist therapist should be mindful to consider factors such as ageism, ableism, and limitations that result from normative life experiences such as limited mobility. An intersectional power analysis might help identify areas where clients may benefit from self-advocacy as well as deciding which assertiveness skills may be most empowering to navigate the future.

## Gaining Recognition of Power through Language

The feminist therapist models and collaborates with clients to help them identify effective communication skills related to power. For example, the therapist can encourage the use of "power" statements. These statements can be framed in the following format: "When I (fill in the blank), I, standing in my power, feel (fill in the blank)." Clients could also examine, "I feel no power when I (fill in the blank)". By regularly framing dialogues in this manner, feminist therapists can help clients gain insight into when power is absent or lacking in their lives.

## Navigating Non-negotiable Power Structures

Power for anyone is not without limits. Although the goals of feminist therapy are for empowerment, there can be some situations that are so oppressive that they cannot be overcome—at least for now. This clinical application of navigation might be used when equal power cannot be shared, as when an aging person is no longer capable of being fully independent because of declining mental or physical acuity and needs caregiving. Navigating and negotiating power from a dependent position is critical to ensure the older adult retains as much agency and autonomy as possible. Having power for a client in these circumstances could include a powerful voice in the decision-making process around their care, their future, and their lifestyle. Even if caretakers have the authority to make decisions on behalf of the elder, the elder should be an active part of the process so that although unequal in decision-making, the process allows the elder to be overruled but not unheard.

## Gerotranscendence as Personal Power

Feminist therapists can use psychoeducation to teach elders about integrity, despair, and gerotranscendence (Erikson, 1997). When describing gerotranscendence, Erikson (1997) stated,

I have found that "transcendence" becomes much more alive if it is activated into "transcen*dance*" which speaks to the soul and the body and challenges it to rise above the dystonic, clinging aspects of our worldly existence that burden and distract us from true growth and aspiration. (p. 127)

Clients and therapists can collaboratively deconstruct burdensome worldly concepts of aging and healthy transen*dance* approaches to death, and where anxiety or fear is empowering or disempowering. Clients can explore any dimensions of gerotranscendence they connect to and what is meaningful to them while gaining a sense of freedom and power.

## Assertiveness Skill-Building

Assertiveness is another underpinning of feminist therapy. It allows for people to take personal power and responsibility in their lives. Identifying how people currently seek power (e.g., passive-aggression, internalizing, self-destruction, aggression, not seeking power at all, or giving up power, etc.) is the first part of each client's process toward assertiveness. A feminist therapist will assist aging persons, often socially and personally overlooked or ignored, to practice assertiveness skills to achieve more agency and autonomy.

## Smash the Patriarchy Question

The "Smash the Patriarchy" question can be a version of "If there were no social, political, or cultural forces acting upon me any longer, I would (fill in the blank)." This question allows people to explore their wants and needs related to aging that are limited by social, cultural, and political norms, constructs, expectations, stereotypes, ageism, and so on. This projective question helps clients identify an ideal world free of constraints that can highlight where they are experiencing deficits in power, choice, and/or meaning.

## Dealing with Grief and Loss

As loss is an expected part of aging, particularly in older adulthood, clinical understanding and of grief and loss is essential for feminist therapists working with this population. The feminist therapist can help a client consider how their intersectional identities impact experiences of loss. As with other feminist analyses, grief rituals can be collaboratively analyzed to prioritize the ones clients identify as most healing and empowering. Feminist therapists may offer cultural traditions or abandon tradition in favor of individual preference for mourning processes. Collaboratively crafting mourning rituals could be deeply meaningful and empowering for clients.

# Feminist Intersectional Applied Case Study

Landon (African American, 86, male) and his White female partner have been together since 1960; they fell in love when interracial marriage was not largely accepted. They never got married, but cohabitated until his partner fell ill with dementia and was moved to a nursing home, where she passed away at the age of 72. They had one child, Amina (African American and White, female), who is now 58. Landon is currently seeking treatment for depressive symptoms. Landon is currently in the last stage of his life and is experiencing a rapid physical decline. He is no longer driving or able to walk without a walker. His night vision is not good, and he is not comfortable going out at night. He now lives with his daughter. The feminist therapist, Julie (age 60, White), hopes she can assist Landon with exploring current and past power in his life, while also considering where he is in terms of integrity and gerotranscendence.

During **Transparency and Validation**, Landon and Julie begin to meet. Julie explains the process of therapy, some of her methodologies and the egalitarian nature of the relationship; she also self-discloses her own age of 60 years. Landon mentions that Julie is close in age to his daughter Amina. Julie acknowledges this and suggests they keep track of any ways in which this age difference helps or hinders their work. Julie works to flatten the hierarchical nature of the therapist/client relationship by asking Landon for his input on presenting concerns of depression, diminishing health, and loss of his partner. She mentions that he is the expert in his life, and her role is to add new dimensions to his experiences to see if he would like to make changes or not. She ensures that the office space is comfortable and accessible for him and his walker. She assures him they will schedule appointments during times when he has transportation. She checks in to make sure that they are focusing on what Landon wants to discuss.

In **Normalizing Aging**, a primary consideration is the notion that gains and loss of power and identity often emerge from aging. Landon identifies his therapeutic issues as arising from aging and loss. Because of this, in the **Review Power in Previous Life Stages**, the feminist intersectional consciousness raising exercise is used to help him consider how his intersectional identities have been impacted by social norms, messages, and expectations over his lifetime. As Landon reflects on his childhood and early adulthood, he can recall the oppression caused by segregation and racism. He was unable to marry his partner, and when interracial marriage became legal, he and his partner opted against it because of opposition from the families.

His intersectional identity as a Black, heterosexual, Baptist, able-bodied man was salient through much of his work life as he recalls struggles to obtain work sufficient to care for his family despite being a skilled laborer. During his parenting years, he recalls the challenges that resulted from having a biracial daughter who was quite light-skinned and often assumed not to be his daughter. There were occasional incidents when White people seemed suspicious about a Black man being with what they saw as a young White girl. He felt angry at these moments but also disempowered to show his anger, attempting not to feed into the existing stereotypes about Black men. He recalls frustration about relying on his wife's income, since she was able to secure a higher wage, and how this led him to feel "emasculated." He recalls being criticized for being with a White woman and experiencing rejection by both the Black and White communities.

Later in life, when his partner fell ill, he recalled the many struggles with being her healthcare proxy and not "being taken seriously." Now as he is aging, he too claims to "not be taken seriously." He believes his health care providers to be dismissive of his complaints and felt the system saw him as less valuable than a White counterpart. He experiences deep grief over the loss of his partner, and many other friends and family members. His daughter will no longer allow him to drive himself, despite being able to see still during the day. He lives with his daughter and misses the autonomy he had, often feeling like a burden to her.

In **Examining Intersectional Identities**, Julie asks Landon to list all his identities and to name them. He identifies as being Black, male, older, and having limited mobility (but not disabled). Julie explains the concept of intersectionality to Landon and asks him about which identities are core intersections for him now or in the past. Landon identifies the intersectional identities of race, gender, and age are most salient to Landon's identity now, and intersections of race and gender as salient in the past.

As part of their work together, Julie asks Landon if he wants to spend some time talking about grief and loss. He wants to talk particularly about the loss of his partner and the loss he experienced while her dementia worsened in the time before she died. In addressing **Dealing with Grief and Loss**, Landon identifies that visiting her grave brings him comfort because he talks to her there, but he is not religious and does not find it helpful to go to church to seek comfort there. He and Julie process ideas about whether he can create his own rituals to mourn. In these discussions, Landon has an idea to create a playlist of songs that mark different points in their lives together. He finds working on this to be both sad and uplifting.

In **Striving for Empowerment**, Landon identifies wanting to work on his relationship with Amina. He is struggling with feeling old and disempowered. Amina is protective of him, but he thinks she does not see what he is still capable of doing. In doing an intersectional power analysis, Landon, interestingly, is able to identify having equal power to Amina much of the time but cites times when she "puts her foot down" and gets frustrated. In response to the Smash the Patriarchy question, Landon replies that he would want to live with his daughter but maintain the right to come and go as he pleases and not have her worry so much. He further states that ideally, his doctors would listen to him when he complains of pain and not write it off as "just part of aging." Julie and Landon work on a combination of **Gaining Recognition of Power** and **Assertiveness Skill-Building** to practice how Landon can work with Amina to feel more of a power balance in their relationship, and how he can talk to his medical providers to treat his concerns seriously.

In order to further Landon's sense of personal power, Julie asks if they can shift their goal toward discussions around gerotranscendence. They explore Landon's connection to spirituality. Landon examines his thoughts about death and feels resolute and comforted in his belief in an afterlife. Landon, who is a gifted carpenter, begins to teach his grandson his skills, and soon finds that he still has a great deal to offer to others. He agrees to join the local senior center and connect with others. After a few weeks, Landon addresses **Advocacy** by becoming a consumer representative at the senior center, advocating for fair treatment of his friends.

Over time, Landon's depressive symptoms lift as he reflects on his life. He acknowledges the many struggles that he has encountered and understands that there were many areas of oppression that limited him throughout his life. He celebrates his triumph even more in the fortitude of loving his partner despite society's bias toward them, and he is proud of their ability to raise a well-adjusted daughter. He acknowledges all that he has to give to others, and enjoys friendships, some autonomy, and his new ability to be assertive and to advocate for himself and others.

# What If?

What if the social positioning of the United States put the elders in the highest esteem due to their wisdom?

What if social norms dictated that decisions could not be made without consulting family or community elders?

What if, culturally and socially, life was valued based on wisdom as opposed to economic success?

What if gender roles and expectations did not serve to shame, emasculate, or label people based on career choices or economic successes?

What if people could live their entire lives in the freedom of "gerotransecdance"?

# References

Ackerman, L. S., & Chopik, W. J. (2021). Cross-cultural comparisons in implicit and explicit age bias. *Personality and Social Psychology Bulletin, 47*(6), 953–968.

Adler, A. (1938). *Social interest: A challenge to mankind.* Faber & Faber.

Administration on Aging. (2024). *2023 profile of older Americans.* https://acl.gov/sites/default/files/Profile%20of%20OA/ACL_ProfileOlderAmericans2023_508.pdf

Bateson, M. C. (2013). Changes in the life course: Strengths and stages. In C. Lynch & J. Danely (Eds.), *Cultural perspectives on aging and the life course.* Berghahn Books.

Berger, R. (2017). Aging in America: Ageism and general attitudes toward growing old and the elderly. *Open Journal of Social Sciences, 5,* 183–198. https://doi.org/10.4236/jss.2017.58015

Black, L. L., & Stone, D. (2005). Expanding the definition of privilege: The concept of social privilege. *Journal of Multicultural Counseling and Development, 33*(4), 243–255. https://doi.org/10.1002/j.2161-1912.2005.tb00020.x

Brinkhof, L. P., de Wit, S., Murre, J. M. J., Krugers, H. J., & Ridderinkhof, K. R. (2022) The subjective experience of ageism: The Perceived Ageism Questionnaire (PAQ). *International Journal of Environmental Research and Public Health, 19*(14), 8792. https://doi.org/10.3390/ijerph19148792

Brothers, A., Kornadt, A. E., Nehrkorn-Bailey, A., Wahl, H. W., & Diehl, M. (2021). The effects of age stereotypes on physical and mental health are mediated by self-perceptions of aging. *The Journals of Gerontology. Series B, Psychological Sciences and Social Sciences, 76*(5), 845–857. https://doi.org/10.1093/geronb/gbaa176

Brown, L. S. (2018). *Feminist therapy* (2nd ed.). American Psychological Association.

Buehler, S. (2021). *What every mental health professional needs to know about sex* (3rd ed.). Springer.

Chang, E. S., Kannoth, S., Levy, S., Wang, S. Y., Lee, J. E., & Levy, B. R. (2020). Global reach of ageism on older persons' health: A systematic review. *PLoS ONE, 15*(1), e0220857. https://doi.org/10.1371/journal.pone.0220857

Chasteen, A. L., & Cary, L. A. (2015). Age stereotypes and age stigma: Connections to research on subjective aging. In M. Diehl & H.-W. Wahl (Eds.), *Subjective aging: New developments and future directions* (pp. 99–119). Annual Review of Gerontology and Geriatrics. Springer Publishing Company.

Chaudhuri, A. (2023, Feb. 16). *Whatever happened to middle age? The mysterious case of the disappearing life stage.* https://www.theguardian.com/science/2023/feb/16/whatever-happened-to-middle-age-the-mysterious-case-of-the-disappearing-life-stage

Chuang, S. (2019). Generation Xers' performance and development in midlife transition. *Human Resource Development International, 22*(1), 101–112. https://doi.org/10.1080/13678868.2018.1440130

Crenshaw, K. (1989). Demarginalizing the intersection of race and sex: A black feminist critique of antidiscrimination doctrine, feminist theory and antiracist politics. *University of Chicago Legal Forum, 139*(1), 139–167. https://chicagounbound.uchicago.edu/cgi/viewcontent.cgi?article=1052&context=uclf

De Paula Couto, C., Ostermeier, R., & Rothermund, K. (2022). Age differences in age stereotypes: The role of life domain and cultural context. *GeroPsych: The Journal of Gerontopsychology and Geriatric Psychiatry, 35*(4), 177–188.

Edström, M. (2018). Visibility patterns of gendered ageism in the media buzz: A study of the representation of gender and age over three decades. *Feminist Media Studies, 18*(1), 77–93. https://doi.org/10.1080/14680777.2018.1409989

Erikson, E. H. (1997). *Childhood and society.* W. W. Norton. (Original work published 1950)

Erikson, J. M. (1997). *The life cycle completed*. W. W. Norton.

Fernandez-Ballesteros, R., Olmos, R., Perez-Ortiz, L., & Sanchez-Izquierdo, M. (2020). Cultural aging stereotypes in European countries: Are they a risk to active aging? *PLoS ONE, 15*(5): e0232340. https://doi.org/10.1371/journal.pone.0232340

Flett, G. L., & Heisel, M. J. (2021). Aging and feeling valued versus expendable during the COVID-19 pandemic and beyond: A review and commentary of why mattering is fundamental to the health and well-being of older adults. *International Journal of Mental Health and Addiction, 19*(6), 2443–2469. https://doi.org/10.1007/s11469-020-00339-4

Freund, A., Napolitano, C., & Knecht, M. (2017). Life management through selection, optimization, and compensation. In N. A. Pachana (Ed.), *Encyclopedia of geropsychology*. Springer. https://doi.org/10.1007/978-981-287-082-7_130

Generation Menopause. (n.d.) *The GenM invisibility report*. https://gen-m.com/wp-content/uploads/2021/09/106847-Gen-M-Invisibility-Report-082.pdf

Jackson, S. S., Brown, J., Pfeiffer, R. M., Shrewsbury, D., O'Callaghan, S., Berner, A. M., Gadalla, S. M., & Shiels, M. S. (2023). Analysis of mortality among transgender and gender diverse adults in England. *JAMA Network Open, 6*(1), e2253687. https://doi.org/10.1001/jamanetworkopen.2022.53687

Kaspar, R., Wahl, H. W., & Diehl, M. (2023). Awareness of age-related gains and losses in a national sample of adults aged 80 years and older: Cross-sectional associations with health correlates. *Innovation in Aging, 7*(4), 1–10. https://doi.org/10.1093/geroni/igad044

Knochel, K. A., & Seelman, K. (2020). Understanding and working with transgender/nonbinary older adults. In S. K. Kattari (Ed.), *Social work and health care practice with transgender and nonbinary individuals and communities: Voices for equity, inclusion, and resilience* (pp. 120–133). Routledge. https://www.taylorfrancis.com/books/9780429443176

Kornadt, A. E., Hess, T. M., & Rothermund, K. (2020). Domain specific views on aging and preparation for age-related changes: Development and validation of three brief scales. *Journals of Gerontology: Psychological Sciences, 56*(2), 303–307.

Lachman, M. E., Teshale, S., & Agrigoroaei, S. (2015). Midlife as a pivotal period in the life course: Balancing growth and decline at the crossroads of youth and old age. *International Journal of Behavioral Development, 39*, 20–31. https://doi.org/10.1177/0165025414533223

Lodge, A. C., & Umberson, D. (2013). Age and embodied masculinities: Midlife gay and heterosexual men talk about their bodies. *Journal of Aging Studies, 27*(3), 225–232. https://doi.org/10.1016/j.jaging.2013.03.004

Meagher, M. (2014). Against the invisibility of old age: Cindy Sherman, Suzy Lake, and Martha Wilson. *Feminist Studies, 40*(1), 101–143. https://doi.org/10.1353/fem.2014.0023

North, M. S., & Fiske, S. T. (2013). Act your (old) age: Prescriptive, ageist biases over succession, consumption, and identity. *Personality and Social Psychology Bulletin, 39*(6), 720–734. https://doi.org/10.1177/0146167213480043

Savoie, C., Voyer, P., Lavallière, M., & Bouchard, S. (2024). Transition from driving to driving-cessation: Experience of older persons and caregivers: A descriptive qualitative design. *BMC Geriatrics, 24*(1), 219. https://doi.org/10.1186/s12877-024-04835-3

Teo, R. H., Cheng, W. H., Cheng, L. J., Lau, Y., & Lau, S. T. (2023). Global prevalence of social isolation among community-dwelling older adults: A systematic review and meta-analysis. *Archives of Gerontology and Geriatrics, 107*, 104904. https://doi.org/10.1016/j.archger.2022.104904

Tornstam, L. (2005). *Gerotranscendence—A developmental theory of positive aging*. Springer.

U.S. Centers for Disease Control and Prevention. (2022). *Life expectancy*. https://www.cdc.gov/nchs/fastats/life-expectancy.htm

U.S. Department of Justice. (n.d.). *Red flags of elder abuse*. https://www.justice.gov/elderjustice/red-flags-elder-abuse

Voss, P., Kornadt, A. E., Hess, T. M., Fung, H. H., & Rothermund, K. (2018). A world of difference? Domain-specific views on aging in China, the US, and Germany. *Psychology and Aging, 33*(4), 595–606. https://doi.org/10.1037/pag0000237

Welzel, F. D., Löbner, M., Quittschalle, J., Pabst, A., Luppa, M., Stein, J., & Riedel-Heller, S. G. (2021). Loss and bereavement in late life (60+): Study protocol for a randomized controlled trial regarding an internet-based self-help intervention. *Internet Interventions*, 26, 100451. https://doi.org/10.1016/j.invent.2021.100451

Witten, T. M. (2014). It's not all darkness: Robustness, resilience, and successful transgender aging. *LGBT Health*, 1(1), 24–33. https://doi.org/10.1089/lgbt.2013.0017

Yon, Y. Y., Mikton, C. R., Gassoumis, Z. D., & Wilber, K. H. (2017). Elder abuse prevalence in community settings: A systematic review and meta-analysis. *Lancet Glob Health*. 5(2):e147–e156. https://doi.org/10.1016/S2214-109X(17)30006-2

# 19

# Feminist Intersectional Theory and Privileged Identities

*Joanne Jodry, Kathleen McCleskey, Nicole Jackson Walker, and Ashley Krompier*

*"Privilege" is often a trigger word for the privileged.*

## Social Location Privilege

What is privilege? Brown (2018) defines privilege as "[a] construct that calls attention to how certain social locations systemically confer on those situated in their experiences of power, access to resources, and promises of protection from harm, all of which are unearned" (p. 50). Brown (2018) also suggested that some intersectional identities that experience higher social value and privilege include European descent, which is often associated with having White skin, being heterosexual, being male, having Christian faith, and having a middle-class or higher social status. In addition to these social location privileges, there are many "norms" and "right" ways of being that society grants hierarchical power to, including but not limited to physical ability, "beauty" and health, body type and shape, prestigious educational opportunities, and family legacies and geography with associated wealth, and so on.

These are complicated multiple intersections of privilege and oppression that impact each person's unique identities, and the subsequent value assigned by society. All aspects of social, cultural, and political norms and existing social systems (legal, educational, medical, etc.) are based on these Eurocentric, heteronormative, Christian-dominant, patriarchal norms. People whose identities, thoughts, and beliefs align with these dominant norms are considered to have a social advantage over those who do not align. Those whose identities, thoughts, and beliefs are different from the norms are often marginalized, oppressed, and/or rejected by society, which may impact their psychology and suffering.

# Sociology and Psychology

Many people find it difficult to disagree conceptually with the feminist, multicultural, and social justice desire for equality and equity for all people. So, where is the social natural resistance to creating this ideal society where everyone is seen as equal and equal opportunities are offered to all people without bias, prejudice, and discrimination? Consider the answer through the lens of psychological reactions for which the feminist therapist may be able to have some impact and raise higher consciousness.

One way to think about how people process information is through personal ego realities. The ego organizes the person's reality and decides what to do with new information based on their existing ego system realities (Safran, 2012). One potential automatic ego reaction when hearing about concepts of privilege is for the ego to defend the person's reality by thinking, "I'm not privileged," "I have worked for everything I have," "I did not have it easy," "Other people just want a handout," or "Anyone can work hard and succeed; they are just lazy." Another way to think about this could be the assimilation/accommodation model, where people first try to add new information to existing cognitive schemas and only create new schemas when information cannot fit into an existing one (Cherry, 2023). A person could experience disequilibrium when confronted with concepts of privilege but assimilate the information into current belief structures that privilege does not exist. Such automatic reactions, embedded in patriarchal messages to deny privilege, are common (Knowles et al., 2014; Phillips & Lowery, 2015).

Essentially, sociological concepts of equality and equity become psychologically analyzed through the individual, and the conversation is often stopped due to individual natural psychological resistance. Therefore, someone who may be more privileged than oppressed may resist the concept to such a degree that they will never realize their privilege. This defensiveness can be conscious or unconscious. This natural resistance could be conceptualized as a defensive mechanism against the ego's reality of the ideal self that will not allow the knowledge of the self to be challenged, or as a way to remain in cognitive equilibrium.

Notwithstanding one's privileged or oppressive identity, it is natural for many, if not all, people developing in early life to automatically accept society's embedded messages and norms, no matter how unbalanced they may be, hoping to gain favor or privilege. So many children and subsequent adults move through educational and employment systems, assimilating to unequal, disadvantaged norms in attempts to fit in with the privileged. Therefore, it is natural not to want to give up any perceived favor that one has gained by being the "proof" that anyone can do it if they work hard enough. Once the assimilated beliefs of the oppressive society are embedded, they are hard to challenge because they could threaten the entire self-concept. Hardy (2023) discussed how this belief that "anyone can do it" often leads to internalized devaluation of the oppressed, marginalized people who cannot succeed in the oppressive system, which can also lead to racial trauma.

Additionally, some people react to concepts of privilege as oppression. There are some people who might feel that White males are the most disadvantaged group because of the gender and race affirmative action and equal pay legislation that has attempted to create more equality and equity in society. For example, when the Black Lives Matter (BLM) movement began in 2013, there was a swift social rebuttal of *All Lives Matter* and *Blue Lives Matter* and *Red Lives Matter*, and so on. Why? The Black Lives Matter mission, as stated on their website, "[i]s working inside and outside of the system to heal the past, reimagine the present, and invest in the future of Black lives through policy change, investment in our communities, and a commitment to arts and culture" (BLM, n.d., para 2). What makes this feel so oppressive to White people that they need to rebut the desire for equality and equal social value? Of course, all lives matter, but the point was that historically and presently, society does not view Black lives as mattering equally and is trying to create equality and justice. The automatic psychological resistance to this social concept of equality is again met with an arguably organic, natural psychological response.

A possible reactive response to exploring privilege may be a sense of associated expectations of social blame or social guilt. Reactions such as "I didn't own slaves, so why does this affect me?" or "Get over it already; women have equal rights" might suggest a rejection of the exploration because the client does not want to be associated with hurting others or own any associated assumed blame in the situation. The feminist therapist can view this as a strength. The person does not want to feel guilty for oppressing another person. It is a strength that they may feel oppression is terrible. Removing the associated personal guilt from the person may allow for a more open conversation about the historical legacies that led to today's systems and other social, cultural, and political norms that privilege some and oppress others.

Association with groups can also offer people identity and a sense of belonging and create a sense of safety in the person. Developmentally, different people have been exposed to different levels of privilege and oppression. Some people have been raised embedded with hate or violent groups such as street gangs, religious cults, or racial hate groups. Due to proximity, fate, birthplace, birth circumstances, and the like, a client may have these exclusive us/them bonding thoughts as the core of their identity. Asking someone to examine thoughts that bond them with their safety nets is like asking them to reconsider their existence. The feminist therapist might need to help the client find new identities and safety before examining the old ones. This must be done collaboratively and without judgments.

Lastly, some people feel that they deserve the privilege. They may be conscious of it, and they may believe in White supremacy, women belonging to a specific role(s), and/or social status as a birthright deserved. These clients often prove challenging for the feminist therapist due to divergent personal views between entitlements and equity/equality. The clinical goals and process remain the same—to alleviate suffering and create a higher consciousness for more accessible choices based on expanded awareness. The goal is not to change personal views; it is to offer more options and allow the client to decide with full awareness of their choices.

# Ways to Understand or Misunderstand Privilege

## Implicit and Explicit Bias

Often clients are not conscious of any organic developmental bias because it became embedded in their sense of normal raised in a Eurocentric, heteronormative, Christian-dominant, patriarchal society. Collaborative transparent discussions and psychoeducation on the nature of explicit and implicit bias may be useful. The feminist therapist may want to use self-disclosure to explain how they have been a perpetrator of both types of bias in the past, and perhaps the measures they took to examine them. This could assist the clients in normalizing and understanding the natural reactions of resistance rather than shaming or having the client experience guilt. Living in a society with a dominant culture means that absorbing beliefs of that culture is somewhat inescapable for everyone, including even the most skilled clinician.

## Visible Privilege versus Invisible Privilege

Peggy McIntosh (2003) wrote "White Privilege: Unpacking the Invisible Knapsack" to explain the many unseen ways in which people reap the benefits of their privilege. Many people are unaware of social privileges and see them as "normal"—for example, the ability to find their cultural foods at a supermarket. Pointing out the smaller instead of the larger (and sometimes more controversial ways) that privilege exists allows for a starting point to examine the concept. A therapist might want to inquire by stating, "I am certain that you may not even be aware of some of the ways that privilege is afforded to you without you asking; for example, can you go to the supermarket and buy food from your culture? What would it be like if you had to drive out of town to a special market to find that food?" This subtle discussion is far easier than directly discussing the notion of racism in society, but it may open the client up to the possibility that if they possess some privilege, then more might also exist.

## White Guilt, Fragility, and Tears

The term "White guilt" was first coined by James Baldwin in 1965 in his essay "The White Man's Guilt" (Katz, 1978). White guilt describes a person who processes racial information based on self-focused beliefs related to racial inequality. In other words, White people may see themselves as personally (vs. systemically) responsible for injustice and, therefore, may experience White guilt (Doosje et al.,1998). According to Knowles et al. (2014), White individuals respond to privilege in one of three ways: they will deny the existence of privilege, distance themselves their self-concepts from the privilege, or work to dismantle it. White guilt does not appear effective at promoting equality but may foster a sense of sympathy for others (Iyer et al., 2003). Additionally, Swim and Miller (1999) suggested that White guilt may be associated with stronger beliefs in the existence of White privilege and more significant estimates of the prevalence of discrimination.

DiAngelo (2018) stated, "Socialized into a deeply internalized sense of superiority that we either are unaware of or can never admit to ourselves, we become highly fragile in conversation about race" (p. 2). Di Angelo (2018) refers to this as "White fragility." Hamad (2020) expanded this concept by referring to "White tears" as a reaction to embedded White racial dominance. These "White tears" are often a genuine, organic reaction to any challenge to someone's identity and sense of moral goodness around their views and behaviors related to race (Hamad, 2020). "The kind of distress we are analyzing may feel genuine, but it is neither legitimate nor innocent" (Hamad, 2020, p. 12). These emotional outbursts, often by women, are commonly triggered by racial stress intolerance, and they serve to create a return of White equilibrium (DiAngelo, 2018). The person focuses so heavily on their guilt that they will, in turn, direct attention at themselves and their pain while taking the attention away from an oppressed person (Negra & Leyda, 2021; Lemieux, 2017).

Clinically, feminist therapists must recognize this embedded, often organic, reaction that many White people have when confronted with racial and social inequalities or incongruent internalized moral beliefs. For example, people often do not notice mobility ramps until they need them. Similarly, a White person may not have needed to consider racism or other "isms" because it did not affect them directly, and now they are being confronted with this new thought of privilege. Shaming people who do not understand their reactions only serves to embed the White privilege further. The feminist therapist wants to collaboratively be able to navigate through these difficult avenues of thought while quelling the need for the often-unconscious defensive organic White fragility or White tears.

# Feminist Intersectional Therapy and Social Privilege

Some of the basics of feminist therapy include an intersectional examination of the individual's identities, exploring how they are advantaged or disadvantaged in society and how to navigate the oppressive systems for higher consciousness and optimum personal power. Feminist theory was built on the feminist movement "the personal is political" and may feel more aligned with working with oppression rather than privilege. There could be some personal emotional reactions when working with people who resist or reject examining their privilege. Therefore, it is important, like all therapists, that feminist therapists maintain their self-examination and maintain a level of self-awareness that does not exacerbate the client's resistance.

The feminist therapist must skillfully examine new thoughts collaboratively and monitor the power between the client and themselves while being careful not to trigger a need for client defensiveness. How can that be done? Here are some thoughts to consider when working with clients who are naturally resistant to self-examination of privilege:

- Feminist therapists maintain a congruent, neutral stance, honoring all ways of knowing, even if it creates an emotional reaction in them.
- Move the conversation out of the client's reality to other people's by asking, "What would they say about this topic?"
- Move conversations to a sociological perspective, shifting dialogue from an individual's emotional, psychological relationship to the topic to a wider societal conceptual lens.
- Perhaps discuss current issues and deeply examine a person's beliefs, how they came to believe what they do, and how they feel safe/unsafe in those beliefs (e.g., reproductive rights, affirmative action, etc.)
- Keep personal guilt away from the conversation. If a client personalizes the concept of privilege, address the differences between conceptions and the individual's experience. Perhaps the difference between being guilty and responsible and taking future responsibility could be addressed. When you know better, you do better.
- Collaboratively explore how most people "live in reaction" and explore options to live in higher consciousness action. Without directly discussing privilege, perhaps explore how the client has learned to react throughout their lives.

# Feminist Process of Working with Intersectional Social Privilege

The feminist intersectional therapist must consider many factors when working with natural resistance to the core values many feminist therapists embrace. Like other therapists, feminist therapists' values cannot be imposed in the therapeutic relationship, or that serves as another form of oppression to the client. It is important to remember that a presenting problem would be very unlikely to be social privilege. Therefore, unlike other chapters, this feminist process will not focus on a specific issue or population but will offer possible avenues to raise consciousness among people naturally resistant to examining themselves, especially around areas of social privilege.

## Thought 1: Feminist Therapist Preparation and Self-awareness

The feminist intersectional therapist may be different from another therapist because they combine the underpinnings of feminist theory into their clinical practice. Feminist theory has a history of advocacy and activism to change society toward more equality for gender, racial, and other intersectional oppressed populations. Unlike many different theories, there is a viewpoint of equality. Therefore, the feminist therapist might find it even more challenging to work with clients who resist the examination of privilege than a therapist with other theoretical orientations. So, it is very important that the feminist therapist enters with each client prepared to take a nonjudgmental stance that does not react (implicitly or explicitly) to the client's resistance. Remembering and honoring all ways of consciousness, feminist therapists must genuinely prepare themselves not to push a feminist agenda on anyone. This would serve as another form of social oppression.

## Thought 2: Collaborative Intersectional Examination

Due to the complicated nature of intersectionality, a client would rarely have a complete identity of privilege with no oppression or a full identity of oppression with no privilege. In most situations, a client will likely need to look deeply into the complications of their identities, how they are viewed by society, and how they want to navigate their identities through society in the future. Beginning with clients' oppressions may be more manageable as a starting point.

## Thought 3: Discussion on Sociology

The feminist therapist might serve the client well by creating many frames for topics of higher consciousness. Defensive or resistant clients could be more open to exploration if the clinician moves topics away from what feel like personal threats. The feminist clinician might discuss deeper consciousness topics on conceptual sociological macro levels and then attempt to help clients find congruency between the macro and micro beliefs. Of course, remaining in alliance with feminist principles, the transparency of this exploration process would be shared with the client and done collaboratively.

## Thought 4: Reframing Strengths: Honoring Fears

The feminist therapist might collaboratively reframe organic and natural resistance and defensiveness as strengths. The clients who resist aligning themselves with any privilege or historical legacies of oppression must believe in equality as being the better way of existence. Helping the client realize that they want their sense of self to be viewed as a good, hard-working, right-minded, and knowing person is a strength. The feminist therapist may then help them examine their identities and help the client build upon their strengths, reframing how explored strengths can be scaffolded through new discoveries and challenging themselves. Higher consciousness examination and understandings can lead to more responsibility for beliefs and congruence with less need to defend them.

## Thought 5: What Thoughts Are New?

The feminist therapist may want to ask clients which identities, beliefs, and thoughts are available for examination and which ones are off-limits, helping the client explore their reasons for that list through the therapeutic process and avoid the content. Understanding that perhaps the most fragile identities and beliefs are the ones that clients may want to avoid examining, the feminist therapist might move to the therapeutic process of understanding the fragility rather than addressing the identity/beliefs themselves.

## Thought 6: Reactive versus Active: Exploration of Responses

The feminist therapist might want to review with clients past decisions that they are proud of and ones they regret. They then can examine whether these decisions were reactive or fully inspected and initiated by the client. Did the client seek or need validation for these decisions or not? Collaboratively explore with the client if they would like to live in reaction to others' beliefs/experiences or fully take responsibility for their own beliefs and actions—or somewhere in between. If the client chooses to remain in reaction or chooses a combination, help them delineate the motivations and boundaries around their choices so they are fully conscious.

## Thought 7: Meaning of Life: Advocacy for . . .

Following in the tradition of feminist therapy, advocacy can have healing properties. Alfred Adler highlighted the therapeutic benefit of social interest and suggested that when one engages in community as in service to others, they experience psychological relief from their own suffering (Ansbacher,1992). Advocacy can be a "pop" word associated with liberal thought that could promote defensiveness. So, how might advocacy be helpful for naturally resistant clients? The feminist therapist may want to encourage exploration to help clients find things they care about that transcend themselves. Exploring the existential meaning of life (Yalom, 1980) has healing properties and could move clients beyond focus on the self. The feminist therapist wants to be sure not to attempt to push an agenda on the client and to instead explore the client's passions. It could be possible that the first passions that arise are ego driven. They may be topics close to the client, such as family, or a cause directly affecting them. Helping the client muse with topics they might care about that have no direct connection to them and would give society a better quality of life experience may also move them outside themselves.

## Therapeutic Relationship with Privilege

Feminist therapists emphasize building and maintaining transparent, power-sharing, egalitarian relationships (Brown, 2018). Feminist therapists and clients become a microcosm of a power structure that holds therapeutic healing. The feminist therapist will not only need to address and monitor power as part of the therapeutic process but will also need to flatten any hierarchy assumptions. This can be done through a genuine relationship of modeling equality, placing and honoring the client as the expert in their lives and responsible for their beliefs and actions.

The transparent feminist therapist might need additional skills to keep the language used in therapy socially neutral, avoiding any "pop" words that may trigger a client's defenses. The word "feminist" itself is often a word that can trigger a natural emotional defensiveness. Perhaps explaining the feminist concepts without using the words might serve the client's understanding better. The word "feminist" is often associated with historical constructs of women for women only and even women who hate men. The intersectionality of being socially favored or not can be explained without triggering potentially damaging natural schematic images that cause a natural defensive stance. Words can also be added to "privileged," such as "natural," "normal," "unintentionally," and so on. One might also add "historically" to patriarchal. It may help to initially avoid discussing controversial topics or current events in the media in favor of more generalized examples. For example, perhaps avoid Black vs. Blue Lives Matter movements and instead, perhaps discuss the historic Civil Rights Movement or general beliefs about equality.

What does a feminist therapist do when a client espouses beliefs or practices that are "isms"—oppressive, marginalizing, and even cruel to others? Is it up to the feminist therapist to correct them through reprimanding? Does the therapist ignore an "ism" or oppressive comment? The feminist therapist remains therapeutic and genuine. Process and content are always in therapeutic interplay. It may be helpful to move the conversation to process when this happens. Why do they need to bring up this "ism," and why now? What were they feeling that allowed this to be the next topic of conversation? Helping to identify motives behind the statement can move to a process of understanding where this comment or thought fits into the larger picture of the current discussion at that moment. It is important that the client does not sense agreement about the "ism" from the therapist while skillfully continuing the process of exploration.

When the client is making attempts to exert power over a therapist (challenging age, race, gender, degree, abilities, or even sexualizing, etc.), it usually is best to address this in real time. Although it might seem clear that there is a power dynamic related to identity, social positioning, and the like, do not assume. Again, move to process over content. Be inquisitive; it may not be immediately necessary to directly speak to the gender/age, appearance, and so on. For example, a feminist therapist might say, "I am sensing that we are struggling to share power at this moment. What about our relationship makes you want to exert power in this moment? What can I do to help you feel more empowered at this moment in this relationship?" This type of response is meant to empower the client, not embarrass them, so an answer to the empowerment must be collaboratively found, or it could be viewed as a sarcastic relationship-damaging rebuttal.

Due to the ever-evolving and imperfect nature of humans and changing society, feminist therapists must be mindful of the possibility of saying offensive things to clients by accident. Feminist therapists were also raised in this society, and may impulsively slip into old, less evolved thinking in a reactive moment. Acknowledging and correcting any mistakes immediately model vulnerability and serves to flatten hierarchies.

# Feminist Intersectional Applications for Working with Privilege

## Avoid Pop Words: Inclusive Language

When discussing privilege and oppression, the client and feminist therapist must have a dialogue that flows naturally, and the client must have the space to speak plainly as it is comfortable for them to communicate their experiences. The feminist therapist will speak directly and clearly in a language relatable to the client, being mindful not to use words that may trigger a natural defensive stance. These words could be media-distorted "woke" words like feminist, oppression, White privilege, critical race theory, and so on. Describing concepts or theories is possibly more understandable without conjuring images triggered by words that the cultural, social, and political environment has distorted for personal and political gain.

The clarity in the language the therapist uses during communication surrounding possible sensitive and vulnerable topics is an attempt to encourage the client to feel supported in verbalizing their experiences more directly and vulnerably. The client may use pop-triggering language, and the feminist therapist needs to gain clarity on the client's interpretive meaning of such language. For example, the client might say, "All Lives Matter." This is an opportunity to discover what the client believes the connotation behind that slogan is and why it is meaningful to them. Additionally, the feminist therapist will also gain clarity from the client to ensure that they understand the client's intersectional experiences around privilege and oppression are clearly understood within themselves, in the context of society, and in the session. The goal is for work done in session to consistently support the client and lend a hand in consciousness raising through deepening clarity in language used to describe self, society, and interrelated experiences.

## Understanding Definitions, Images, and Automatic Thoughts

Understanding how a client defines privilege and oppression and what images, automatic thoughts, and emotions these concepts provoke is therapeutically crucial. For example, someone may internalize their privilege as a label describing someone terrible, wrapped up in fear. How this identity is valued in the world may not be congruent with their conscious self and cause natural resistance and inner conflict. Essential to understanding the client's experience is exploring what feelings arise for the clients as they explore their intersectional identities and how they feel a privileged identity will show up when in action out in the world. The feminist therapist may use a two-chair technique to allow the client to express each of their privileged identities, showcasing what they feel the role they play in holding this identity may have in different areas of their life, essentially role-playing how their privilege may look as they venture throughout their days (i.e., at home, at work, in the checkout line buying groceries, etc.), and adjusting as needed in session allowing the client more visibility of self to choose further characteristics that they accurately identify with, consciously, and in ways that are genuinely congruent with themselves. This clinical application may hold value by bringing a heightened awareness to anything that may lie subconsciously or dormant within the client that acts itself out within their privileged roles and identities. Bringing these realizations of privilege and oppression into consciousness and taking responsibility for their empowerment is the goal of this application; it is not helpful for the client to take responsibility in the forms of shame or guilt but rather gain awareness for future choices.

## Acknowledging and Working through Sociological and Psychological Reactions

Emotions are purposeful and often signal to others that something is wrong and needs to be changed. When a person realizes they hold a privileged identity or may have played a role in the oppression of others, they may feel a sense of moral incongruence, guilt, or shame; and, in the absence of the ability to process that new information, may organically reject that role to emotionally self-regulate (Hamad, 2020; DiAngelo, 2018). White fragility and White tears may come into play. The privileged person may, in turn, direct attention to themselves and their pain while taking the attention away from the person who is oppressed. A skilled feminist therapist might explore socially embedded reactivity and inquire about what thoughts and actions the person would like to take to shift any possible moral incongruence away from themselves and instead explore ways to possibly share power with oppressed persons.

## Intersectional Exploration of Privilege

The feminist therapist may want to work alongside the client to explore the different identities that make up their sense of self. When exploring the different identities that the client holds, it will be important for the therapist to note which identities are assumed first and are more confidently embraced; which identities the client may be unsure of or less attached to; and which identities are outright denied, vilified, or described with shame or guilt language, in terms of themselves and/or of others. Working with the client in this technique may involve the client listing, in order of importance, which identities they most identify with and which identities they least identify with.

Additionally, it will be important to explore which aspects of the client's identity the client feels are privileged and which are oppressed. The feminist counselor should acknowledge if a client identifies themselves with all privileged or all oppressed identities as well, as this will indicate an opportunity for deeper therapeutic exploration to take place. This exercise should provide the client space for possibly the first time to express themselves and begin to see clearly, with the support of the feminist therapist, the internalized elements that define who they are in addition to unprocessed or unconsciously chosen beliefs, stereotypes, fears, and so on, that have gotten woven into their current construction of self. This feminist clinical application might help clients understand and see what barriers arise for them and what may be necessary to reach their desired state of wellness.

The feminist therapist must also be prepared to process the identities the client identifies as privileged without any emphasis on guilt. The client must feel they are in a safe space to speak freely, so deconstruction and reconstruction of frameworks about identities can possibly occur later if chosen. If the client senses judgment, they may retreat into defensiveness. When done supportively, the feminist therapist will use this technique as a steppingstone to help the client lean into the vulnerable and positive unknown space of ego expansion. Creating space for the client to see their identities creates an opportunity for further understanding of self, self in relation to society, societal influence on self, and full conscious acknowledgment and acceptance of identities. This process may be quite uncomfortable for the client, even if they are willing to be exploratory with their intersectional identities. Care must be taken to remind the client that they are encouraged to express who they are and that there will be no repercussions, judgment, or shame administered in the therapeutic space.

## Empowered Choices of Self

After exploring intersectional identities, the feminist therapist may want to collaboratively explore the client's feelings around the "self" and their power to choose how to perceive their identities and role expectations. They can discuss which identities are immovable and must be navigated, which ones they want to embrace, and what needs to happen to be congruent to their higher consciousness. The feminist therapist creates a space for the client to consciously choose perceptions around their intersectional identities and take responsibility for their current life's issues and narrative. Empowerment may be gained through clarity of self and consciously making choices about beliefs of life and self. Through this process, the feminist therapist may observe some inconsistencies/incongruencies between the client's narrative to describe their self, their life, experiences, and how they feel about society separate from themselves and within society. Questions may be asked to explore how the client's macro system, present and past, as well as their family of origin and society's norms and beliefs, have become entangled into what may currently be a more unconscious passive acceptance of external and internal norms.

The feminist therapist may explore the following with their client:

- Does the client truly understand the impact of their own intersectional identities?
- When did they realize their identities and roles?
- What memories come to mind for clients regrading privileges and/or oppressions related to their identities or roles?
- How do they speak about these identities?
- What can the client recall of people closest to them feeling or relaying about those with such identities or roles?
- Do they define any of these identities/roles as "good" or "bad," "better" or "worse" than others or than the other identities they hold?

The focus will be on helping clients align their macro and micro beliefs. For the feminist therapist, authentically expressing unconditional positive regard while processing possible incongruencies that may arise for the client in this process must be handled with transparency. A deconstruction and reconstruction of identity may occur during this time and the space must feel safe and nonthreatening.

## Navigating Natural Reactive Resistance

Clients who have been through experiences where they have fallen victim to circumstances that were out of their control, including traumas and abuse, may have an even greater propensity to experience resistance and fear when acknowledging the realities that come with being privileged. Defensiveness often suffocates people's ability to be open when they feel personally scrutinized or worry that something may be taken from them. The defensive dialogue that may arise can be clinically productive as it allows the client to explore within a safe therapeutic relationship, where they can better learn what their defenses are trying to defend. The client can gain the ability to consciously reframe the story they tell themselves about privilege, practice new skills, and develop more congruence internally without the need to defend the ego. This feminist exploration encourages clients to challenge themselves and take responsibility for their perceptions and choices.

It is always valuable for the feminist therapist to explore the client's worldview. This can include exploring their history to get an understanding of how their needs have been met throughout life, where they may perceive having been stunted or wronged in life, whether those feelings have been generalized to a group, system, or have they been internalized, how they feel about their needs being met today, and their self-efficacy around their ability to provide their needs for themselves.

Questions to consider could include the following:

- What events did the client experience where they felt wronged, or were victims of an event(s)?
- Do they hold resentment, or have they healed the wound of injustice done to them?
- Did the client grow up having their primary needs met?
- Did their parents and grandparents grow up having their primary needs met?
- Were clients able to feel safe growing up?
- Do they feel safe now?
- How do they feel around those who look different than they do?
- Does the client live life primarily in fear or in a scarcity mindset?
- Does the client feel currently victimized in life?
- Do they feel angry about perceived or real victimization?
- Who does the anger primarily get taken out on?
- Have they generalized those feelings to a whole group or systems?
- How do these feelings possibly restrict them from finding freedom, taking responsibility, and feeling content with their lives?
- How does the client feel about their ability to get what they need today?

## Strengths and Criticisms of Working with Resistance

The feminist therapist must skillfully, through self-awareness, remain compassionately present with naturally resistant clients, not imposing their feminist values on them, and exploring identities and beliefs with them. It may seem incongruent to some feminist therapists to work with such clients, but the actual foundation of feminist theory includes not creating a new oppressive agenda of telling clients how to think. The only agenda is higher consciousness. Some clients with full awareness may choose non-compassionate, non-empathetic life stances. Feminist principles honor all ways of knowing and being and must consider therapeutic goals achieved.

Lastly, due to the demystifying and transparent collaboration relationship, feminist therapists may be viewed as less intelligent, less professional, and even less effective. A naturally resistant client may believe that the medical model is more structured and, therefore, more effective and use that belief as part of their natural defense mechanisms. The feminist therapist may want to address this early in the relationship.

# What If?

What if all clinicians saw all defensiveness as natural or organic strengths?

What if the social and political landscape valued all people equally and there were no hierarchies of social privilege?

What if people of color were the political majority and banded together politically? What would that political party look like?

What if White people all embraced the notion of White privilege?

What if all therapeutic settings accepted feminist principles over the medical model?

# References

Ansbacher, H. L. (1992). Alfred Adler's concepts of community feeling and social interest and the relevance of community feeling for old age. *Individual Psychology: Journal of Adlerian Theory, Research & Practice*, 48(4), 402–412.

Baldwin, J. (August 1965). "The white man's guilt." *Ebony Magazine*.

Black Lives Matter. (n.d.). About Black Lives Matter. https://blacklivesmatter.com/about/#vision

Brown, L. S. (2018). *Feminist therapy*. Oxford University Press.

Brown, L. S., & Walker, L. E. A. (1990). Feminist therapy perspectives on self-disclosure. In G. Stricker & M. Fisher (Eds.), *Self-disclosure in the therapeutic relationship* (pp. 135–154). Plenum Press. https://doi.org/10.1007/978-1-4899-3582-3_10

Cherry, K. (2023). *Adaptation in Piaget's theory of development*. https://www.verywellmind.com/what-is-adaptation-2794815#:~:text=Not%20surprisingly%2C%20the%20accommodation%20process,changing%20a%20deeply%20held%20belief

DiAngelo. R. (2018). *White fragility*. Beacon Press.

Doosje, B., Branscombe, N. R., Spears, R., & Manstead, A. S. R. (1998). Guilty by association: When one's group has a negative history. *Journal of Personality and Social Psychology*, 75(4), 872–886.

Hamad, R. (2020) *White tears, brown scars*. Catapult.

Hardy, K. V. (2023). *Racial trauma*. W. W. Norton.

Iyer, A., Leach, C. W., & Crosby, F. J. (2003). White guilt and racial compensation: The benefits and limits of self-focus. *Personality and Social Psychology Bulletin*, 29(1), 117–129. https://doi.org/10.1177/0146167202238377

Katz, J. (1978). *White awareness: Handbook for anti-racism training*. University of Oklahoma Press.

Knowles, E. D., Lowery B. S., Chow R. M., & Unzueta M. M. (2014). Deny, distance, or dismantle? How White Americans manage a privileged identity. *Perspectives on Psychological Science*, 9, 594–609.

Lemieux, J. (2017). *Weinstein, White tears and the boundaries of Black women's empathy*. https://cassiuslife.com/33564/white-women-dont-look-out-for-black-victims/amp/

McIntosh, P. (2003). White privilege: Unpacking the invisible knapsack. In S. Plous (Ed.), *Understanding prejudice and discrimination* (pp. 191–196). McGraw Hill.

Negra, D., & Leyda, J. (2021). Querying "Karen": The rise of the angry white woman. *European Journal of Cultural Studies*, 24(1), 350–357. https://doi.org/10.1177/1367549420947777

Phillips, L. T., & Lowery B. S. (2015). The hard-knock life? Whites claim hardships in response to racial inequity. *Journal of Experimental Social Psychology*, 61, 12–18.

Safran, J. D. (2012). *Psychoanalysis and psychoanalytic therapies*. American Psychological Association.

Swim, J. K., & Miller D. (1999). White guilt: Its correlates and relationship to attitudes about affirmative action. *Personality and Social Psychology Bulletin*, 25, 500–514.

Yalom, I. D. (1980). *Existential psychotherapy*. Basic Books.

# PART FOUR

# Feminist Academic and Future Evolution

# 20

# Feminist Intersectional Pedagogy in Higher Education: Clinical Mental Health Focus

## Kathleen McCleskey, Donnette Deigh, Amber Sutton, and Joanne Jodry

*Education systems reflect the hierarchical power structures found in other patriarchal systems. Feminist educators seek to disrupt traditional power hierarchies and ensure that all voices are heard and valued.*

## Feminist Intersectional Pedagogy

Applying feminist intersectional theory in educational settings may be one of the most challenging implementations of the theory due to current educational systems born and evolved from historical legacies of Eurocentric, heteronormative, Christian-dominant, patriarchal constructs. Traditional public educational systems in the United States are grounded in structural hierarchies, government oversights and regulations, and social and political norms often based on geographical culture. Education systems also often underpin classroom management with behavioral techniques of rewards and punishments. Although feminist pedagogy might serve to benefit every level of learning, the constraints of the traditional oppressive school settings may force feminist pedagogical application to higher education where there is more academic freedom and where students are legal adults. This allows for more expansive feminist conceptualization; it is hoped that educators at every level can find pieces of this conceptualization that may be implemented within their specific systems.

Feminist intersectional pedagogy seeks to de-emphasize hierarchies and rejects oppressive social, cultural, and political norms in any system (De Santis & Serafini, 2015) while questioning equity and equality within the systems and even within the individual classrooms. With these conflicting educational conceptualizations and modalities, how does a feminist academic remain authentic to their values and provide the best educational opportunities to their students in a patriarchal system?

Developing intentional critical thinking within higher education classrooms and systems is crucial in feminist intersectional pedagogical approaches (Sinacore et al., 2013). These approaches emphasize cultivating students' critical thinking skills to question and challenge existing social and cultural norms, power dynamics, and inequalities in the academic landscape and beyond. As students learn the roots of these Eurocentric, heteronormative, Christian-dominant patriarchal systems, they may collaboratively seek ways to improve systems so everyone has equal opportunities. Teaching this critical thinking might be best served as a sociological model as opposed to a psychological model. By encouraging students to engage critically with their learning environment, educators can raise consciousness and empower them to become agents of change, giving them tools to make choices on how to navigate cultural, social, and political structures.

Inclusivity is another key aspect of feminist intersectional educational conceptualization. Feminist educators aspire to create a learning environment and educational relationships that honor and value all intersectional diverse perspectives, histories, and backgrounds (Sinacore et al., 2013). By fostering a culture of inclusivity, as opposed to tolerance, educators can ensure that all students feel respected, represented, and supported in their educational journey. Feminist instructors monitor students for any exclusivity of certain students' needs and address that through feminist mentorship and modeling. If the teacher puts the students in high esteem, sometimes the students follow. Reprimanding students who are excluding others may be contraindicated in a feminist inclusive model.

*An example of an important note:* Critically examining historical legacies of privilege and oppression has no intention of making students who hold privilege feel guilty or inadequate. Arguments have been made against teaching critical race theory (see, e.g., Briscoe & Jones, 2024), which is sometimes taught in higher education, due to the distress it might cause a privileged person or due to unjustly labeling systems as racist or sexist. This is an example of taking sociological concepts and making them psychologically personal. A feminist professor must be skillful in clarifying this distinction to students and helping them to understand the difference.

## Academic Freedom

In higher education, university professors are protected by having academic freedom, which is not offered to all educators. However, there are boundaries and restrictions associated with these freedoms. According to American Association of University Professors (AAUP) policies,

> the freedom to teach includes the right of the faculty to select the materials, determine the approach to the subject, make the assignments, and assess student academic performance in teaching activities for which faculty members are individually responsible. Faculty members are entitled to freedom in the classroom in discussing their subject, but they should be careful not to introduce into their teaching controversial matters which are unrelated to their subject, or to persistently introduce material which has no relation to the subject. This doesn't mean teachers should avoid all controversial materials. As long as the material stimulates debate and learning that is germane to the subject matter, it is protected by freedom in the classroom. (AAUP, n.d., para. 3)

At the same time, feminist educators need to be sure to connect areas such as these, which might be "controversial" in the political arena, to the professional and academic foundations of their helping professions and to ensure that students are free to engage in frank, honest conversations around all ideas.

# Feminist Intersectional Pedagogical Underpinnings

## Egalitarian Relationship–Collaborative Learning

In a classroom where feminist intersectional pedagogy guides the educational journey, the principles of mutual respect, shared decision-making, and equal partnerships are at the forefront. This approach emphasizes the value of every individual's voice, experiences, and perspectives, fostering collaboration and cooperation in both teaching and learning (Ares, 2008; Magen-Nagar & Shonfeld, 2018; Weinberger & Shonfeld, 2020). Although there is an organic hierarchy since the instructor has the knowledge to provide to the student and has an evaluative role, the instructor holds every student in high regard and in a position of honor for navigating their particular intersectional lived experience. Through the lens of feminist pedagogy, collaborative learning becomes an interactive and engaging experience where students actively participate in shaping their educational path. This pedagogical approach promotes teamwork, knowledge sharing, and the collective creation of meaning.

By creating a sense of community and cooperation, feminist pedagogy challenges traditional power structures and creates a more democratic and inclusive learning environment (Crabtree et al., 2009). "Feminist pedagogy is marked by the development of nonhierarchical relationships among teachers and students and reflexivity about power and relations, not only in society but also in the classroom" (Crabtree et al., 2009, p. 5). Critical components of feminist pedagogy include a focus on encouraging and empowering open and respectful communication that values diverse viewpoints. "With respect to objectives and outcomes, feminist pedagogy seeks not only to enhance students conceptual learning but also to promote consciousness-raising, personal growth, and social responsibility" (Crabtree et al., 2009, p. 6). Shared and distributed leadership is also emphasized, which enables collaborative decision-making. This feminist intersectional framework recognizes and values diverse forms of knowledge and experiences, and students are prompted to critically reflect on power dynamics, intersectional social inequalities, and systemic injustices. Ultimately, feminist pedagogy aims to empower students to actively shape their learning experiences and advocate for community, social, and educational change.

## Taking Ownership of Education and Learning

In concert with the egalitarian relationship, feminist pedagogy encourages active student participation in shaping learning experiences. Students advocate for themselves and challenge traditional power dynamics in the academic environment (Doyle, 2023; Webb et al., 2002). This approach focuses on self-directed learning, critical thinking, and the autonomy to independently shape one's educational trajectory.

In this framework, self-reflection plays a crucial role by encouraging individuals to delve into their beliefs, values, and biases. By engaging in this introspective process, individuals can gain a deeper understanding of themselves and how these internal factors influence their learning experiences. The promotion of critical thinking skills is central to feminist pedagogy.

These skills enable individuals to question, analyze, and challenge dominant narratives, power dynamics, and inequalities in educational settings (De Santis & Serafini, 2015). By fostering a critical mindset, learners are empowered to deconstruct existing systems and explore alternative perspectives.

Empowering students toward self-advocacy and assertiveness is another way to help students find personal agency and take responsibility for their education. This involves empowering individuals to assert their needs, interests, and learning goals within the often-oppressive educational system. This may include seeking resources, support, and accommodations to ensure an inclusive and supportive learning environment for all learners. It may also involve conversations with professors, which some students initially find intimidating and daunting.

Collaborative learning is also emphasized within this pedagogical approach (Sinacore et al., 2013). Caughie and Pearce (2009) said collaborative learning was "difficult to develop because of the conservative pedagogical bias of most faculty because they don't lead to prestigious publications but most of all because they exist within a field where the dominant model is dualistic, individualistic, and competitive" (p. 34). However, by highlighting the importance of collaboration, peer support, and community building, students are encouraged to engage with others to enhance their learning process and expand their knowledge base. This collaborative ethos fosters a sense of belonging and mutual support among learners.

## Intersectionality

Intersectionality plays a vital role in fourth-wave feminist educational discourse, acknowledging that all students carry multiple social and cultural identities, such as gender, race, class, socioeconomic status, and sexuality, intersecting and shaping their educational experiences (De Santis & Serafini, 2015). Understanding these intersecting identities and their privilege or oppression is crucial for addressing the unique challenges and barriers that students from diverse backgrounds may experience within the educational system. Recognizing how intersectional identities can impact how students interact with academic material is important. By recognizing how these intersecting factors shape individuals' learning journeys, educators can create more inclusive and equitable educational environments that cater to all learners' diverse needs and experiences. Feminist intersectional principles recognize the importance of creating a level playing field where every student can thrive and succeed without marginalization, oppression, discrimination, or bias. This may involve the feminist instructor advocating for equal and just educational opportunities for all individuals.

Another aspect of feminist pedagogy is the creation of safe and inclusive spaces within the classroom where diverse perspectives are welcomed, respectful dialogue is promoted, and the well-being of every student, especially those from marginalized groups, is safeguarded (Ratts, 2017). Freedman (2009) suggested, "The creation of a safe space to talk rested upon the ability to listen" (p. 122). By embracing an intersectional perspective, feminist educators can better understand the unique complex dynamics of social inequalities and power structures. Furthermore, feminist pedagogy challenges traditional power dynamics by encouraging students to critically examine their privileges and biases and the systemic structures of power and oppression that influence societal norms (Busse et al., 2024). Through this critical self-reflection, students can develop a heightened awareness of social injustices and consider their roles in perpetuating or challenging inequities.

In addition, building empathy and solidarity among students from diverse backgrounds is crucial for fostering a sense of community and shared responsibility for creating a more just society (Ratts, 2017). Educators can cultivate a supportive and understanding culture within the educational environment by promoting mutual respect and allyship. Lastly, feminist pedagogy emphasizes the importance of incorporating diverse perspectives through educational materials and resources (Simon et al., 2022). By including readings, case studies, and guest speakers that represent a variety of experiences and voices, educators can ensure that all students feel validated, heard, and valued in the educational discourse. This inclusive approach helps to broaden students' understanding of social issues and encourages them to engage critically with different viewpoints.

## Flexible Assignments or Outcome Measurements

In feminist intersectional pedagogy, empowering students is a key component (Webb et al., 2002). One way to empower students can be to collaborate with them on assignments and assessment methods. This can help create an inclusive and empowering learning environment (Soffer et al., 2019) that recognizes individual differences and caters to diverse learning styles. One of the principles of incorporating flexibility in education is promoting personalized learning. By allowing students some freedom to tailor assignments to their interests, strengths, and goals, educators encourage a sense of ownership in the learning process (Soffer et al., 2019). This personalized approach hopes to motivate students and foster a deeper connection to the course material.

Consistent with the conceptualization of feminist pedagogy, educators may consider offering multiple pathways for achievement. This could involve offering students various options to demonstrate their understanding of the material, such as written essays, presentations, creative projects, or collaborative group work (Soffer et al., 2019). By providing diverse assessment methods, feminist educators ensure that different learning styles and preferences are accommodated, promoting a more inclusive learning environment. Furthermore, encouraging self-reflection and self-assessment plays a significant role in feminist pedagogy. By prompting students to evaluate their progress, set goals, and reflect on their achievements, educators foster self-awareness and metacognition among learners (Soffer et al., 2019). This approach can empower students to take control of their learning experiences and become more actively engaged in their academic journey.

In addition, negotiated assessment criteria are employed as a collaborative effort between feminist educators and students to establish transparent and equitable evaluation standards (De Santis & Serafini, 2015; Soffer et al., 2019). This collaborative approach ensures that assessment processes are fair, accountable, and aligned with the student's needs and expectations. Lastly, providing flexible deadlines and extensions can be another important aspect of feminist pedagogy. By recognizing students' diverse responsibilities and needs, educators can support student well-being and enhance overall success by offering adaptable deadlines, extensions, or alternative methods to demonstrate learning (Soffer et al., 2019). Incorporating flexibility in assignments and assessment methods within feminist pedagogy promotes inclusivity and empowerment and enhances student engagement, success, and overall well-being in the educational setting.

Flexibility can also create a collaborative dynamic of problem-solving. For example, students and the professor can converse about what is and is not working in terms of classroom learning or assignment learning. Students can be invited to brainstorm ideas on how to improve the planned activities and assessment activities. This can lead to creative, collaborative, and cooperative adjustments to syllabi or classroom instruction that may also heighten student investment in the educational process.

## Using Experiential Knowledge and Learning

Within feminist intersectional pedagogy, educators aim to offer students a transformative learning journey by integrating diverse forms of experiential knowledge and implementing holistic experiential learning theory (Fromm et al., 2021; Kolb, 1984). This method can enhance student's understanding of societal issues, power structures, and real-life encounters. By appreciating experiential knowledge gained from personal experiences, emotions, and interactions, educators enable students to participate in critical analysis and impact social progress.

One key aspect of this pedagogical approach is the emphasis on centering lived experiences. Students are encouraged to reflect on their experiences, identities, and viewpoints to recognize how societal structures and power dynamics influence their lives and relationships (Webb et al., 2002). Students deepen their understanding of social justice issues and intersectional identities through reflective practices and critical self-analysis. Moreover, a collaborative and participatory learning environment is fostered where students can share their experiences, knowledge, and insights. By co-constructing knowledge and meaning together, students engage in a collective learning journey. The application of experiential learning cycles guides students through stages of experiencing, reflecting, conceptualizing, and experimenting, leading to critical reflection and action rooted in their experiences (De Santis & Serafini, 2015). Integrating community engagement further enhances the learning process. Students can apply classroom knowledge in real-world contexts by incorporating community-based learning experiences, service-learning projects, and activism opportunities. This hands-on approach empowers students to contribute meaningfully to social change efforts and advocate for equity.

Through the incorporation of diverse forms of experiential knowledge and experiential learning theory, feminist educators equip students with a profound understanding of social justice issues. This approach nurtures empathy, solidarity, and empowerment to champion equity and social change within their communities and beyond. By upholding the core tenets of feminist pedagogy, which celebrate diverse perspectives, challenging traditional power structures, and fostering inclusivity, educators cultivate a more equitable and enriching educational experience for all (Fromm et al., 2021).

## Privilege and Marginalization in Student Populations

Privilege and marginalization are significant concepts that impact student populations in educational settings (Busse et al., 2024; Crabtree, et al., 2009; Ratts, 2017; Simon et al., 2022). The principles of feminist intersectional pedagogy are instrumental in addressing these issues by fostering a learning environment that prioritizes equity, inclusivity, and social justice. Educators who adopt a feminist pedagogical approach strive to create a classroom that values and respects all students' diverse, intersectional identities and experiences, particularly those who have historically been marginalized or oppressed.

## Amplifying Marginalized Voices

In higher education, it is now more crucial than ever to listen to the voices of marginalized communities. From the insightful works of Loes et al. (2018), Mansfield and Welton (2018), and Tewell (2019), the call for feminist educators to design curricula that not only acknowledges but actively supports social action and justice resonates powerfully. Research has illuminated that teaching methodologies that embrace and amplify students' cultural identities have the potential to impact their educational experiences profoundly. By expanding students' worldviews, fostering motivation for social justice, and encouraging critical analysis through social, political, and economic lenses (Chung & Bemak, 2013), educators can pave the way for a transformative educational experience.

Central to this transformative approach is creating a learning environment characterized by safety and respect. By nurturing discussions around differences in culture and politics, educators can cultivate a space where diverse voices are heard and valued. Furthermore, the imperative of decolonizing education, as advocated by Silva and Students for Diversity Now (2018) and Singh et al. (2020), emerges as a cornerstone of this narrative. By challenging traditional power structures and narratives within educational frameworks, feminist educators can actively work toward creating a more inclusive and equitable learning environment for all. Feminist educators are responsible for championing marginalized student's voices and creating spaces where all students feel seen, heard, and empowered. By weaving together the threads of cultural identity, social justice, and decolonization, feminist pedagogy may pave the way for a more inclusive and transformative educational landscape.

## Addressing the Student Holistically

As feminist educators, it is crucial to recognize and address the holistic needs of students, as emphasized by McDougall (2019). One key aspect is understanding the challenges they may face outside of the classroom that can impact their learning and well-being. This includes recognizing and addressing any problems they may face at home or work. At home, the adult learner may be dealing with challenges related to their families, including their children. Balancing the demands of parenting with academic responsibilities can be overwhelming, and providing support and resources to help manage this juggle is crucial for their success.

For students also employed, strained work relationships or high-pressure situations can create stress and affect their focus on academic pursuits. Offering guidance on effective communication and conflict resolution may help alleviate these issues. Additionally, the student may be dealing with illness or family needs requiring attention and care. Health concerns or family emergencies can disrupt their academic routine and impact students' mental well-being. Providing accommodations, such as flexible deadlines or referrals to counseling services, can assist them in navigating these challenges while staying on track with their studies. By addressing these aspects of the student's life, educators can create a supportive and understanding environment that promotes their holistic well-being and academic success.

## Mental Health Needs of Students

More than 60% of college students met the criteria for at least one mental health problem during the 2020–2021 school year (Lipson et al., 2022). Feminist educators must carefully balance the demands of teaching (what happens inside the classroom) with the realities of students' lives (outside of the classroom). Part of feminist pedagogy lies in creating a culture of well-being that welcomes the totality of our students' identities, including mental health diagnoses, survivorship and trauma, caretaking responsibilities, and so on. While educators cannot become therapists or case managers for students, they must be mindful of how these experiences may appear in educational spaces. There are ways to build feminist trauma-informed classrooms that increase connection, strengthen learning ability, and encourage bravery and compassion between faculty and students. Some techniques can include providing accessible resource guides (including on-campus and off-campus assistance) at the beginning of the semester and revisiting them as needed, providing clear syllabi, including self-care plans as graded assignments or as optional practice tools, using mindfulness exercises to open or close classes (with permission of all students), doing temperature checks / scaling questions at the beginning of classes, and providing snacks, hand sanitizer, and/or tissues. Small human touches can mean a great deal to students coping with their needs.

# Feminist Pedagogy in Clinical Mental Health Training Programs

One of the strengths of feminist pedagogy in clinical mental health training programs, found throughout different academic disciplines, is that it mirrors many of the relational dynamics and concepts taught in the helping professions. For example, these students must learn how to consider systemic contexts when doing client conceptualization and separate what is systemic from what is psychological. By fostering a feminist critical mindset, clinical mental health trainees can be encouraged to deconstruct and decolonize theories, modalities, and underlying therapeutic assumptions. Through transparent discussions of these concepts, students can better understand and apply them to themselves, their peers, and their educational systems, which will model how to do the same kinds of assessments and conceptualizations with their current and future clients.

A feminist pedagogical approach can provide clinical trainees with lived experience in applying these concepts and dynamics before and during client work. An inclusive environment can create empathy and understanding among classmates and cultivate empathy for current or future clients. From a feminist perspective, this process mirrors the goal of students being inclusive in clinical settings. In addition, helping professions have moved over time to embrace social justice and multiculturalism, and this is built into professional codes of ethics and competency documents as well as in academic scholarship (see, e.g., Hailes et al., 2020; NASW, 2021; Ratts et al., 2016). These are necessary topics in clinical training programs for working with clients and align with feminist principles.

Ultimately, feminist pedagogy aims to empower clinical students to shape their learning experiences and actively advocate for community, health, and educational change. This active learning process can be seen as a parallel process of feminist therapy, where each person has their areas of expertise and works together, using all their resources, toward the common goal of client healing. In clinical mental health training programs, students can also practice learning how to seek information, find resources, and ask for instructor assistance, which may be similar to skills they will use with clients and clinical supervisors. Meaningful skills grounded in feminist pedagogy can be modeled and connected to later work as clinicians.

# Addressing SES/Class, Race, Gender among Helping Professions

In the realm of helping professions such as social work, counseling, psychology, education, and healthcare, the intricate dynamics of socioeconomic status (SES)/class, race, and gender play a pivotal role in shaping individuals' experiences of privilege and marginalization (LaMantia et al., 2015; Marecek, 2016; Pasque & Nicholson, 2023; Simon et al., 2022). When viewed through the lens of feminist pedagogy, it becomes evident that a deeper exploration of these intersections is essential to comprehending and addressing the complex power dynamics, oppression, and inequalities that impact both practitioners and the individuals they serve.

## Socioeconomic Status (SES)/Class

The influence of SES and class dynamics on individuals' access to resources, opportunities, and support systems cannot be understated. Mental health practitioners must acknowledge the socioeconomic disparities and systemic barriers that may hinder clients' well-being and utilization of services. Class privilege has also emerged as an issue in clinical training programs. Miller et al. (2021) describe several hidden costs of clinical counseling training, from admissions fees to required credentialing examinations. A compelling discussion centers on unpaid internships, which are common in many programs. Unpaid field placements also impact the ability to have or to keep a full-time job while in training. The cost of a master's or doctoral degree can incur large student debt. Class privilege may also intersect with other privileges—students identifying as female and/or BIPOC may be most impacted by graduate school debt (Pyne & Grodsky, 2019). Feminist instructors and administrators can advocate for more inquiry into current and future students' barriers to attending or completing clinical training programs and to seek solutions to create more diversity of all kinds, including class diversity.

## Gender

In clinical training programs, gender may be an area of focus for various reasons. For example, data (given as male/female binaries) show a large gender split regarding helping professionals, all favoring females. Ratios for social workers are reported as being 81.1% women and 18.9% men (DataUSA, 2017a), for mental health counselors are reported as being 77.1% women and 22.9% men (DataUSA, 2022 figures), and for psychologists as 71.8% women and 28.2% men (DataUSA, 2017b). Therefore, gender diversity is likely in training programs, with more students identifying as female than male. Transgender and nonbinary students may be more visible in programs now but likely remain a minority. At the same time, women may not be equitably represented in positions of power within leadership roles (see, e.g., Clay, 2017). A feminist educator should be aware of and sensitive to the gender ratios in training rooms and be able to facilitate conversations about that; in addition, in reflecting on intersectional identities, including gender, trainees should be invited to reflect on ways that their gender could impact creating and maintaining helping relationships with clients.

## Monitoring Power in the Classroom

When monitoring power in the feminist pedagogical spaces, faculty in clinical mental health programs have an advantage from being trained in group work modalities. Instructors can consider how group work facilitators attend to content and process on an ongoing basis. Using this awareness, a feminist instructor can attend to dynamics such as who speaks more, less, or not at all, what topics inspire discussion, what topics do not, and so on. The instructor may then ask students to reflect on those dynamics through the lens of how power is, or is not, being shared. Or the instructor could notice out loud what they are seeing, and they may then ask students their thoughts and reactions. Similarly, understanding group dynamics can help create and maintain brave spaces for difficult dialogues. Learning to facilitate and have productive, healthy, and frank discussions about multicultural and social justice topics helps students navigate similar dialogues in academia and other systems they will interact with, including with clients.

## Self-Assessments of Dispositions

As part of clinical training to be mental health professionals, professional dispositions are regularly assessed by faculty (Homrich & Henderson, 2018), particularly in some places such as clinical classes. This serves dual purposes. For faculty and supervisors, assessing dispositions is an integral part of the gatekeeping requirement for programs that train mental health professionals. Trainees must be able to understand and show evidence of core professional behaviors tied to working with clients, such as keeping information confidential or being able to accept feedback on their performance from instructors and supervisors. Giving students this regular dispositional feedback can help identify areas of strength and areas where further development is needed. Typically, this assessment has occurred in one direction. A feminist instructor, however, can collaborate with students on these assessments. Students doing self-assessments of dispositions may be more invested in the process. They will also receive more training in reflecting on skills, strengths, and areas of growth—a helpful skill for their entire career in mental health. Assessments by students can be compared to those of faculty to look for agreement or areas of disagreement. Lastly, students can collaborate with instructors by giving feedback about what dispositions are assessed and how academic programs assess them—this can provide an avenue for programs to evolve this critical process over time by incorporating students' voices and ideas into program evaluation and development.

## Mental Health of Students

The mental health of all students is important; it is particularly pertinent in clinical mental health training programs as helping professionals are responsible for discussing mental health issues, including trauma. Social work graduate students have been found to be 3.3 times more likely to have four or more adverse childhood experiences (Thomas, 2016), and 93% of counselors-in-training have been found to report at least one traumatic experience in their lives (Conteh et al., 2017). While not all students coming into the helping profession do so because of personal experience, past trauma can act as a motivation for students wanting to help others. Feminist instructors must be skilled at balancing inclusiveness, including of personal mental health issues, while also providing gatekeeping to clinical professions.

## Title IX Reporting

Colleges and universities have Title IX reporting requirements that obligate designated persons to report instances of sexual harassment or misconduct to a Title IX office (Flaherty, 2015). In mental health professional training programs, faculty, in our experience, fall under this required reporting designation. This can be confusing for students who may be inclined to share personal information in classes or in papers, or with professors in person, due to the reflective nature of classes in our clinical training programs. It is therefore critical that students know, before they disclose any of this information, that we may be or are required to report it to a Title IX office. Including this information on course syllabi as well as verbally discussing it in first class meetings is akin to informed consent with clients—students need to know what can happen to personal information before they disclose it to faculty.

## Professionalism

Clinical mental health training programs have required professional behaviors in terms of professional ethics, and they may also have expectations in terms of other professional behaviors, including professional dress. As the concept of what constitutes professional presentation evolves, feminist educators can help students learn to navigate professional expectations without losing their cultures, values, and authenticity. They can also advocate for inclusive practices in defining professional presentation and can create or support clothing pantries for professional attire that may help students without the means to purchase new clothing.

# Feminist Intersectional Model of Pedagogy in Higher Education

## Collaboration on Decisions

As stated before, a foundation of feminist pedagogy is creating a collaborative learning environment (Webb et al., 2002). Ideally, this could include starting a course by collaborating with students on learning goals and objectives as well as on content and assessments. This could be difficult in clinical mental health training programs where curricula are typically required by accrediting bodies and where there may be requirements from university administration. In these cases, a feminist educator can include as much required content and assessment as needed but still leave some areas for flexibility where collaboration can occur with students.

## Course Development Considerations

There are several factors that a feminist educator can consider in terms of flexibility and collaboration. For example, if a class requires a reflection assignment, the instructor could collaborate with students about the format of the assignment, which could be a traditional paper, a videorecording, a photovoice assignment, and so forth. Students could generate options the instructor may not have thought of. If possible, the instructor and students could pick more than one option so that students could use a format that aligns with their comfort, creativity, and motivation. This kind of flexibility may not be possible for all assignments, but including collaborative elements where one is able can lead to a more active learning community. Similarly, if possible, some course time can be unscheduled so that students can brainstorm topics they would like to cover as part of the course.

Deadlines are another place where a classroom community approach can be helpful. An instructor can consult with students about deadlines and see if adjustments are possible based on feedback. Similarly, if students express challenges with an approaching deadline, a feminist instructor can open a conversation to explore moving the deadline. This is not suggesting that only student needs are considered—in a power-sharing learning community, everyone's needs are considered, including the instructors. If there are pedagogical reasons for a deadline, or if moving a deadline would unduly burden an instructor, then having a transparent conversation about that can at least explain the reasons for the deadline.

## Setting the Classroom Egalitarian, Inclusive Tone

Implementing feminist pedagogy requires transparency about process and content. A feminist educator can begin a course by sharing their feminist teaching philosophy and giving examples of what that means. The instructor can both discuss and model honoring all students, wanting all students to be heard, and recognizing that students may have different requirements to feel safe to share their thoughts. Part of this discussion could include inviting students to help develop class rules for respectful dialogue.

## Power Monitoring in the Classroom

It is critical for the feminist educator to monitor power dynamics in the classroom and to be willing and able to focus on those as necessary. It can be helpful to attend to dynamics such as who speaks more, less, or not at all, what topics inspire discussion, what topics do not, and so on. The instructor may choose to ask students to reflect on those dynamics through a power-sharing lens of how power is being shared (or not). Or the instructor could notice out loud what they are seeing and ask students their thoughts and reactions. It is also important to be transparent about power monitoring; a feminist instructor can ask students their views of how power sharing is working through verbal conversations or through written evaluations, including anonymous ones. If students report that power does not seem to be shared either with the instructor or among classmates, the instructor can determine the best way to respond; this will likely differ depending on the situation. If, for example, one student dominates discussion, a private discussion may be helpful to collaboratively reflect on how that may be impacting power sharing in the classroom. Because part of feminist power sharing involves centering voices that have been marginalized, a feminist instructor will be vigilant that oppressive cultural or patriarchal dynamics that occur in broader society do not get recreated in the classroom.

## Self-evaluation

Because feminist pedagogy prizes both reflection and power sharing, there are many ways that an instructor can consider adding self-evaluations into grading. Students can grade their own effort, process, and product in terms of an assignment, or they could identify the areas of learning that stood out to them and how that impacted their learning process. Whether asking students to participate in grading or solely in reflexive practice, student self-evaluations can be part of a feedback loop both for individual students and for the instructor to continue to refine the collaborative learning environment.

## Looking Forward

One of the things that students can take away from feminist pedagogy is the experience of becoming more active learners. For some students, it could be the first time they have been asked their opinions not only about course content but also about course structure and expectations. This process can help students become more active learners in other classes, too, even if not taught from a feminist pedagogical lens. Students may find themselves better able to self-evaluate and self-advocate in future academic environments.

# Sample Assignments or Components for Feminist Pedagogy

## Pre-course Introductions

Prior to the beginning of a semester (particularly for a new group of students), a feminist educator could send out a voluntary introduction form. In the spirit of transparency, the educator could choose to fill out the questions as well and share with the students as a practice of modeling the act (not asking students to do something that you as an educator are not willing to do). Information asked for could include the following: an identification of the student's identities and social locations, chosen name and preferred pronouns, hopes for what they will get from the course, what has worked for them in previous educational experiences, what has not worked for them in previous educational experiences, and any other information they would like to share. Answers to these prompts could be turned in only to the instructor, or they could be shared in an online discussion board. Either way, this activity may cue students that their identities and educational experiences are valued.

## Shared Instruction

Looking at the syllabus schedule and based on course content, students can select a date where they lead that day's topic (perhaps a 15-minute activity and/or discussion). Students can have creative freedom on how they wish to present this material to their peers and will also provide potential prompts to help encourage conversation. This activity models power sharing in that the students are also responsible for the learning that takes place, and the feminist educator relinquishes the need to be "expert."

## Identity Journals

An instructor can incorporate self-reflexive journals as an assignment or can work with students to develop other formats that encourage creativity, ownership of the material, critical thinking, and acknowledge skill sets beyond the traditional paper model. The projects would focus on identity work and how the student's various identities and positions impact their work with clients, including their intersectional identities. For example, questions or assignments can be answered in the form of infographics (using a platform such as Canva), mind maps, audio recordings, poetry, photography, and so on. This process also raises the question—what are other ways we can share and exchange information that center accessibility, different ways of knowing, and different ways of doing?

## Brave Spaces

While feminist instructors need to co-create safe spaces for students to feel comfortable to participate in class at all, they also need to co-create brave spaces to engage in dialogues about potentially challenging topics. Arao and Clemens (2013) discuss the need for brave spaces for discussing diversity and social justice as these conversations are not always emotionally comfortable (safe) but are critical for clinical mental health trainees to experience. Learning to facilitate and have productive, healthy, and frank talks helps students to navigate potentially difficult dialogues not only in academia but also in other systems they will interact with. These discussions can help foster a culture of respect and self-reflection.

## Flexibility in Assignments

As discussed earlier, finding places to provide flexibility in assignments can be a way to respond holistically to students instead of viewing them only in their student role. The balance may come in determining what assignments are required based upon competencies, accreditation boards, and so on., vs. places feminist educators can be flexible.

## Regular Check-Ins

Also discussed earlier is the strategy of attaining regular feedback from students. In part, this practice models the ability to ask for and to receive feedback (beyond simply the university-level evaluations). This can be done using anonymous polls as check-ins on the progress and process of the class, mid-term evaluations, end-of-the-semester evaluations, and using immediacy to discuss what is happening at the moment. Information sought can be very open-ended (What do you wish we would do more of? Less of?) or more specific (When we talk about privilege and marginalization, what is that like for you? How can we make those discussions more meaningful?).

# Challenges of Feminist Intersectional Pedagogy

In addition to some of the previously discussed potential challenges of using a feminist intersectional pedagogical approach, it is also worth noting that in order to share power with students, feminist educators have to relinquish some of the traditional (and perhaps comfortable) authority that comes from traditionally being seen as the expert in the room. It is worth continued self-reflection for feminist educators to ponder their comfort with that.

Students may also be uncomfortable, at least initially, with a feminist approach. Students are often used to the traditional, hierarchical educational structure, so being asked to take on a new role may be both unexpected and uncomfortable. We have sometimes found that some students see us as less credible if we do not quickly supply them with "the" answer and instead initiate a dialogue to discern what answer or answers are available to choose from. In addition, students who are GPA-focused may be curious, and perhaps concerned, about how their collaborating on assignments and procedures might reflect in their grades. These are valid concerns, and feminist educators can welcome these kinds of discussions in class or with individual students.

Lastly, it can be challenging to create a more egalitarian and collaborative dynamic in an environment founded on hierarchies. Feminist faculty need to work within the traditional academic culture while also carving out spaces where they can transform traditional education. This is no easy feat, especially for feminist educators who find themselves alone in these pursuits and perhaps unsupported in them by people who have power over them.

# What If?

What if all education was free in all settings?

What if traditional grading was not used? How could other assessments change education?

What if students and instructors could collaborate on and co-create classes beforehand?

What if students were able to construct their assignments and rubrics?

# References

American Association of University Professors. (n.d.). *FAQs on academic freedom.* https://www.aaup. org/programs/academic-freedom/faqs-academic-freedom#:~:text=Academic%20freedom%20 is%20the%20freedom,%2C%20donors%2C%20or%20other%20entities

Arao, B., & Clemens, K. (2013). From safe spaces to brave spaces: A new way to frame dialogue around diversity and social justice. In L. M. Landreman (Ed.), *The art of effective facilitation* (pp. 135–150). Stylus Publishing.

Ares, N. (2008). Appropriating roles and relations of power in collaborative learning. *International Journal of Qualitative Studies in Education, 21*(2), 99–121. https://doi. org/10.1080/09518390701256472

Briscoe, K., & Jones, V. (2024). Challenging the dominant narratives: Faculty members' perceptions of administrators' responses to critical race theory bans. *Equality, Diversity and Inclusion: An International Journal, 43.* 459–480. https://www.emerald.com/insight/content/doi/10.1108/EDI-01-2023-0040/full/html

Busse, E., Krausch, M., & Liao, W. (2024). How the "neutral" university makes critical feminist pedagogy impossible: Intersectional analysis from marginalized faculty on three campuses. In S. B. Donley & M. Johnson (Eds.), *Intersectional Experiences and Marginalized Voices* (pp. 30–53). Routledge.

Caughie, P. L., & Pearce, R. (2009). Resisting "the dominance of the professor": Gendered teaching, gendered subjects. In R. D. Crabtree, D. A. Sapp, & A. C. Licona (Eds.), *Feminist pedagogy: Looking back to move forward.* Johns Hopkins University Press.

Chung, R. C. Y., & Bemak, F. (2013). Use of ethnographic fiction in social justice graduate counselor training. *Counselor Education and Supervision, 52*(1), 56–69. https://doi.org/10.1002/j.1556-6978.2013.00028.x

Clay, R. A. (2017). Women outnumber men in psychology, but not in the field's top echelons. *Monitor on Psychology, 48*(7), 18. https://www.apa.org/monitor/2017/07-08/women-psychology

Conteh, J. A., Huber, M. J., & Bashir, H. A. (2017). Examining the relationship between traumatic experiences and posttraumatic growth among counselors-in-training. *The Practitioner Scholar: Journal of Counseling and Professional Psychology, 6,* 32– 46. https://research.wright.edu/ws/portalfiles/portal/40590893/Examining%20the%20Relationship%20between%20Traumatic%20 Experiences%20and%20Post.pdf

Crabtree, R. D., Sapp, D. A., & Licona. A. C. (2009). *Feminist pedagogy: Looking back to move forward.* Johns Hopkins University Press.

DataUSA. (2017a). *Social workers.* https://datausa.io/profile/soc/social-workers

DataUSA. (2017b). *Psychologists.* https://datausa.io/profile/soc/psychologists

DataUSA. (2022). *Mental health counselors.* https://datausa.io/profile/soc/mental-health-counselors#:~:text=The%20workforce%20of%20Mental%20health,Mental%20health%20 counselors%20is%20White

De Santis, C., & Serafini, T. (2015). Classroom to community: Reflections on experiential learning and socially just citizenship. In T. Penny Light, J. Nicholas, & R. Bondy (Eds.), *Feminist pedagogy in higher education: Critical theory and practice* (pp. 87–112). Wilfrid Laurier University Press. https://doi.org/10.51644/9781771120975-006

Doyle, T. (2023). *Helping students learn in a learner-centered environment: A guide to facilitating learning in higher education.* Taylor & Francis.

Flaherty, C. (2015, February 3). Endangering a trust. *Inside Higher Ed.* https://www.insidehighered.com/news/2015/02/04/faculty-members-object-new-policies-making-all-professors-mandatory-reporters-sexual

Freedman, E. B. (2009). Small group pedagogy: Consciousness-raising in conservative times. In R. D. Crabtree, D. A. Sapp, & A. C. Licona (Eds.), *Feminist pedagogy: Looking back to move forward.* Johns Hopkins University Press.

Fromm, J., Radianti, J., Wehking, C., Stieglitz, S., Majchrzak, T. A., & vom Brocke, J. (2021). More than experience? On the unique opportunities of virtual reality to afford a holistic experiential learning cycle. *The Internet and Higher Education, 50,* 100804. https://doi.org/10.1016/j.iheduc.2021.100804

Hailes, H. P., Ceccolini, C. J., Gutowski, E., & Liang, B. (2021). Ethical guidelines for social justice in psychology. *Professional Psychology: Research and Practice, 52*(1), 1–11. https://doi.org/10.1037/pro0000291

Homrich, A. M., & Henderson, K. L. (2018). *Gatekeeping in the mental health professions.* American Counseling Association.

Kolb, D. A. (1984). *Experiential learning: Experience as the source of learning and development.* FT Press.

LaMantia, K., Wagner, H., & Bohecker, L. (2015). Ally development through feminist pedagogy: A systemic focus on intersectionality. *Journal of LGBT Issues in Counseling, 9*(2), 136–153. https://doi.org/10.1080/15538605.2015.1029205

Lipson, S. K., Zhou, S., Abelson, S., Heinze, J., Jirsa, M., Morigney, J., Patterson, A., Singh, M., & Eisenberg, D. (2022). Trends in college student mental health and help-seeking by race/ethnicity: Findings from the national healthy minds study, 2013–2021. *Journal of Affective Disorders, 306,* 138–147. https://doi.org/10.1016/j.jad.2022.03.038

Loes, C. N., Culver, K. C., & Trolian, T. L. (2018). How collaborative learning enhances students' openness to diversity. *The Journal of Higher Education, 89*(6), 935–960. https://doi.org/10.1080/00221546.2018.1442638

Magen-Nagar, N., & Shonfeld, M. (2018). Attitudes, openness to multiculturalism, and integration of online collaborative learning. *Journal of Educational Technology & Society, 21*(3), 1–11. https://go.openathens.net/redirector/liberty.edu?url=https://www.proquest.com/scholarly-journals/attitudes-openness-multiculturalism-integration/docview/2147859942/se-2

Mansfield, K. C., & Welton, A. (2018). Listening to student voice: Toward a more holistic approach to school leadership. *Journal of Ethical Educational Leadership,* (1), 1–18.

Marecek, J. (2016). Invited reflection: Intersectionality theory and feminist psychology. *Psychology of Women Quarterly, 40*(2), 177–181. https://doi.org/10.1177/0361684316641090

McDougall, J. (2019). "I never felt like I was alone": A holistic approach to supporting students in an online, pre-university programme. *Open Learning: The Journal of Open, Distance and e-Learning, 34*(3), 241–256.

Miller, C., Fachilla, F., & Greene-Rooks, J. (2021). *Exploring class privilege in counselor education.* https://ct.counseling.org/2021/02/exploring-class-privilege-in-counselor-education

National Association of Social Workers. (2021). *Code of ethics.* https://www.socialworkers.org/About/Ethics/Code-of-Ethics/Code-of-Ethics-English

Pasque, P. A., & Nicholson, S. E. (Eds.). (2023). *Empowering women in higher education and student affairs: Theory, research, narratives, and practice from feminist perspectives.* Taylor & Francis.

Pyne, J., & Grodsky, E. (2019). Inequality and opportunity in a perfect storm of graduate student debt. *Sociology of Education, 93*(1), 20–39. https://doi.org/10.1177/0038040719876245

Ratts, M. J. (2017). Charting the center and the margins: Addressing identity, marginalization, and privilege in counseling. *Journal of Mental Health Counseling, 39*(2), 87–103. https://doi.org/10.17744/mehc.39.2.01

Ratts, M. J., Singh, A. A., Nassar-McMillan, S., Butler, S. K., & McCullough, J. R. (2016). Multicultural and social justice counseling competencies: Guidelines for the counseling profession. *Journal of Multicultural Counseling and Development*, 44(1), 28–48. https://doi.org/10.1002/jmcd.12035

Silva, J. M., & Students for Diversity Now. (2018). #WEWANTSPACE: Developing student activism through a decolonial pedagogy. *American Journal of Community Psychology*, 62(3-4), 374–384. https://doi.org/10.1002/ajcp.12284

Simon, J. D., Boyd, R., & Subica, A. M. (2022). Refocusing intersectionality in social work education: Creating a brave space to discuss oppression and privilege. *Journal of Social Work Education*, 58(1), 34–45. https://doi.org/10.1080/10437797.2021.1883492

Sinacore, A. L., Ginsberg, F., & Kassan, A. (2013). Feminist, multicultural, and social justice pedagogies in counseling psychology. In C. Z. Enns & E. N. Williams (Eds.), *The Oxford handbook of feminist multicultural counseling psychology* (pp. 413–431). Oxford University Press.

Singh, A. A., Appling, B., & Trepal, H. (2020). Using the multicultural and social justice counseling competencies to decolonize counseling practice: The important roles of theory, power, and action. *Journal of Counseling & Development*, 98(3), 261–271. https://doi.org/10.1002/jcad.12321

Soffer, T., Kahan, T., & Nachmias, R. (2019). Patterns of students' utilization of flexibility in online academic courses and their relation to course achievement. *International Review of Research in Open and Distributed Learning*, 20(3). https://doi.org/10.19173/irrodl.v20i4.3949

Tewell, E. (2019). Reframing reference for marginalized students: A participatory visual study. *Reference & User Services Quarterly*, 58(3), 162–176. https://www.jstor.org/stable/26788549

Thomas, J. T. (2016). Adverse childhood experiences among MSW students. *Journal of Teaching in Social Work*, 36(3), 235–255. https://doi.org/10.1080/08841233.2016.1182609

Webb, L., Allen, M., & Walker, K. (2002). Feminist pedagogy: Identifying basic principles. *Academic Exchange Quarterly*, 6, 67–72.

Weinberger, Y., & Shonfeld, M. (2020). Students' willingness to practice collaborative learning. *Teaching Education*, 31(2), 127–143. https://doi.org/10.1080/10476210.2018.1508280

# 21

# Feminist Research: A Fourth-Wave Frame for Inquiry

## *Amber Sutton, Eunae Han, Takeesha Hawkins, and Candace N. Park*

*Authentic feminist research that honors the narrative over statistical probability often does not fit into the patriarchal constructs of "good research" and becomes marginalized in academia and society.*

## What Is Feminist Research? What Makes Research Feminist?

Feminists have long led the crusade of challenging conventional research roles, methods, and purposes. Given the debate spanning decades about what constitutes feminist research, this chapter offers a collective interpretation from a group of interdisciplinary and self-identifying feminist researchers and practitioners on what we believe to be important distinctions between feminist research and other mainstream or traditional approaches. The very nature of feminist research invites complexity, embraces the stewardship of intersectionality, and rejects monolithic thinking. Feminist scholarship and writing can be transgressive and liberatory, and it can be an asset in aiding clinical practice.

Just as there is no one definition of feminism across various perspectives, there is no one definition of feminist research. It has been simply defined as research guided by feminist theory(ies) with a central argument being that feminist research adopts critical perspectives with the intention to bring to the surface voices that are often excluded and to unearth systemic mechanisms that organize and exert power (Frisby et al., 2009; Gustafson et al., 2019). Feminist research moves beyond a fixed identity or doctrine and critiques inequality and inequity with the aim of social justice (Goodkind et al., 2021). Feminist research is a discovery process responsible for delving deeper to find out not only what needs to change but how to change it (Kelly et al., 1994; Westmarland, 2001). At the core of feminist research lie questions about who controls resources, structures, and discourses, discourses that have tended to be racist, sexist, and homophobic (Hartman, 1990; Staller, 2016). While there is not one universal definition of feminist research, several principles and ethics are repeatedly mentioned throughout the literature aimed at resisting oppressive and discriminatory scholarship practices that can prevent knowledge from being buried, silenced, or ignored (Staller, 2016). As Leavy and Harris (2019) discussed in detail, feminist theories are used across numerous disciplines, which establishes space for feminist research to be conducted from multiple epistemological and theoretical perspectives. Feminist epistemology and ethical obligations will have a direct impact on the methodological decisions for any study. This includes all decisions related to study design, data collection and generation, analysis, and methods of trustworthiness.

There are many truths and many ways of knowing as each discovery contributes to the greater knowledge base and has the potential to deepen our understanding, which can directly strengthen our clinical practice (Hartman, 1990). Feminist research acknowledges there are many knowers: researchers, practitioners, and clients and the production of our research is not simply for production's sake but in the service of our clients and communities. Most recently, Goodkind et al. (2021) noted the following feminist principles for research and praxis and summarized findings into three areas: conceptual, epistemological, and political.

## Conceptual Principles of Feminist Research

As stewards of intersectionality, fourth-wave feminist researchers call for an expansion beyond dichotomous thinking (e.g., man/woman, nature/nurture) that embraces and attempts to make sense of multitudinous identities and complex realities (Goodkind et al., 2021). The intersectional perspective reminds the researcher that we all have multiple facets of our identities and experiences but that social categories have developed their meaning with each other (Crenshaw, 1991; Hancock, 2013; Goodkind et al., 2021). This perspective is foundational to the research paradigm, as the questions we ask are often more important than the answers, and the value we choose to place on relationships and connections to promote equity is in direct response to hierarchy and oppression (Collins, 2019).

## Epistemological Principles of Feminist Research

Feminists have demonstrated the importance of positionality and the partiality of all perspectives (Collins, 1986; Haraway, 1988). Knowledge has traditionally been measured by how objective it is deemed to be and that if reliability, objectivity, and validity rules are followed, then "truth" will be discovered, that there is one way, and if the research does not follow those rules, it is criticized and dismissed (Westmarland, 2001). Epistemology is another branch of philosophy that concerns the study of knowledge, what is considered knowledge, and how knowledge is determined. Feminist epistemology is the systematic study of how gender influences our knowledge, how we have come to know and understand the world around us, and how we can justify what we know (Anderson, 2020). Further, it highlights and addresses how the dominant understanding of knowledge (1) ignores the experiences of women and other subordinate groups, leaving them disadvantaged, and (2) requires reform to support the needs and interests of these individuals and groups. Although there are varying feminist epistemological views, the central concept shared is situated knowledge, which is understood to be knowledge specific to the knower (Anderson, 2020). This concept is consistent with one of the central concepts of feminist theory, honoring an individual's ways of knowing, in that knowledge is seen as determined from the perspective of the knower.

Feminist research relies heavily on our humility to learn, unlearn, and relearn and must include radical transparency and reflexivity regarding who we are and how this impacts the research we choose to conduct. This unlearning includes what bell hooks (2000) refers to as the "taught" self, including some of the academic beliefs we have internalized relating to knowledge production such as what counts as knowledge and who counts as a knower (Gustafson et al., 2019). Reflexivity is a cornerstone of good quality feminist research and includes questions such as: What does the author bring to the research project in terms of past experiences, relationships, interests, and identities that have a bearing on the project and the participants? (Gringeri et al., 2010). Reflexivity calls us to get in touch with the stories beneath our skin and make visible the intertwining of scholarship and self.

The work makes room for nontraditional research paradigms, methods, and processes recognizing that the methodologies that we choose to analyze our worlds directly shape the truths we find (Collins, 2019; Goodkind et al., 2021). Feminist research acknowledges that complete objectivity is impossible and that through the act of interpreting data, the researcher is therefore incorporating subjectivity (Westmarland, 2001). There is always some degree of subjective interpretation regardless of the method, and knowledge can never be regarded as universal.

## Ontological Principles of Feminist Research

Ontology is a branch of philosophy that explores the nature of reality. Feminist ontological perspectives assert that "reality" is essentially unknowable due to the influence of gendered experiences (Maruska, 2017). This understanding is a direct challenge to a positivist view of reality that would suggest there is an objective reality that can be determined through quantifiable means, a stance often taken in White, Western cultures and research (Leavy & Harris, 2019). Feminist ontology rejects the notion of objective reality and affirms multiple realities exist due to intersecting experiences. Feminist ontology assumes that knowledge formation occurs relationally, which is consistent with feminist epistemology.

## Political Context of Feminist Research

Feminist research adds a political component that resists individualizing systemic-level failures and rather promotes that individual and structural change are interdependent. Recognizing that individual problems have social roots in Eurocentric, heteronormative Christian-dominant, patriarchal constructs, conducting and disseminating feminist research asks us to engage in collective action toward consciousness raising and have the courage to take a stand by challenging accusations of partiality and bias (MacKinnon, 1989; Goodkind et al., 2021). Feminist research acknowledges power differentials and aims to minimize these.

# Feminist Theoretical Perspectives

The exploration of how intersectional identities such as gender, ability, sexuality, race, and so on, influence what is known has evolved and can be conceptualized and discussed from three different perspectives: feminist empiricism, feminist standpoint theory, and feminist postmodernism/poststructuralism.

# Feminist Empiricism

Empiricism is an epistemological perspective that suggests knowledge is derived from experience, specifically sensory experience (e.g., evidence, data, and facts; Hundleby, 2011). Feminist empiricism took what was traditionally an androcentric epistemological approach and reconceptualized it from a feminist framework. Because of this renegotiation of terms, so to speak, feminism and empiricism have often had a contentious relationship (Code, 1998). Nevertheless, contemporary feminist empiricists assert that research conducted from this methodological perspective eliminates gender bias while achieving objective knowledge due to the presence of individuals and the totality of their intersectional identities in all phases of research (Leavy & Harris, 2019).

Empirical feminist research is conducted to better understand the experiences of intersectionally minoritized individuals influenced by oppression utilizing more traditional methods such as surveys, observations, and interviews. Although critics of feminist empiricism take issue with the adherence to methods and epistemologies traditionally associated with positivist worldviews, feminist empiricists counter that their presence is what best situates them to fight bias in research. This argument, specifically, is utilized by standpoint feminists, among others.

## *Standpoint Feminism*

Standpoint feminism is a subset of the larger standpoint theory (and a broad categorization within itself; Gurung, 2021; Naples & Gurr, 2014), which posits "that a standpoint arises when an individual recognizes and challenges cultural values and power relations that contribute to subordination or oppression of particular groups" (Wood, 2009, p. 397). Generally speaking, a standpoint is a position or viewpoint formed by a group's experience in the world based on social positioning (Gurung, 2021). For standpoint theorists, however, this more narrowed definition is expanded and situated within the larger social context reflecting political conscientiousness.

Consistent with feminist theory, feminist standpoint theory in research emphasizes knowledge that is established from those experiences that are common among marginalized groups. Standpoint feminism values transparency in the researcher's perspective and position in the world and rejects the idea of objective knowledge, as seen in feminist empiricism (Leavy & Harris, 2019). Further, although it is not tied to any particular emphasis within social sciences, standpoint feminist theory does value women's perspectives and assumes they are distinct from those of men. It emphasizes how social ideologies that affect women and girls disproportionately influence their knowledge and understanding of the world (Wood, 2009). Additionally, standpoint feminism assumes that inequality in society is structured by uneven power differentials, resulting in systemic and structural disparities between members of dominant and nondominant groups.

Both empirical feminists and standpoint feminists have been instrumental in breaking down barriers that kept scientific communities from departing from traditional positivist approaches to research (Leavy & Harris, 2019). Doing so has provided opportunities for understanding other means of knowledge acquisition, including post-positivist approaches. However, standpoint feminism is not without its criticisms. One such criticism that suggests that women's experiences are distinct from men's is a return to essentialism, as if there is one way of being for each, perpetuating a dualistic approach that is seen as inadequate for understanding and honoring differences. Additionally, this only examines gender and not any deeper complexities of intersectional oppression.

## *Postmodernist/Poststructuralist Feminism*

Feminist postmodernist and poststructuralist approaches in research directly challenge the notion of an essentialist understanding of gender. They explore how language is created and utilized to uphold the essentialist and simplistic view of woman and man as binary options and emphasize the importance of context influencing and forming multiple realities (Frost & Elichaoff, 2014). Instead of seeking a universal understanding of what it means to be woman/man, feminist postmodernists and poststructuralists strive to highlight the variation of women's experiences and how intersectional identities are formed. It is critical to conceptualize the complexities of intersectional identities and positionality beyond only examining gender.

Postmodernist feminism brings language and how it is used to the forefront, offering its role as integral to constructing reality versus reporting reality (Leavy & Harris, 2019). It rejects the notion of an objective reality, instead seeking to understand the multiple realities across and among multiple identities, seeking to dismantle categorizations of identity in general (Frost & Elichaoff, 2014). Because language is central to postmodern feminist approaches in research, discourse analysis is frequently utilized in research across different fields of study. Critics of this theory would suggest that too much emphasis has been placed on the philosophical nature of the arguments with too little being accomplished to address real-world issues (Leavy & Harris, 2019). Additionally, the idea that feminism would reject the understanding of "woman" as a category of analysis and understanding is quite controversial in and of itself (Anderson, 2020).

Sharing many of the same values as postmodernist feminism, poststructuralist feminism acknowledges the social construction of realities and how power influences the perpetuation of certain realities (Frost & Elichaoff, 2014). Post-structuralism "shows how it is that power works not just to shape us as particular kinds of being, but to make those ways of being desirable such that we actively take them up as our own" (Davies & Gannon, 2005, p. 312). In research, poststructuralist feminism examines dominant constructions of reality (e.g., male, straight) that serve to perpetuate the status quo of dominant power interests (Frost & Elichaoff, 2014). Knowledge is viewed as fluid and unfixed, influenced by the material and social surroundings. Sharing criticisms similar to postmodernist feminism, this fluidity is often viewed as problematic in the scientific community (Leavy & Harris, 2019). However, theorists would counter, that is the point.

# The Qualitative vs. Quantitative Debate

A place of pain for many feminist researchers has been the ongoing ranking rather than the linking of qualitative and quantitative methods. There is not one way of knowing that can explore all the vast and varied territory/social problems and issues. Neither method is "hard" nor "soft," they are simply methods, and their success depends upon the researcher employing them (Westmarland, 2001). Feminist researchers can view these as complementary to one another rather than oppositional. Feminist research is certainly not the only way to conduct research, but it is one way and within this idea, there is space for variety that welcomes and promotes healing among and between feminist researchers.

There is a need for large-scale studies in which variables can be reduced to measurable units and results translated into the language of statistical significance and a need for in-depth and thick descriptions grounded in the context of a single case, a single instance, or even a brief exchange (Hartman, 1990). Essentially, different feminist issues will call for different research methods, and if they are applied from a feminist perspective, there is no need for dichotomous qual vs. quant debates (Westmarland, 2001). Once again, feminist research calls us to resist this dichotomy and embrace other ways of knowing and doing including multi-method and mixed-method approaches as well. What does the study call for and what method(s) do we use to best answer the questions?

# Ethics in Feminist Research

Feminist research may be conducted from a variety of paradigms. Nevertheless, there are shared constructs across approaches. Inherent within feminist research is a determination toward social and political justice and activism that centers the experiences of those impacted by the process and outcomes of research practice (Leavy & Harris, 2019). Given the nature of this sentiment, it is widely acknowledged that feminist research is considered value-laden and promoted as such. The acknowledgment of an emphasis on elevating different voices, recognition of the role of authority and power in relationships and experiences, and the commitment to the communities served are all inherently value-laden, and those values naturally permeate the understanding and practice of ethics within feminist research.

Feminist researchers have been intent on addressing ethics within the practice of research for decades. This is in part due to the shared concern with issues of power and politics in a global society (Edwards & Mauthener, 2012; Williams, 2010). Not limited to feminist research, it has been suggested that there is no real distinction between feminist ethics and the broader understanding of ethics in research when considering best practices (Brennan, 1999; Kelly, 2020). Given the understanding that ethical principles are based on morality, and morality can vary by culture and environment, ethical practice can be questioned based on how one defines "good" human behavior (Iphofen, 2009). To address this factor, Edwards and Mauthner (2012) provided a conceptualization of feminist research through multiple models of research ethics (i.e., deontological ethics model, utilitarian ethics model, virtue ethics, and feminist ethics of care).

Pertaining to feminist ethics in practice, feminist researchers not only conceptualize through a feminist lens what many would consider standard research protocols and issues of governance (Bell, 2014), they also incorporate additional measures to ensure consistency with feminist values. For example, reflexivity is not simply viewed as a method within feminist research, as much as it is considered an ethical obligation to examine and reexamine the influence of power within the methodology (Leavy & Harris, 2019). Additionally, Bell (2014) highlighted multiple key aspects that feminist researchers must give attention to for consistent ethical practice:

> Do no harm (beneficence); confidentiality, privacy, and anonymity; informed consent; disclosure and potential for deception (e.g., relating to overt or covert research practices); power between researcher and subject; representation or ownership of research findings; and ensuring respect for human dignity, self-determination, and justice, including safeguards to protect the rights of vulnerable subjects. (p. 85)

Bell continues, stating that the researcher must demonstrate engagement with the items listed above when seeking formal approval (e.g., institutional review board) for research and/or adherence to professional standards.

# Benefits of Applying Feminist Research from Multiple Perspectives

## From the Feminist Researcher's Perspective

Feminist research allows researchers to obtain benefits in several ways: (a) to increase their awareness regarding location as a researcher, (b) to expand their research endeavor beyond a discipline, (c) to facilitate inclusive research participating environments, and to respect the individuals and communities that are historically marginalized.

Across the methods that researchers adopt, an essential aspect of feminist research is to be mindful of the position of the researcher throughout the entire research process. In other words, the essence of feminist research is not the methodologies employed but rather the way those methodologies are applied to achieve feminist goals (Letherby, 2011; Wigginton & Lafrance, 2019). Feminist researchers are expected to actively increase their self-awareness and openly recognize it in their written work on how their own attributes and social context may impact the way they interpret their data (Naples & Gurr, 2014). For instance, Wigginton and Lafrance (2019) request researchers contemplate methodological considerations for critical feminist research such as curiosity regarding research questions such as "Whose interests are served in asking this question?" and reflexivity to think of how the researcher's personal experiences or identities may shape the selection of topics they are interested in.

Another benefit for feminist researchers is to collaborate across various disciplines. Of course, certain aspects of feminist methodology demonstrate discipline-specific characteristics that are employed within a particular academic field, while others possess a broader applicability that transcends disciplinary boundaries (Fonow & Cook, 2005). Nevertheless, feminist research emphasizes collaborative, nonhierarchical, and reflexive methodologies. Researchers can communicate under feminist research beyond their discipline and facilitate collaborative academic conversation. Given that feminist research aims to decolonize structural oppression, interdisciplinary work is encouraged to serve various underserved populations.

The ultimate goals of feminist research include illuminating the experiences of underserved individuals. Feminist researchers strive to perceive the world from the eyes of their research participants and gain a deeper understanding of how their social positions shape their experiences within society (Aranda, 2018; Wilson, 2023). Thus, feminist researchers employ both quantitative and qualitative approaches in their methodologies and use active and intentional listening skills with their participants. To feminist researchers, their research projects are not "about" research participants, but they are doing the research "with" their research participants. Research participants who are especially historically marginalized often feel a lack of sense of community connectedness. Thus, participatory action research (PAR), which shares common threads with feminist research, is an approach that empowers members of historically marginalized communities to come together, collaborate, and actively tackle issues together (Smith et al., 2010).

## From the Research Participant's Perspective

Feminist research offers research participants multiple advantages, including (1) raising their consciousness and voices in the process of research, and (2) obtaining necessary knowledge that aligns with their life issues through research outcomes. As feminist research highlights the importance of the research process, including generating research questions, location of the researcher and power dynamic, data collection, and finding distribution, participation in feminist research projects allows research participants to raise their consciousness around societal oppression and to center their experiences as valued knowledge. Feminist research underscores the research questions that are beneficial to research participants and inherently works to facilitate consciousness raising, which will benefit both researchers as well as research participants. Moreover, an egalitarian relationship with the researcher and connection with other research participants can offer empowering experiences. This process can also allow space for them to discuss their life issues and facilitate change through action or advocacy.

Feminist research outcomes are beneficial for research participants, given that the focus of feminist research is to obtain a better understanding of the experiences of research participants—diverse people and historically marginalized populations. A feminist perspective works under the assumption that knowledge is shaped by one's social context that marginalizes certain voices. Thus, feminist researchers strive to prioritize the voices of marginalized people and their experiences of oppression and to uncover previously concealed insights about their lives (Campbell & Wasco, 2000).

Research topics on feminist professionals' service is another area that is beneficial to clinicians and needs to be expanded. Professionals who adopt a feminist approach in their helping can gain a better insight into their service through feminist research outcomes exploring feminist helping professionals. Clinicians who are interested in feminist practice sometimes find themselves not knowing the specific techniques and the way to employ feminist therapy. Providing specific guidance for feminist counseling is beneficial for research participants who are helping professionals, which feminist research aims to achieve.

## Models of Feminist Research

Interlocking oppressive systems and intersecting identities play major roles in identity development (Rosenthal & Lobel, 2016) as well as the epidemiology of common diseases and treatment outcomes (Shai et al., 2021). The importance of examining the role of intersecting oppressions and identities has been affirmed by the increase in the utilization of intersecting frameworks by researchers across disciplines (Rosenthal & Lobel, 2016). Feminist research processes should be collaborative, nonhierarchical, and reflexive. Researchers operating from this approach have a goal and duty to be cognizant of how the production of knowledge is influenced by social, political, historical, and gendered processes (Wilson, 2023). This form of research is grounded in and committed to social justice and equality. Davis and Hattery (2018) reinforce that beyond theory, feminism must be used to rectify inequalities and guide our actions.

### A Feminist Research Model

1 *Research Topic Exploration:* Choose a research topic by identifying a gap in the literature or gap in perspective from an intersectional lens. Explore current research to identify what and whose voices are missing from the production of knowledge in academia. What experiences are not being discussed and what voices are missing from those experiences?

2 *Reflexivity:* The feminist researcher spends time exploring their own intersectional identities, their desire to research chosen topics with chosen populations, and any power or privilege issues that may uncover.

3  *Research Question Formulation (if applicable):* Construct research questions centering on the chosen population, their experiences, and their voices.

4  *Research Method:* Choose a research method that will adequately answer the research question(s) and best articulate the experiences and voices of the chosen population. Ensure that the method will account for participants' intersectional identities and is in tune with their needs.

5  *Recruit Participants:* Seek out participants and populations that are missing from the current productions of knowledge in academia; rapport building begins here. Honor and include participants by going to them, meeting them where they are, and increasing their access to be included in the research study.

6  *Transparent Informed Consent:* Include egalitarian dynamics, and the right to withdraw at any time. Consider an opportunity for appropriate self-disclosure for transparency and collaboration.

7  *Data collection:* Explore what means of collecting data would best aid in meeting the needs of the participants. How can this process be accessible and convenient for participants? (Examples include locations such as community centers, churches, and local libraries; also consider providing resources and offering incentives). This is one way to include and honor participants during the research process.

8  *Member checking:* Use member-checking in quantitative and qualitative approaches. Provide participants with a copy of their transcripts, survey, or questionnaire. Ensure that each participant feels as though they have been able to fully answer questions and articulate their lived experiences.

9  *Data Analysis:* Consider an intersectionality self-analysis of identities before data analysis.

   a  Do a bracketing check for biases explicit and implicit

   b  Utilize an inclusive data analysis method that allows for the expansive exploration of the participants' experiences. How does the method amplify their voices and experiences?

10  *Interpret data:* Draw conclusions using feminist theory that is inclusive and representative of participants' experiences and voices. Utilize this process to honor and validate participants and their lived experiences.

11  *Recommendations:* For future research, consider suggesting feminist intersectional inclusivity and research geared toward centering participants' needs, voices, and lived experiences.

## Feminist Research Model Imagined

1  Identify who and what experiences are missing from research focusing on oppressed and marginalized voices.

2  Once marginalized individuals, groups, or experiences are identified, collectively ask:

   a  What don't we know?

   b  What do you think we should know?

   c  How might knowing this help?

   d  What needs should we learn more about?

3 Missing voices/participants led: How and to what extent are you interested in collaborating on new knowledge?

4 Missing voices/participants: How could collaborating on new knowledge benefit you/ your community?

5 Engage and collaborate with the community on co-developing a research question or a survey to explore further the experiences of those individuals and experiences that are missing from research.

6 Reciprocity- Engage research participants to participate in answering the research question(s) and/or survey while giving back to those who aid in new knowledge. Potential ways to give back to people and communities that aid in new knowledge:

    a For each survey completed, $1 will be donated back to the community. For each survey completed or interview completed, individuals get to choose which community organization they would like to direct their participation funds to.

    b Reference 2.d to identify community needs as reimbursement or act of reciprocity.

7 Member check: participants view words, qualitative and quantitative responses to ensure that what they intended to relay is what is relayed.

8 Who analyzes the research? Does it need to be analyzed?

    a Organize research data without analyzing it?

    b Describing missing voices, experiences, and identified needs.

    c Collaboratively analyzing the research with participants.

9 Disseminate Research: How do we ethically and responsibly share knowledge? Examples might include a blog, social media, podcast, town hall meetings, a free book, YouTube, and creating mentorship programs with experts and people with life experiences.

# Challenges of Feminist Research

Feminist research is not immune to challenges or ethical dilemmas. The mere process of scholarly research and writing is steeped in academic privilege and conventional dissemination practices. For example, researchers must adhere to the regulations of IRB/ethics boards, funders, and journal editorial boards (Gustafson et al., 2019). Access is controlled and limited beginning with IRB protections to traditional academic channels such as peer-reviewed journals, making it difficult to reach broader audiences, including practitioners. We acknowledge that in many ways, the academy excels in maintaining the status quo and that researchers make decisions within systems that dictate the *how*, the *why*, and the *what*. These models offer options and opportunities to infiltrate existing spaces but also encourage the creation of new ones that do not exist. After all, at the core of feminist research, there is a call for feminists to become subversives, to disrupt, and to question. Ultimately, feminist researchers must decide how to claim the space needed to research, practice, and disseminate while befriending systems designed to exclude them.

In addition to navigating these structures, feminist researchers risk scholarly respectability and credibility in terms of producing political knowledge that is not considered scientific. Although a tenet of feminist research is to produce transformative work, academic environments have tended to not take this type of research as seriously as compared to more traditional approaches. Feminist research can meet practical challenges as well, such as time. As with most research, feminist research is not a linear or simple process as there can be significant ethical dilemmas in balancing the interests of the researcher and the interests of the participants and the greater community. The goals, methods, collaborative nature, attention to care, and intentionality take time, planning, and energy to execute, which can often rub against publication deadlines, tenure and promotion expectations, funding sources, conference venues, and the like.

A possible perceived weakness of feminist research is that these practices are too heavily influenced by political bias and a drive for advocacy. Although advocates acknowledge and embrace these factors as inherently within feminist ideology, critics would suggest that this may compromise the objectivity and neutrality of the research (Harding, 1986). This critique can also expand to concerns about methodological rigor (Ramazanoglu & Holland, 2002). Some find the potential influence of such a bias in feminist research practices worrisome, particularly related to sample representativeness, validity, and reliability.

## Strengths of Feminist Research

The power of feminist research is its intentional regard for the complexity of difference and relationality. Positioning the participants as collaborators addresses the power dynamics attached to the traditional researcher-participant dichotomy and puts the voices of the community/partners at the center of the work itself (Harding, 2020). This type of research invites various dissemination venues that can highlight the important work while also increasing accessibility (a social justice issue). Feminist research can provide opportunities to pause and reflect on one's own experiences, which is a crucial part of healing and similar to that of the clinician's role. Feminist research involves emancipatory practices and collaborations that can lead to further action. It challenges norms and centers perspectives and praxis of historically ignored voices. Through the legitimization and recognition of the knowledge produced in feminist research, we can challenge structures of inequality, injustice, and oppression that have the potential to produce meaningful change (Harding, 2020). The very act of collaboratively writing this chapter is a prime example of what it means to do feminist research from conception to ideation to implementation. The collaborative writing process is inherently and yet intentionally feminist.

## What If?

What if all knowledge sources were equally valued no matter how obtained?

What if all knowledge was free and accessible to everyone?

What if there was no hierarchy of preferred research methodologies?

What if feminist research was sought after in the academy?

What if there were no social barriers or hierarchies between researchers and participants?

What if all research considered intersectionality?

# References

Anderson, E. (2020, spring). Feminist epistemology and philosophy of science. In E. N. Zalta (Ed.), *The Stanford encyclopedia of philosophy*. Stanford.

Aranda, K. (2017). *Feminist theories and concepts in healthcare: An introduction for qualitative research*. Bloomsbury Publishing.

Bell, L. (2014). Ethics and feminist research. In S. N. Hesse-Biber (Ed.), *Feminist research practice: A primer* (2nd ed., pp. 73–106). SAGE.

Brennan, S. (1999). Recent work in feminist ethics. *Ethics, 109*, 858–893.

Brown, L. S. (2018). Feminist therapy (2nd ed.). American Psychological Association. https://doi.org/10.1037/0000092-000

Campbell, R., & Wasco, S. M. (2000). Feminist approaches to social science: Epistemological and methodological tenets. *American Journal of Community Psychology, 28*, 773–791. https://doi.org/10.1023/A:1005159716099

Code, L. (1998). Feminist epistemology. In *The Routledge encyclopedia of philosophy*. Taylor & Francis. https://www.rep.routledge.com/articles/thematic/feminist-epistemology/v-1/sections/feminism-and-empiricism; https://doi.org/10.4324/9780415249126-P020-1; https://plato.stanford.edu/archives/spr2020/entries/feminism-epistemology

Collins, P. H. (1986). Learning from the outsider within: The sociological significance of black feminist thought. *Social Problems, 33*(6), s14–s32. https://doi.org/10.2307/800672

Collins, P. H. (2019). *Intersectionality as critical social theory*. Duke University Press.

Crenshaw, K. (1991). Mapping the margins: Intersectionality, identity politics, and violence against women of color. *Stanford Law Review, 43*(6), 1241–1299. https://doi.org/10.2307/1229039

Davies, B., & Gannon, S. (2005). Feminism/post-structuralism. In B. Somekh & C. Lewin (Eds.), *Research methods in the social sciences* (pp. 318–325). SAGE.

Davis, S. N., & Hattery, A. (2018). Teaching feminist research methods: A comment and an evaluation. *Journal of Feminist Scholarship, 15*(15), 49–60.

Edwards, R., & Mauthner, M. (2012). Ethics and feminist research: Theory and practice. In T. Miller, M. Birch, M. Mauthner, & J. Jessop (Eds.), *Ethics in qualitative research* (2nd ed., pp. 14–28). SAGE.

Fonow, M., & Cook, J. A. (2005). Feminist methodology: New applications in the academy and public policy. *Signs: Journal of Women in Culture and Society, 30*(4), 2211–2236.

Frisby, W., Maguire, P., & Reid, C. (2009). The "f" word has everything to do with it: How feminist theories inform action research. *Action Research, 7*(1), 13–29. https://doi.org/10.1177/1476750308099595

Frost, N., & Elichaoff, F. (2014). Feminist postmodernism, poststructuralism, and critical theory. In S. N. Hesse-Biber (Ed.), *Feminist research practice: A primer* (2nd ed., pp. 42–72). SAGE.

Goodkind, S., Kim, M. E., Zelnick, J. R., Bay-Cheng, L. Y., Beltrán, R., Diaz, M., Gibson, M. F., Harrell, S., Kanuha, K., Moulding, N., Mountz, S., Sacks, T. K., Simon, B. L., Toft, J., & Walton, Q. L. (2021). Critical feminisms: Principles and practices for feminist inquiry in social work. *Affilia, 36*(4), 481–487. https://doi.org/10.1177/08861099211043166

Gringeri, C. E., Wahab, S., & Anderson-Nathe, B. (2010). What makes it feminist?: Mapping the landscape of feminist social work research. *Affilia, 25*(4), 390–405. https://doi.org/10.1177/0886109910384072

Gurung, L. (2021). Feminist standpoint theory: Conceptualization and utility. *Dhaulagiri Journal of Sociology and Anthropology, 14*, 106–115. https://doi.org/10.3126/dsaj.v14i0.27357

Gustafson, D. L., Parsons, J. E., & Gillingham, B. (2019). Writing to transgress: Knowledge production in feminist participatory action research. *Forum Qualitative Sozialforschung Forum: Qualitative Social Research, 20*(2). https://doi.org/10.17169/fqs-20.2.3164

Hancock, A. M. (2013). Empirical intersectionality: A tale of two approaches. *UC Irvine Law Review, 3*(2), 259–296.

Harding, N. A. (2020). Co-constructing feminist research: Ensuring meaningful participation while researching the experiences of criminalised women. *Methodological Innovations, 13*(2), 1–14. https://doi.org/10.1177/2059799120925262

Harding, S. (1986). *The science question in feminism.* Cornell University Press.

Haraway, D. (1988). Situated knowledges: The science question in feminism and the privilege of partial perspective. *Feminist Studies, 14*(3), 575–599. https://doi.org/10.2307/3178066

Hartman, A. (1990) Many ways of knowing. *Social Work 35*(1), 3–4.

hooks, b. (2000). *Feminist theory: From margin to center.* Pluto Press.

Hundleby, C. (2011). Feminist empiricism. In S. N. Hesse-Biber (Ed.), *Handbook of feminist research: Theory and praxis* (pp. 28–45). http://scholar.uwindsor.ca/philosophypub/31

Iphofen, R. (2009). *Ethical decision-making in social research: A practical guide.* Palgrave Macmillan.

Kelly, L., Burton, S., & Regan, L. (1994). Researching women's lives or studying women's oppression? Reflections on what constitutes feminist research. In M. Maynard & J. Purvis (Eds.), *Researching women's lives from a feminist perspective* (pp. 27–48). Routledge.

Kelly, M. (2020). Putting feminist research into practice. In M. Kelly & B. Gurr (Eds.), *Feminist research in practice* (pp. 1–12). Rowman & Littlefield.

Leavy, P., & Harris, A. (2019). *Contemporary feminist research from theory to practice.* The Guilford Press.

Letherby, G. (2011). Feminist methodology. In W. Vogt & M. Williams (Eds.), *The SAGE handbook of innovation in social research methods* (pp. 62–79). SAGE.

MacKinnon, C. A. (1989). *Toward a feminist theory of the state.* Harvard University Press.

Maruska, J. H. (2017). Feminist ontologies, epistemologies, methodologies, and methods in international relations. Oxford research encyclopedia of international studies. https://oxfordre.com/internationalstudies/view/10.1093/acrefore/9780190846626.001.0001/acrefore-9780190846626-e-178

Naples, N. A., & Gurr, B. (2014). Feminist empiricism and standpoint theory: Approaches to understanding the social world. In S. N. Hesse-Biber (Ed.), *Feminist research practice: A primer* (2nd ed., pp. 14–41). SAGE.

Rader, J., & Gilbert, L. A. (2005). The egalitarian relationship in feminist therapy. *Psychology of Women Quarterly, 29*(4), 427–435.

Ramazanoglu, C., & Holland, J. (2002). *Feminist methodology: Challenges and choices.* SAGE.

Rosenthal, L., & Lobel, M. (2016). Stereotypes of black American women related to sexuality and motherhood. *Psychology of Women Quarterly, 40*(3), 414–427. https://doi.org/10.1177/0361684315627459

Shai, A., Koffler, S., & Hashiloni-Dolev, Y. (2021). Feminism, gender medicine and beyond: A feminist analysis of "gender medicine." *International Journal for Equity in Health, 20,* 1–11.

Smith, L., Rosenzweig, L., & Schmidt, M. (2010). Best practices in the reporting of participatory action research: Embracing both the forest and the trees. *The Counseling Psychologist, 38*(8), 1115–1138. https://doi.org/10.1177/0011000010376416

Staller, K. M. (2016). The many ways of knowing Ann Hartman: Themes of power, subjugation, and narration. *Qualitative Social Work, 15*(4), 447–456. https://doi.org/10.1177/1473325016652531

Westmarland, N. (2001). The quantitative/qualitative debate and feminist research: A subjective view of objectivity [28 paragraphs]. *Forum Qualitative Sozialforschung / Forum: Qualitative Social Research, 2*(1), Art. 13, http://nbn-resolving.de/urn:nbn:de:0114-fqs0101135

Wigginton, B., & Lafrance, M. N. (2019). Learning critical feminist research: A brief introduction to feminist epistemologies and methodologies. *Feminism & Psychology,* 1–17, https://doi.org/10.1177/0959353519866058

Williams, J. (2010). Doing feminist demography. *International Journal of Social Research Methodology, 13*(3), 197–210.

Wilson, G. (2023). Research made simple: An introduction to feminist research. *Evidence-Based Nursing, 26*(3), 87–88. https://ebn.bmj.com/content/26/3/87.abstract

Wood, J. T. (2009). Feminist standpoint theory. In *Encyclopedia of Communication Theory* (pp. 397–399). SAGE Reference Online.

# 22

# The Future of Feminist Theory: Fourth Wave or Fifth Wave?

## *Joanne Jodry, Kathleen McCleskey, Nicole Jackson Walker, and Ashley Krompier*

*The future of feminist intersectional theory is in our collective hands.*

## Feminist Waves of Movement

The feminist movement has been delineated and described as "waves." Although the movement has never disappeared, it has peaked and become more visible during these waves. Perhaps it should be "crests" instead of waves. Each "wave" has specific markers and iconic heroic foremothers associated with it, as seen in chapter 1. So, what are the tipping points, delineations, or events that trigger the next wave's arrival?

Baumgardner (2011) suggested that there was a wave "0" that began "[m]ore than 500 years before the Senaca Fall women's liberation meeting in 1848" (para. 7) in the United States, driven by the Iroquois and Cherokee mothers who created an egalitarian society with gender equality. There were also movements in 1400s Europe that challenged patriarchy much earlier than the recognition of the first wave of feminism (Baumgardner, 2011).

The *first wave*, in full swing in the early part of the 20th century, began with the suffragist movement to obtain the right for women to vote. This ended in legislation granting women the right to vote. The *second wave* originated decades later with the women's movement of the 1960s, culminating with some important legislative progression with the Equal Pay Act of 1963 (focused on gender pay equality and opportunity) and the Equal Rights Act of 1964 (focused on nondiscrimination based on race, color, religion, sex, or national origin). Martin Luther King Jr. (1965) spoke at UCLA about legislation, saying, "It may be true that the law cannot change the heart, but it can restrain the heartless." The Equal Rights Amendment (first introduced in 1923) was finally ratified by the Senate 49 years later in 1972 but failed to pass through the House of Representatives. It is yet to be ratified by Congress (as of 2024). Additional legislation focused on equality and other women's issues that promoted more legal equality, such as the Equal Credit Opportunity Act (1974) and the Family Violence and Prevention Services Act (1984). The second wave was also the time (1960) when the Federal Drug Administration first approved oral birth control. Baumgardner (2011) said, "These feminists declared that they were the experts—not male doctors, shrinks, religious leaders, fathers, or husbands—when it came to abortion, rape, pregnancy, and female sexuality" (para. 12).

The feminist clinical theory began during this second wave. In this feminist wave, gender was the main focus of therapeutic change, recognizing that women had different mental health needs and responses to oppressive traditional therapeutic treatment that had been developed and often administered by Eurocentric men. The Association of Women in Psychology declared it was a time of rejecting the status quo in mental health: "Sexist psychotherapy and psychotherapists were among the targets for change" (Tiefer, 1991, p. 15). The focus of this "radical" or "reformist" clinical feminist was creating new therapeutic constructs for women to heal patriarchal oppressive wounds while recognizing their own power and expertise. Brown (2018) said, "Feminist practice during this period focused on identifying what were seen as women's unique and special treatment needs as well as on the person of the woman therapist" (p. 24).

Some suggest that the *third wave* of the feminist movement began with Walker in 1992, who declared the third wave had arrived in *Ms. Magazine*. Due to the work of the second-wave feminists, young females had more rights and opportunities; however, the first two waves of the feminist movement lacked inclusiveness and consideration for multiple oppressions, intersectionality, multiple injuries, and even discrimination.

The third wave seems to have shifted to a more individual feminist experience over the collective force of women banding together. Baumgardner (2011) stated, "A Third Waver might say, 'Every time I make a move, I make a woman movement'" (para. 17). Although there was interplay and empathy between the civil rights movement and the women's movement, it is important to recognize that first- and second-wave feminist movements focused more on equalizing rights for White heterosexual women's experiences. Acknowledging and embracing ideas around social and clinical intersectionality and multiple oppressions seemed to have created a paradigm shift and cultural change to the third wave.

Some people felt/feel resentment or disrespect between the second-wave and third-wave feminists. Rampton (2015) reported,

> The third wave does not acknowledge a collective "movement" and does not define itself as a group with common grievances. Third-wave women and men are concerned about equal rights but tend to think the genders have achieved parity or that society is well on its way to delivering it to them. The third wave pushed back against their "mothers" (with grudging gratitude) the way children push away from their parents in order to achieve much-needed independence. (p. 6)

The women between the first and second wave probably did not have as much chance to interact with each other as the second- and third-wave women. It may be natural for new generations to feel like they marginalize each other, but that is a way of separating feminists. Finding new ways to fight the oppressive patriarchy needs to be united throughout the generations.

The third wave of feminist therapy faced additional criticisms from within the feminist therapy community. hooks (2015) reminds us that

[w]omen in lower-class and poor groups, particularly those who are non-white, would not have defined women's equality as women gaining social equality with men, since they are continually reminded in their everyday lives that all women do not share common status. (p. 19)

Brown (2018) stated, "These criticisms arose in part because of the Eurocentric quality of the different feminist theorists whose work had begun to predominate feminist therapy discourse" (p. 28). Feminist therapy recognizing intersectionality, multiple oppressions, and embracing diversity began to shift feminist therapy "from the margin to the center" (hooks, 2015). New multicultural, intersectional, social justice–focused clinical psychological conceptualizations that align with third-wave feminist therapy have deeply influenced the growth and evolution of feminist therapy (e.g., social justice theory, multicultural theory, decolonization theory, racial trauma theory, etc.).

## Fourth-Wave Feminist Theory or Therapy?

Many suggest or believe the *fourth wave* has already arrived (Brown, 2018; Cochrane, 2013; Baumgardner, 2011). Others are still contemplating its arrival (Smithsonian Institution, 2020). We endorse that we are currently in the fourth wave of feminism. There seems to be a new identification as feminist emerging, as Rampton (2015) indicated, "Part of the reason a fourth wave can emerge is that these millennials' articulation of themselves as 'feminist' is their own; not a hand-me-down version from grandma" (p. 7). Brown suggested, "The current fourth wave of U.S. feminists are increasingly global in their awareness and attentive more than ever to matters of social location; as a result, they challenge even more deeply essentialist remnants of earlier construction of feminism" (p. 139). Baumgardner (2011) suggested that the markers of a fourth-wave transition began around 2008 and can be seen in the tech-savvy generation and the immersion in social media platforms, Barack Obama and Hillary Clinton as political candidates, blogs with feminist messages, and popular songs of power and independence. As stated by Cochrane (2013), "It's defined by technology: tools that are allowing women to build a strong, popular, reactive movement online. Just how popular is sometimes slightly startling" (para. 3).

Related to fourth-wave feminist therapy, Brown (2018) also pointed to the influence of the transgender, gender nonconforming, and gender-queer influence in feminist therapy. According to Brown (2018), "This radical subversion of cultural norms of sex and gender, including those upheld by the older generation of feminist therapists, may herald things to come in feminist therapy theorizing" (p. 140). Rampton, in 2008, asked, "Will the fourth wave materialize and in what direction" (p. 7)? As the fourth wave is forming or even just beginning, maybe we can consider the words of accomplished greatness: "The future depends entirely on what each of us does every day; a movement is only people moving" (Steinem, n.d.).

## What Now for Feminists?

*The authors of this chapter offer some of our current thoughts about the future hopes, new conceptions, and projections for the fourth wave of feminism and feminist therapy and its potential to impact continuing changes for lasting social justice for all.*

## Reacting to the Backlash

With a new wave of activism and discourse, there has also come a pushback against both recent and established socially and legislatively progressive gains. Women's right to autonomy over their bodies has been reversed; LGBT+ and transgender people's rights have been challenged; affirmative action has been eliminated; there has been pushback toward diversity, equity, and inclusion efforts; and normalized political figures sexualize women, minimize sexual assault, and mock social identities. Explanations for these political and cultural backlashes include "anti-wokeness" and social media and political influence by political and social conservatives (see, e.g., Young, 2023). No matter the root, it is a clear indicator that although the second wave of legislation moved toward codifying equality for all, the internal psychological desire for equality was not widespread enough in all people to stop the rise of oppressive, divisive cultural and political backlash. Martin Luther King Jr. (1962) stated in his speech at Gross Pointe, Michigan, "It may be true that morality cannot be legislated, but behavior can be regulated." This fourth wave of feminism must again be successful in beginning to regulate behavior.

Since many important gains of equal rights legislation are being reversed, is it time to take note of the second-wave feminists and organize again with the new tools of technology? There are examples of organizing done in response to cultural, legal, or political shifts during the fourth-wave period. Black Lives Matter (BLM) was formed in 2013 by Alicia Garza, Patrisse Cullors, and Opal Tometi, who created a movement to bring awareness to injustice in the Black community and helped bring national awareness of this to consciousness. The organization for the Women's March in 2017 began immediately after the election of a candidate whose policy positions promoted oppression and a lack of empathy for others; the organizers were a diverse group including Bob Bland, Carmen Perez, Linda Sarsour, and Tamika Mallory. Tarana Burke started the MeToo movement in 2008 to raise awareness about sexual violence toward girls of color and to provide support and resources to victims. In 2017, the hashtag #metoo went viral, illustrating how many people, worldwide, experience sexual violence.

Is it time for the fourth-wave feminist intersectional movement to combine inspiration from these recent movements and strategies from second-, third-, and fourth-wave feminists to begin a new era of feminist protest? Whatever direction the fourth wave takes, it must include refighting for the already fought-for legislative rights, to both restore those rights to current and future generations and to honor the people who previously won these battles.

## Feminist Clinical Therapy of the Future

No matter which feminist "wave" is currently happening, feminist therapy needs to adapt and remain current and inclusive. Brown (2018) states, "Feminism continues to change, and as it changes, feminist therapy will reflect those transformations" (p. 139). What are some projected feminist clinical hopes for the next wave? Is it time for feminist clinicians to take the lead in the movement?

## Legislation Doesn't Change Hearts: Feminist Therapists Do

Martin Luther King Jr. (1968) said in a speech, "I'll be the first to say that we will never have a truly integrated society, a truly colorless society until men and women are obedient to the unenforceable." Although there have been many legislative victories in the fights for sex, gender, race, religion, age, ability, and intersectional equality, associated social and cultural norms did not saturate throughout the country. The continuing patriarchal culture has illustrated the embedded lack of desire for equality through divisive backlashes to equality legislation and accepted hate speech by politicians and the media. This can also be evidenced by the fact that, more than a century later, the ERA is still not ratified, indicating that gender quality is not a national priority and illustrating that political, social, and cultural norms are not "obedient to the unenforceable" as King (1968) suggested. The question becomes this: How can feminist therapy play a role in healing the fears, hate, anger, and inner wounds of people who live in and potentially perpetuate an unjust society? Can feminist therapists impact the larger culture through clinical practice, advocacy, and positive social change?

Feminist therapy has traditionally focused on examining Eurocentric, heteronormative, Christian-dominant, patriarchal oppressive forces and helping people find empowerment within the oppressive system created by the patriarchy. Healing comes from recognizing, imagining, and navigating one's ideal self and life through raised consciousness, assertiveness, advocacy, experiencing power-sharing egalitarian relationships, and so on. This helps the individual who is injured by oppression, but it does not focus on the perpetrator. People who are privileged, entitled, and superior-minded, who grab power, take advantage of, and hurt others to gain favor for themselves—these may be people for whom and with whom feminist theorists need to find strategies to approach deep and frank discussions of equity and equality. Chapter 19 of this book will offer some ideas about working with privileged and naturally resistant clients.

## Cultural Changes and Shifting Norms

But should we go further? The progression of equality and connected shifting social and cultural norms have left some people feeling left behind, not finding where they can fit into society. Some of these shifts may be embedded in aspirational expectations. For example, why is not going to college seen as unequal to going to college? Some shifts may be connected to people being reduced to their visible singular identities. It may be psychologically easier to resent or dismiss a person or a group for being rich, male, or holding any other privileged identity. However, taking a reductionist lens on fellow human beings is not situating them into all their societal contexts—it is taking cognitive shortcuts.

Understanding the complexity of intersectionality and multiple oppressions has been a required addition to feminist discourse to understand often-overlooked people more deeply. Should the next step include compassion and empathy for anyone who feels abandoned or reviled, even people with privileges? Should the next step for feminists be to help move to a compassionate understanding of how fear, hate, and a need for oppressive superiority may grow? This is not meant to dismiss harmful actions from anyone or minimize oppression or marginalization of anyone. We are simply wondering how to help everyone to feel a part of the conversation about shifting cultural norms.

## Next Waves in Feminist Therapy: A Shift in Focus onto the Oppressor

Steinem (n.d.) said, "Empathy is the most radical of human emotions." In terms of empathy and polarization, the picture is not so straightforward. Crawford (2014) says that ongoing conflicts are connected to low levels of trust and empathy. Indeed, "Empathy may be both a mirror and potential antidote to individual and institutionalized fear in world politics" (p. 538). Fear, or any emotion, can become encoded into policies, laws, and so on, by those in power, wherein emotionality is "replaced with the language of justification, beliefs, and reasons" (Crawford, p. 546).

Increasing empathy could help in reducing conflicts between groups. However, empathy does not necessarily override beliefs, so a person may have empathy for someone and still believe they brought harm upon themselves and, therefore, "deserve it." Interestingly, high levels of empathy have increased negative feelings toward a political out-group, which seems counterintuitive. Simas et al. (2020) report, "Those predisposed toward empathic responding, our results suggest, are more likely to dislike their partisan 'opponents' and perhaps even enjoy their suffering or failures" (p. 267). In the next wave of feminist therapy, perhaps there can be a focus on empathy toward one's out-group while simultaneously understanding the contribution of perceived lack of power in the face of institutionalized fears in order to help heal a polarized society.

Should the next generation of feminist therapists focus on areas of society that grow perpetrators who lack empathy toward out-groups and who have a hollow sense of inner power? Dobash and Dobash (1979) explored the notion that victimizing behavior is indeed embedded in a wider social and cultural context rooted in patriarchy. For the feminist psychotherapist, the idea that victimization will not end until there is a cultural shift is significant. If the problem of oppression, polarization, bigotry, bias, or violence in all forms is rooted in culture, then should we not work to understand the culture and those who have bought into it as a method for disrupting the culture? Should the next step for feminists be to help move to an understanding with compassion of how fear, hate, and the need for oppressive superiority grows?

Perhaps the next wave of feminist therapists could focus on helping those who are the knowing or unknowing perpetrators of oppression or even hate. It seems clinically manageable to conceptualize that "hurt people, hurt people." Or perhaps it is helpful to conceptualize a cultural narcissism (Paris, 2013). In other words, in today's society people are more concerned with themselves than social commitments to their larger communities, and this is at the root of personal and social oppression challenges. Paris (2013) suggests an "anti-narcissistic psychotherapy," one that is focused on empathy and social connectedness; perhaps the fourth wave of feminist theory is a vehicle to explore that. Should the onus of change lie with the victims of oppression or with the oppressors? What would be the motivation to share power and flatten hierarchies for the privileged person?

Consider that feminist intersectional theory might, through the process of consciousness raising, have a greater appeal to the perpetuator of social privilege and oppression than many of the other theoretical approaches. For example, a cognitive behavioral approach might overly emphasize the internal "irrational thoughts" or "misperceptions" in one's thoughts and seek to change behavior due to consequences. Contrastingly, feminist intersectional therapy asserts that the client is neither right nor wrong but often living in reaction to oppressive cultural, social, and political norms. Understanding the psyche of the often-unknowing oppressor and being able to collaboratively help them work through their challenges with understanding by utilizing empathy, not personalizing, and consciousness raising is potentially the healing factor of both the oppressed and the oppressor. The perpetuator of oppression is likely similarly impacted by the same organic natural assimilation to the Eurocentric, heteronormative, Christian-dominant, patriarchal ecosystems, only with more privilege and less need to explore. Alas, all are victims of the same patriarchal system, some to a lesser or greater extent, and all are unconsciously living out their roles in that system.

# Impact of Technology

Technology continues to develop and impact almost every part of life. How technology impacts individuals, systems, and clinical mental health work will be of great interest to fourth-wave feminist therapists. One of the most significant areas of technological impact is social media. Brown (2018) says, "[T]he power and visibility engendered in social media will lead to even more lasting cultural changes than were possible in the past 5 decades" (p. 139). Social media can be connecting or rejecting (APA, 2024). It can help spur protest (Gerbaudo & Treré, 2015) and result in isolation (APA, 2024). Social media is used professionally and personally. It may be used for recreation or news, and if used for news, consumers will also be exposed to fake news masquerading as actual news (Olan et al., 2022).

The psychological impacts of social messages shared in real-time have great implications for continuing to perpetuate the privileged patriarchal-embedded messages. When thoughtful media communication is crafted with care and shared, it could create a ripple of positivity by serving as a spark for expanded thought and consciousness raising and serve as a bridge to greater mental health awareness and stigma reduction (Vaingankar et al., 2022). When inaccurate and harmful messages are frequently shared and consumed by the brain, the effects can cause heightened anxiety; fear; confusion; isolation; a decrease in functioning at work, school and/or home; physical health problems; and other real implications on general cognitive wellness (Bhatt et al., 2022; Cherney & Legg, 2020).

Social media sits in a powerful and privileged seat, determining the type of connection administered to connection-seeking people. With this knowledge, feminist therapists must consider what their clients are exposed to and how they engage with powerful platforms and technologies. Additionally, a feminist therapist, while observing their privilege of influence, should ponder what kind of message and impact they want to have and share on social media. For positive movement and change to occur, they need to be clear on what shared purpose or goal they are trying to achieve. If a post or message were to go viral, it would be important to reflect on who or how the message may *harm* and who or how the message may *help*. How can something that starts digital move from the screen into action? Where can advocacy and community be encouraged through the connecting tool technology now provides? Influence and the notion of connection today come with greater costs and implications through the ever-growing social gathering places we call platforms today. Social media and its use have grown so quickly that it is hard (for us, at least) to predict the possible ways it could be used positively or negatively in the near and far future; fourth-wave feminism must be attuned to its developments.

Generative artificial intelligence (AI) is also a new technology that is developing exponentially. ChatGPT launched a free version on November 30, 2022, and since then, generative AI has become ubiquitous. AI applications are now found in customer service, in medicine, and in academia, to varied levels of enthusiasm. As with social media, generative AI has both positive and negative applications. For example, generative AI programs have been developed to write clinical progress notes. However, they require session recordings or transcripts to do so, which raises ethical concerns about client confidentiality and relying on nonhuman software to use critical thinking about client issues (ACA, 2024; Weisman, 2023).

As with social media, predicting how generative AI will become added to or even integral to areas of life in the coming years is challenging. Fourth-wave feminists must keep a keen eye on AI use, its impact on clients' experience with these technologies, social, cultural, and political impacts on existing patriarchal norms, and how society may use the technology to gain power in the socially constructed hierarchies. Lastly, the feminist therapist must be mindful of the evolving impact in the clinical mental health field.

## Mainstream Feminist Therapy: Critical Thinking for All

For fourth-wave feminist therapists, researchers, and academic educators, is it time that feminist therapy is taught at the same frequency as cognitive behavioral therapy? Although feminist therapy has been included in many theoretical compilation textbooks, it still seems to be an afterthought or addendum (Jodry, unpublished dissertation, 2011).

What keeps feminist therapy from becoming more centered as a chosen theory in practice? "Feminist therapy has its clinical roots in the humanistic psychotherapies that were practiced by many of its initial adherents before they engaged with the Women's Movement at the end of the 1960s" (Brown, 2018, p. 11). Many of the more traditional humanistic theories lack clear technical applications (such as person-centered theory or existential theory) and rely on necessary therapeutic underpinnings and the quality of conditions on the therapeutic relationship. This seems to also hold true for feminist clinical theory as well.

An issue that is different from traditional humanistic theories is that there is no one founder of feminist theory to go to for applications. The beauty of the feminist collective remains true to the values of feminist therapy but, at the same time, makes conceptualization and application to the budding clinical therapist difficult. One goal in the conceptualization of this book is to make feminist therapy more clinically user-friendly for feminist therapists in hopes that the theory becomes more saturated throughout the mental health world.

## Is the Term "Feminist Therapy" Too Gendered?

The word "feminist" is directly associated with gender, which makes the breadth and depth of fourth-wave feminist theory hard to explain to the typical client, student, or member of the public. Although feminist therapists have moved to an intersectional understanding of privilege and oppression, and often, feminist therapy is a gold standard when working with men, the word "feminist" has a connotation of the second wave, the gendered focus of women working with women on women's issues. Does this hold the theory back from therapeutic market saturation and from clinical acceptance? Should the fourth-wave feminist clinicians consider other options that would move this theory away from the word "feminist"? One idea, based on Bowen's (2006) family therapy concept of "differentiation" from the family of origin, was to call feminist theory "Patriarchal Differentiation" which essentially describes the aims of feminist therapy. After much discussion with many people, it seemed too disrespectful and not honoring enough of the feminist foremothers to build on their feminist construction of the therapy to eliminate the word "feminist." Hence, this book title is now *Feminist Intersectional Therapy*. The hope is that a nonbinary gender acceptance in the larger culture allows future therapists and clients to recognize that everyone is both feminine and masculine intersectionally and that "feminist" stops being exclusive to women.

## Revisiting the Unconscious

If fourth-wave feminist therapy is going to be able to address privilege, feelings of superiority, and power seekers, feminist clinicians may have to revisit the often-rejected psychoanalytic theories. Psychoanalytic theory is often not mainstreamed in most academic settings due to the sexist history of its foundations, the insurance companies' demand for evidence-based treatments, time-limited therapy, and the general lack of understanding of its application. However, it may be beneficial for feminist therapists to gain an in-depth understanding of psychoanalytic defense mechanisms (Safran, 2012) and Adler's (1927/2009) striving for superiority, social interest, and so on, to take feminists into the next wave of increased understanding of the unconscious social, cultural, and political quests to gain or retain unequal power rather than sharing it.

## Feminist Therapy Economic Networks

As part of the fourth wave of feminist therapy, feminists might hope to see increased feminist economic equality and justice by moving toward equalizing the many *wage gaps* that are generated by gender, race, sexuality, and other oppressive capitalistic values (see, e.g., Gould & deCourcey, 2023; U.S. Department of Labor, 2020). Feminist therapists need to support each other in all work settings to gain equal pay and support unions that insist on wage analyses for them and for their clients. Isn't it time for this to happen already? The Equal Pay Act was passed in 1963. "Title VII of the Civil Rights Act of 1964, the Age Discrimination in Employment Act of 1967 (ADEA), the Americans with Disabilities Act of 1990 (ADA), the Rehabilitation Act of 1973, and the Genetic Information Nondiscrimination Act of 2008 (GINA)" (U.S. Equal Employment Opportunity Commission, n.d., para. 1) all give equal protection to workers on the basis of race, sex, age, ability, gender, national origin, or genetics, yet pay gaps persist. How long should it take to become equal? What role can feminist therapists play? Perhaps discussions about this can start in academia?

## Musings about Possible Near and Far Futures for Feminist Intersectional Therapy

As science continues to advance with medical breakthroughs, is it probable that lifespan will continue to lengthen? If this becomes a reality, who will have access to such medical treatment? How would a longer lifespan impact those living longer as well as those who were younger? Would some choose to live longer and others not? How could longer-lived individuals impact resources, both public and private? How could that impact the family?

Climate change and climate justice are another area connected to resources. If weather were to destabilize more and more, who would be most affected? Who would have the resources to endure, and who would not? Other environmental issues such as water supplies, use of fossil fuels, carbon emissions, and so on, could set up societies of "haves" and societies of "have-nots."

For fourth-wave (and beyond) feminists, there could be a call to question if global concerns and universal human concerns will continue to intersect and join with the Eurocentric, heteronormative, Christian-dominant, patriarchal societal, cultural, and political concerns and oppressions, further deepening inequalities. Do feminist therapists want to find ways to connect to these kinds of broader areas outside of the therapy room? Would clients want to?

# What If?

What if humans one day have prolonged lifespans and are able to put off ultimate death at a rate that once was unimaginable? What if, through the expansion of technology and medical science, humans become able to eliminate death altogether? If humans were to conquer what is currently an inevitable fate of far future death, hypothetically, human birth would also become impossible to continue. Simultaneously, what would happen to religious concepts like God, heaven, hell, and reincarnation? People could alter and reconsider the traditional concepts around God in various ways. From that vantage point, is it possible that human existence as we know it could drastically change in the future? If birth were to end due to overpopulation concerns, how would sexuality be experienced once it is not tied to reproduction? How would gender be experienced? If birth ended, would most people biologically evolve to become LGBT+ oriented to adapt for civilization to survive? How would such changes impact how religion is experienced? Could some people have a sense that an evolution like this could change the way God is experienced or even threaten the existence of God. Or not? And if God's function, role, involvement in one's life, and related themes come into question, wouldn't there be many areas of society then that would evolve and change into something new, too? Would religion still exist? How would people make meaning if death is removed?

What if over many generations we all end up with the same skin tone and physical features that remove discrimination regarding concepts of race?

What if there was a new feminist mantra to add to "The Personal Is Political" or the "Political Is Personal"? What would it be?

What if the fourth wave of feminist therapy took a new direction? Where would you want to see it go?

What if empathy became part of the school curriculum everywhere? What kind of impact could that have? Would it matter?

What if everyone truly had equal power? What would the world be like?

What if the rights already won (women's right to bodily autonomy, affirmative action, etc.) are not returned? How will that change the future for oppressed people?

What if feminist therapy were to become more saturated among therapists? Would anything be different socially?

# References

Adler, A. (2009). *Understanding human nature*. Oneworld. (Original work published 1927)

American Counseling Association. (2024). *Further recommendations for the future of AI*. ACA https://www.counseling.org/resources/research-reports/artificial-intelligence-counseling/further-recommendations

American Psychological Association. (2024). *Potential risks of content, features, and functions: The science of how social media affects youth*. https://www.apa.org/topics/social-media-internet/youth-social-media-2024

Baumgardner, J. (2011). *F'em: Goo goo, gaga, and some thoughts on balls*. Seal Press.

Bhatt, A., Hilliard, J., & Parisi, T. (2022). *Social media addiction*. Addiction Center. https://www.addictioncenter.com/drugs/social-media-addiction

Bowen, M. (2006). The use of family theory in clinical practice. *Comprehensive Psychiatry*, 7(5), 345–374. https://doi.org/10.1016/S0010-440X(66)80065-2

Brown, L. S. (2018). *Feminist therapy* (2nd ed.). American Psychological Association.

Cherney, K., & Legg, T. J. (2020). What is social media addiction? *Healthline*. https://www.healthline.com/health/social-media-addiction

Cochrane, K. (2013). *All the rebel women: The rise of the fourth wave of feminism*. Guardian Books.

Crawford, N. C. (2014). Institutionalizing passion in world politics: Fear and empathy. *International Theory*, 6(3), 535–557. https://doi.org/10.1017/S1752971914000256

Dobash, R. E., & R. Dobash. (1979). *Violence against wives: A case against the patriarchy*. Free Press.

Dutton D. G. (1986). The outcome of court-mandated treatment for wife assault: A quasi-experimental evaluation. *Violence and Victims*, 1(3), 163–175. https://doi.org/10.1891/0886-6708.1.3.163

Gerbaudo, P., & Treré, E. (2015). In search of the "we" of social media activism: Introduction to the special issue on social media and protest identities. *Information, Communication & Society*, 18(8), 865–871. https://doi.org/10.1080/1369118X.2015.1043319

Gould, E., & deCourcey, K. (2023). Gender wage gap widens even as low-wage workers see strong gains. *Economic Policy Institute*. https://www.epi.org/blog/gender-wage-gap-widens-even-as-low-wage-workers-see-strong-gains-women-are-paid-roughly-22-less-than-men-on-average/?gad_source=1&gclid=EAIaIQobChMIo7PMnpWligMVRUH_AR0ssznEEAAYAyAAEgLq_fD_BwE

hooks, b. (2015). *Feminist theory: From margin to center*. Routledge.

Jodry, J. (2011). *The future of feminist theory in professional counseling: Reaching for a multicultural pinnacle* [Unpublished doctoral dissertation]. Argosy University, Tampa.

King, M. L., Jr. (1962). *The future of integration*. Speech presented at the Park Sheraton Hotel, New York City.

King, M. L., Jr. (1965). *The future of integration*. Speech presented at the University of California, Los Angeles.

King, M. L., Jr. (1968). *I've been to the mountaintop*. Speech presented at the Mason Temple, Memphis, TN.

Olan, F., Jayawickrama, U., Ogiemwonyi Arakpogun, E., Suklan, J., & Liu, S. (2022). Fake news on social media: The impact on society. *Information Systems Frontiers*, 26, 443–458. https://doi.org/10.1007/s10796-022-10242-z

Paris, J. (2013). Why people seek psychotherapy. In *Psychotherapy in an age of narcissism*. Palgrave Macmillan. https://doi.org/10.1057/9781137291394_4

Rampton, M. (2015). *Four waves of feminism*. https://www.pacificu.edu/magazine/four-waves-feminism (accessed August 2, 2024).

Safran, J. D. (2012). *Psychoanalysis and psychoanalytic therapies*. American Psychological Association.

Simas, E. N., Clifford, S., & Kirkland, J. H. (2020). How empathic concern fuels political polarization. *American Political Science Review*, 114(1), 258–269. https://doi.org/10.1017/S0003055419000534

Smithsonian Institution. (2020). *Smithsonian American women's history museum*. Retrieved from Smithsonian Institution. https://womenshistory.si.edu/

Steinem, G. (n.d.). *Gloria Steinem Quotes (marriage, equality, age)*. https://quotlr.com/author/gloria-steinem (accessed August 2, 2024).

Tiefer, L. (1991). A brief history of the association of women in psychology: 1969–1991. *Psychology of Women Quarterly*, 15,635–649. https://doi.org/10.1111/j.1471-6402.1991.tb00436.x

U.S. Department of Labor. (2020). *Fiscal year 2020 Department of Labor budget in brief*. Retrieved from U.S. Department of Labor. https://www.dol.gov/sites/dolgov/files/general/budget/2020/FY2020BIB.pdf

U.S. Equal Employment Opportunity Commission. (n. d.). *Genetic information discrimination*. https://www.eeoc.gov/genetic-information-discrimination

Vaingankar, J. A., van Dam, R. M., Samari, E., Chang, S., Seow, E., Chua, Y. C., Luo, N., Verma, S., & Subramaniam, M. (2022). Social media–driven routes to positive mental health among youth: Qualitative enquiry and concept mapping study. *JMIR Pediatrics and Parenting*, 5(1), e32758. https://doi.org/10.2196/32758

Walker, R. (1992). Becoming the 3rd wave. *MS: Spring 2002*, 12(2), pp. 86–87.

Weisman, H. (2023). Making therapy documentation easier: A comparison of AI note automation tools for private practice therapists. https://www.linkedin.com/pulse/making-therapy-documentation-easier-comparison-ai-hannah-weisman-phd/

Young, I. M. (2023). *Justice and the politics of difference* (2nd ed.). Princeton University Press.

# INDEX

psychotherapy 29, 114, 130, 131, 219, 243, 368, 372
PWUS. *See* "person who uses substances"

Queer people 199–200
queer theory 252–53
question formulation, research 361

race 6, 7, 19–20, 59, 141; CRT 22–23, 236–38, 240, 245, 326, 336; ethnicity, gender and 85, 123, 138, 198, 222, 310
racial identity development 54, 236, 238
racism 128, 151, 156, 244, 309, 314; sexism and 22, 54, 55, 100, 104, 133, 234, 336, 354; White people and 3, 23, 85, 236, 322; White supremacy culture and 22–23, 236–38, 240, 245
Rampton, M. 368, 369
rappers, Black women 8
Ratts, M. J. 235, 255, 256
Real Freedom of Choice 169, 174
recapitulation 93, 98, 106
recommendations, research 361
recovery-cultural analysis 138–39, 141
redlining 237, 243
Reflection–Generational Mentoring, supervisory stage 220–21
reflective journaling, positionality analysis and 272
reflective practices 155, 226, 228, 272, 340
reflexivity 222, 355, 360
Rehabilitation Act (1973) 375
relational power 73, 81, 82, 204
relationships 36–37, 83, 94, 124, 151, 159, 257–58; clinicians and clients 42, 44–46, 88–89, 114, 136, 209, 215; couple, relationship and family therapy model 113–23; feminist intersectional model example 120–23; feminist intersectional therapy 239; feminist therapeutic 9, 39, 76, 130, 164, 166, 184, 235, 254, 255–56; mentor–colleague supervisory stage 220; polyamorous 113, 120, 206, 207, 208; power dynamics in 72–73; triad 113, 120–23, *121*. *See also* egalitarian relationships; therapeutic relationship
religion 36, 128, 179, 191; PRC 180, 185, 198–99; spiritual development and 187–88. *See also* Christianity
reporting: confidentiality and mandatory 45–46; laws and mandatory 42, 270–71; Title IX 344–45
reproduction 6, 47, 53, 59, 253, 299, 376

research, feminist: benefits from multiple perspectives 359–62; challenges of 362–63; ethics in 358; models of 360–62; participants 359–60, 361; theoretical perspectives 355–57; what makes 353–55
resistance 55, 185, 186, 203, 294, 355, 358; of clients to feminist ideology 124; navigating natural reactive 329–30; strengths and criticism of working with 330
revelation, feminist identity model 14
Rich, Adrienne 252–53
rights 55, 252, 367, 371; civil 4, 6, 20, 27, 326, 368, 375; of women 4, 5, 6, 27, 75, 142, 234
Riot Grrrl movement 7
Rizzuto, A. M. 181
role induction 73, 76, 97, 133, 218, 290
role play 102, 119, 259, 273, 278, 280, 294, 327
Rossier, J. 112
Roush, K. L. 7, 14, 103
Russin, S. E. 153

SAIGE. *See* Society for Sexual, Affectional, Intersex, and Gender Expansive Identities
SAMHSA. *See* Substance Abuse and Mental Health Services Administration
Sarsour, Linda 370
science, technology, engineering and mathematics. *See* STEM
"The Second Feminist Wave" (Lear) 5
second-wave feminism 5–6, 7, 368, 370
Sedgwick, Eve Kosofsky 253
Seelman, K. 308
self 82, 122, 128, 143, 270, 274, 355; of clinicians 88, 97, 105, 154–55, 209–10, 235, 239, 255, 271–73, 323–24, 330; consciousness and 101, 167–68, 174; empowerment of 98, 328–29
self-advocacy 75, 79, 259, 292, 294, 299
self-analysis 170, 174, 239, 340, 361
self-assessments 272, 273, 339, 344
self-awareness 170, 183, 229, 271, 272, 339, 359; of clinicians 155, 235, 239, 255, 323, 324, 330; empowerment and 91, 142; importance of 40, 48, 76, 113; intersectional 222, 225, 226
self-awareness/first impressions exercise 222, 226
self-care 27, 37, 103, 273, 342
self-compassion 135, 272, 273
self-deprecation 25, 30, 80
self-development strategies, for clinicians 154–55

# ABOUT THE CONTRIBUTORS

## Editors

**Joanne Jodry**, EdD, DMH, LPC, LCADC, is a middle-aged, middle-class, cisgender, heterosexual, Buddhist, of French/Irish heritage, White female who was raised and lives on the New Jersey Shore. She has identified as a feminist for most of her adult life after being exposed to it in graduate school. She is an Associate Professor and the Program Director for the Clinical Mental Health Counseling program at Monmouth University, New Jersey. She holds two terminal degrees, one focused in counseling and one focused in spirituality. Her research areas of interest include feminist theory and spiritual healing applications (particularly Buddhist psychology and drama therapy).

For personal meaning, Joanne is passionate and involved with the nonprofit *One Life to Love*, where she leads a group of higher education students every year to Delhi, India, to learn from the beautiful children who have survived poverty, hunger, and deplorable conditions to be cared for and loved @onelife2love. In addition to her academic work, she has a private practice grounded in feminist theory.

**Kathleen (Kat) Armstrong McCleskey**, PhD, NCC, is a middle-aged, middle-class, cisgender, married, child-free, of Scots/Irish heritage, White female Episcopalian. She lives on a farm in central Virginia with her husband, many cows, and a variety of woodland animals. She grew into a second-wave feminist after her mother brought *Ms. Magazine* into her childhood home. She evolved into a third- and fourth-wave feminist through graduate school, professional experience, and personal life. She has tried to be a squeaky wheel, inquiring about missing voices in academia and in clinical work.

She is an Associate Professor of Counselor Education at Longwood University in Virginia. Her research has, for many years, focused primarily on various applications of feminist theory to clinical training, supervision, and applications with clients. She has also focused scholarship on human sexuality and on death studies.

Her nonacademic interests include gardening, knitting, spending time in nature, and spending time with her extraordinary husband, Pierce. As she ages, she is more and more like her mother and thinks that is just fine.

**Joanne and Kat** have been presenting together on feminist theory since 2005, when they met at a university. Although they met in the academy, the feminist conversations, support, conceptualizations, and friendship sustained living many states apart. They have consistently presented together at national conferences, always on feminist theory applications. This book is a product of that friendship. Along with 29 old and new feminist friends, we have collectively experienced creating *Feminist Intersectional Therapy: Fourth-Wave Clinical Applications*.

# Contributors

**Kristina S. Brown**, PhD, LMFT, AAMFT approved supervisor, is a middle-aged, middle-class, cisgender, heterosexual, Catholic, German-American, first-generation U.S. citizen, White female who was born and raised in San Diego and Los Angeles, California. She has lived in Boulder, Colorado; San Diego, California; Syracuse, New York; Springfield, Missouri; and now lives in her "empty nest" in the Chicago Loop with her amazing husband, Tucker, of 30 years and their two polydactyl cats, Cameron and Ferris.

She is a Professor and the Chair of the Couple and Family Therapy Department at Adler University. She is a feminist qualitative researcher with a broad focus on the experiences of women across identities as represented in her scholarly work and her role as editor in chief of the *Journal of Feminist Family Therapy*. Her specific areas of interest are varied including the impact of COVID-19 on couples and families, sexual harassment (#metoo) in higher education, the experiences and treatment of endometriosis, infidelity, and other projects such as tattoos in academia.

She especially thanks her mother, Barbara Schelbert, who raised her as a feminist, her PhD student, Kayla Harris, and MA students, Luisa Blanco and Sophie Tobin, for their support on this project and is most grateful for and proud of her two young adult children—Taylor and Kyle—who are staunch feminists in their own right.

**Ann M. Callahan**, PhD, LCSW, is a White, middle-aged, middle-class, cisgender, gay Christian woman who lives in Tennessee after many moves as part of a military family. She continues to grapple with what defines "feminism" and how this informs her own experience of spirituality and religion. She is a Professor of Social Work and founding Director of the Master of Social Work Program at Eastern Kentucky University. Her primary research area is on spiritually sensitive social work in hospice, palliative, and long-term care. In addition to her academic work, she is heavily involved in serving others as part of the Episcopal Church.

**Liz Curtis**, MA, LPC, LCPC, CAADC, NCC, is a cisgender, heterosexual, agnostic, middle-class, married, child-free White woman who lives in an inner-ring suburb of Detroit. She has identified as a feminist for her entire adult life and thanks her graduate professors at the University of Detroit Mercy for encouraging her to pursue academic projects that broadened her understanding of feminist theory as it applies to the counseling field. Her past research includes applications of feminist theory to graduate counseling program curriculums. She currently has a virtual private practice and is dual licensed in the states of Michigan and Illinois. In her private practice she has a strong focus on addiction work, non-cishet populations, and trauma work via EMDR, all through a feminist lens. Visit lizcurtispsychotherapy.com to learn more.

**Darcie Davis-Gage**, PhD, LMHC, is a middle-aged, cisgender, rural, Unitarian, Belgium heritage, White female who was raised on a small farm in the Midwest. She is a Professor in the Department of Counseling and Student Personnel and Director of the Blue Cross Blue Shield of Minnesota Center for Rural Behavioral Health at Minnesota State University, Mankato. Her research interests include trauma and compassion fatigue, career and occupational stress, and rural mental health and wellness. In addition to her academic work, she founded the Tenacity Institute for First Responders where she provides counseling and consulting services.

**Laura Dawson-Fend**, PhD, NCC, LPC, is a mid-career, middle-class, cisgender, heterosexual, agnostic, of Scottish/English heritage, White female raised in southeastern New Mexico. Laura has lived in the United States and Germany and identifies with aspects of the Latino culture she was raised around in New Mexico. Laura has always been a champion of the disenfranchised and oppressed and learned to identify with the term feminism in graduate school. Laura was raised with conservative roots but never fully identified with those values dominant in her rural upbringing.

Laura has been licensed as a clinical mental health therapist since 2011 and has, at times, been licensed as an addiction counselor. After a six-year break from therapy to stay home with her children and support her husband's military career, Laura returned to the paid workforce as an Adjunct Counseling Professor for New Mexico Highlands University. Eventually, she joined the faculty at Thomas Jefferson University in East Falls, Philadelphia, as an assistant professor of community and trauma counseling. Laura's research areas include areas of sexual assault, complex trauma, human trafficking, and other issues that impact social determinants of health and the ability of people and communities to thrive.

**Donnette Deigh**, PhD, LCPC, NCC, CRC, CEAP, is a cisgender, heterosexual, Christian, African American, second-generation Sierra Leonian female who was raised and currently lives in the District of Columbia, Maryland, and Virginia (DMV) area. She had identified as a Black feminist for most of her life but studied it more during her graduate studies. She is an Assistant Professor in Alliant International University's Master of Arts in Clinical Counseling (MACC) program and an approved supervisor in Maryland.

Donnette has been dedicated to helping underserved populations increase their quality of life through teaching, research, and service. Her scholarship interests include vision boards, social justice and advocacy, multiculturalism, wellness, counselor identity and development, cross-racial supervision/mentorship, Black mental health, and academic achievement. In addition to being an educator, she is a social scientist and has a culturally responsive counseling and consulting practice.

**David Julius Ford Jr.**, PhD, LCMHC (NC), LPC (VA, NJ), NCC, ACS, is a cisgender queer, Christian, Black man from rural North Carolina. He lives in Ocean, New Jersey. He is Chair/Associate Professor in the Department of Professional Counseling at Monmouth University. His research interests lie in supporting Black male students at PWIs, Black and Brown queer people of color, and those impacted by HIV/AIDS. He has also published works around religiosity/spirituality and queer/trans people, barriers Black male counseling faculty face getting tenure, and wellness among queer Black men. He is a classically trained pianist and had the honor of taking a class taught by the late Dr. Maya Angelou.

**Eunae Han**, PhD, NCC, NCYC (South Korea), LPC associate (TX) is a feminist scholar and counselor educator who identifies as a woman, cisgender heterosexual, immigrant, able-body, and Korean. She is currently an Assistant Professor in the Counseling and Special Education Department at the University of Texas at El Paso. Before coming to the United States to pursue her doctoral degree, she worked as a certified counselor for over three years in South Korea. She actively continues her clinical practice as an EMDR-trained counselor in the United States.

Her research interests, which emerged from her clinical experiences, include feminist approaches to counselor education, trauma-informed counseling and supervision, and researcher identity/research mentoring. She aims to assist women's mental health through effective counseling, teaching, research, and advocacy. Dr. Han believes it is important to incorporate multicultural and social justice perspectives—particularly feminist approach—into her roles as a researcher, educator, and advocate. She also values her professional identity as a counselor and counselor educator and enjoys working as a data analyst on a research team.

**Takeesha Hawkins**, PhD, LMFT-S, is a middle-class, cisgender, bisexual, spiritually Christian, early middle-aged, multicultural Black female raised in small town in rural Arkansas. Raised by a single teenage mother, she became a first-generation college student. She has identified as a Black feminist since being exposed to the works of bell hooks after graduate school. Her dissertation and future research interest include conducting feminist research, the Superwoman role, and Black Feminism. Located in Houston, Texas, she co-owns a private practice where her therapeutic work is deeply grounded in feminist theory.

**Nicole Jackson Walker**, EdD, MA-LPC, LCADC, BC-TMH, HS-BCP, is a middle-aged, middle-class, cisgender, heterosexual, Unitarian Universalist, of African American/Italian heritage, biracial female who was raised and lives in central New Jersey. She has, in mid-life, become exposed to feminist thought and has readily become a staunch supporter of it. She is a Full Professor and the Program Coordinator for the Human Services Program at Brookdale Community College, and an Adjunct Professor at Monmouth University, New Jersey. Her research areas of interest include applications of feminist theory, attachment theory, healing centered teaching pedagogy, and couples counseling. In addition to her academic work, she has a private practice grounded in attachment theory and supported by feminist theory.

**Justin Jordan**, PhD, LPC, LSATP, is an Assistant Professor of Counseling at Longwood University in Farmville, Virginia. He is a 39-year-old, cisgender, heterosexual, White male. He grew up in Virginia and currently lives there with his wife and two sons. His clinical experience includes public agency and private practice counseling with adult and teen clients, with much of that work involving substance use struggles. His current research focuses on professional identity of counselors who treat substance use, and harm reduction. He also specializes in working with LGBTQ+ clients and has developed a social justice orientation aligned with feminist counseling as an advocate for this population and other marginalized groups. Justin is passionate about bringing humanistic, feminist, and flexible approaches to substance use counseling.

**Ashley Krompier** is a master's student at Monmouth University studying clinical mental health counseling. Her passion for nature, art, spirituality and feminism have shaped her and guided her direction within the counseling profession. She is drawn to nontraditional modalities of healing, existential thought, feminist theory, end-of-life counseling, and spirituality in counseling. Ashley identifies as a heterosexual, cisgender, Italian, and spiritually centered Jewish woman. She loves to cook, paint, and explore the beauty found in nature, quaint towns, and within culturally rich communities. Ashley finds fulfillment through her passions and contributing to community.

**Dominique Maywald**, DSW, RYT200, LICSW-S, LCSW-CSW, is a Black, queer, middle-class woman of Creole and African American heritage. She is a Christian raised in Long Beach, California, now residing in Birmingham, Alabama. Dominique is a U.S. Army veteran, having served eight years as a combat medic. She is currently an Assistant Professor in the Social

Work Department at Jacksonville State University, Alabama, where she centers her teaching on cultural humility and anti-oppressive frameworks to transform social work education.

Her research delves into human rights applications in social work, clinical uses of attachment theory, anti-oppressive social work practices, and the distinct experiences of marginalized social workers and clients. Committed to holistic well-being, Dominique leads community-based vinyasa and yin yoga classes, blending her passion for social justice with practices that promote healing and self-care.

**Emily R. Miller** is a current professional counseling graduate student, MS anticipated January 2025, with an MA in English literature specializing in women's, gender, and sexuality studies. She identifies as a White, middle-class, cisgender, queer Jewish feminist woman. Her previous degree's studies focused on gender, sexuality, and power in contemporary literature as well as Holocaust and genocide studies. As a counselor, Emily's areas of interest lie in gender-based violence, spirituality, existential theory, and trauma healing. She loves to travel, read, volunteer, paint, and practice yoga.

**Mariah Moran**, PhD, LCSW, enjoys multiple professional identities including clinician, academic, teacher, and therapist. She discovered feminist theory in graduate school and several concepts within the theory resonated more deeply when she began practicing as a clinician. Specifically, the importance of relationship emerged as a central theme across all aspects of development, psychological and interpersonal growth, and healing. Dr. Moran integrates the principles of relationship, connection, and mutual growth across her work. This work extends to various topics that honor the continual, iterative, and transformational development of self. It includes mental health, loss and grief, building and repairing relationships, social work education, mind-body well-being, and geographic mobility.

**Chase Morgan-Swaney**, PhD, LPCC-S (OH), LMHC (WA), NCC, CCMHC, ACS, is a White, gay, neurodivergent, cisgender man who was raised and lives in Ohio. He has identified and practiced as a feminist for most of his career after being exposed to it by his doctoral internship supervisor and mentor, Dr. Jessica Headley. Dr. Chase is a Senior Lecturer in the School of Counseling and College of Health and Human Sciences at the University of Akron, Ohio. His scholarship focuses on LGBTGEQIAP+ issues in counselor education, preparation, and training. In addition to his academic work, Dr. Chase is a clinical counselor, supervisor, and administrator in a private group practice.

**Amy Nourie**, MS, is currently a PhD candidate at the University of South Florida School of Social Work. She identifies as a feminist, cisgender, culturally Jewish woman, mother, and member of the LGBTQ+ community. As a native New Englander, Amy lives in Florida and is very politically active. Amy spent most of her career in child welfare and continues to focus on this area in her research, as well as sexual minority foster youth, young adults aging out of foster care, feminist theories, and social welfare history. She also loves to travel, bake, and spend time with her two adorable cats.

**Candace N. Park**, PhD, LPC-S, NCC, is an Associate Professor and the Director of Departmental Operations in the Department of Counseling at the University of the Cumberlands, as well as the owner of a small private practice. Dr. Park identifies as a middle-aged, White, cisgender, heterosexual woman of European descent with a rural, Christian upbringing. Raised by a single mother after the divorce her parents and subsequent death of her father, she gravitated toward feminist thought at an early age. Her exposure to feminist theory and therapy during graduate school has shaped her worldview and professional approach ever since.

Dr. Park has taught a wide range of courses, including marriage, couples, and family counseling; human sexuality; addiction; grief and crisis counseling; counseling theory; clinical supervision; and qualitative research. She has also guest lectured, presented, and published extensively on topics such as feminist theory and therapy, ethics, supervision, gatekeeping, multicultural counseling and social justice advocacy, grief and loss, and program assessment. Her research interests focus on gatekeeping, grief and loss, and the intersection of reproductive rights and mental health. Her feminist perspective not only informs her teaching and research but also her mentorship, where she encourages emerging counselors and counselor educators to explore and embrace diverse perspectives.

At the time of this writing, Dr. Park is able-bodied and economically secure. She resides in southeast Louisiana with her husband, two children, and four dogs. Outside of her professional work, she enjoys spending time with her family, traveling, tending to her orchids, and being outdoors as much as possible.

**Ronee Rice** is an Assistant Professor of Psychology at Tiffin University. She graduated with her PhD in counselor education and supervision from the University of Toledo in 2024, where her dissertation focused on exploring the prevalence of sexual harassment experienced by counselors. Dr. Rice holds a bachelor of science in psychology and a master of arts in counseling with a clinical counseling concentration from Heidelberg University. She is a licensed professional counselor in Ohio with experience in private practice, college counseling, and school-based mental health. Dr. Rice's clinical and research interests include providing advocacy and support services to survivors of abuse, sexual violence, harassment, and relationship violence.

**Janys Murphy Rising** (she/they) is a licensed mental health counselor in Washington state with two decades of clinical experience, and 14 years of teaching graduate level counselors-in-training. Dr. Murphy Rising is a seasoned instructor and practicum and internship supervisor, with experience working in private counseling practice as well as mental health and substance use agencies. Their expertise ranges from children and adolescents to adults on issues from substance including co-occurring disorders. Dr. Murphy Rising received their PhD in counselor education from Oregon State University. They are also a substance use disorder professional (SUDP), an accredited child mental health specialist (CMHS) and an approved supervisor in Washington State.

Dr. Murphy Rising has led research on yoga intervention on counselors with compassion fatigue, and has published on career counseling resources for lesbian, bisexual, transgender, and questioning youth. They have presented at numerous conferences and colloquia on topics including spirituality in counseling, motivational interviewing, treating suicidal patients, self-care and counselor identity, trauma and the brain, and the Enneagram. In their spare time, they enjoy gardening, yoga, podcasting, studying the Enneagram, and spending time with their spouse and two cats.

**Janine Rowe**, MSEd, LMHC, is a White, cisgender, heterosexual woman with Swedish and Italian ancestors, whose socioeconomic privilege has given her access to quality education, resources, and networks and facilitated her academic and personal development to incorporate feminist, constructivist, and intersectional principles in her work as a therapist. She is a PhD candidate in counselor education at the University of Rochester in Rochester, New York.

**Barbara J. Shaya**, PhD, LPC, is a heterosexual, middle-aged, Jewish woman. She was raised in Michigan by middle-class Protestant grandparents who taught that her voice and choices matter. Barbara, her husband, and three children lived in Shanghai, China for three years, and currently reside in Michigan. Barbara has aligned with feminist-oriented therapy. She currently has a private practice specializing in survivors of gender-based violence.

**Carol Klose Smith** (she, hers), PhD, LPC, NCC, ACS, is a middle-aged, middle-class, cisgender, heterosexual, Chrisitan of Irish/German heritage. She is a White female who grew up in central North Dakota and identifies as a "farm girl." She began her professional career providing counseling services to individuals who experienced interpersonal violence or childhood trauma and uses a person-centered approach. Currently, she works as an Associate Professor at Viterbo University in La Crosse, Wisconsin. Research areas include career counseling, clinical supervision, and trauma.

**Valerie Stolicker**, MS, LPC, is a licensed professional counselor with a master of science in counseling education from Longwood University and a bachelor of science from Central Michigan University. She has extensive experience in private practice, specializing in areas such as sexuality, LGTBQIA issues, anxiety, depression, eating disorders, substance abuse, gender identity, play therapy, social skill-building, and LGTBQIA issues. Currently running her own practice, Creative Vision Counseling, Valerie has also worked as a substance abuse and emergency services clinician with Region Ten in Charlottesville.

Her diverse background also includes roles in educational support and residential counseling, providing a strong foundation for her therapeutic work. A committed member of the Virginia Counselor Association, Valerie has presented at numerous conferences, sharing her expertise on topics like empowering clients in uncertain political climates and using art therapy techniques with male clients. She serves as the current president of the Piedmont Chapter of the Virginia Counselor Association and is also a member of the American Counseling Association.

**Madalyn Stott**, BSW, resides in Central Alabama, working at a youth-provider program for a local nonprofit organization while completing her MSW. She is a is a White, heterosexual, agnostic, female, graduate student in her early twenties who was born in Southern California. She has held interest in feminist prose and poetry since adolescence and has since expanded that interest to include applications of feminist theories in life and practice. She obtained her BSW at Jacksonville State University and is currently completing her MSW at Jacksonville State University in their advanced standing program. Madalyn holds academic and research interests such as anti-fat bias in social work practice and the history/current state of Alabama's incarceration systems.

**Michelle Sunkel** is the Director of MSW Social Work Program and Assistant Vice President of Student Success for Academic Affairs at Colorado Mesa University. Dr. Sunkel earned her MSW from San Diego State University and a master of bioethics from a consortium of European universities: Katholieke Universiteit Leuven, Belgium; Radboud Universiteit Nijmegen, Netherlands; and Universita degli Studi di Padova, Italy. She earned her DSW from Capella University. Dr. Sunkel holds the following practice licensures: licensed independent clinical social worker (MN), licensed clinical social worker (CO), and has a license in addiction counseling (CO). Dr. Sunkel has 17 years of clinical experience and has worked in higher education for the past 12 years.

Dr. Sunkel has specialized within psychiatric social work, forensic social work, crisis intervention, trauma, and addictions. Dr. Sunkel has volunteered in Uganda, working with human trafficking victims and HIV/AIDS patients; Finland, specializing in school districts; and Belgium, Netherlands, and Italy, training in bioethics across multiple religions and cultures. Additionally, Dr. Sunkel has developed an MSW extern program to provide clinical oversight to the social workers, social work case managers, and the psychiatric social workers. Dr. Sunkel is the cochair of the ethics consultation team and assists in ethical consultations for a hospital.

**Amber Sutton**, PhD, LICSW-S, is a cisgender, middle-class, White female who was raised and lives in Alabama. As a mother, recovering academic, first-generation student, and trauma survivor, she understands the critical importance of intersectionality and applying feminist theory to further examine lived experiences. She has been a practicing social worker for over 12 years and was an Assistant Professor of Social Work at Auburn University at Montgomery where her research focused on intimate partner violence and advocate support. Most recently, Amber has left the academy and is now a full-time feminist psychotherapist in private practice.

**Olivia Turner**, BA, is as a cisgendered White woman of European descent from a lower middle-class socioeconomic background. Olivia was raised in the South of England, later moving to Wisconsin, in the United States. Olivia is a first-generation university graduate and an emerging professional in the counseling field. Feminist ideology has always resonated with Olivia, she has identified as a feminist from an early age. Olivia is a University of Wisconsin-Madison alumna, who graduated with a bachelor's degree in psychology with minors in criminal justice and gender and women's studies. Olivia is in her final year in the clinical mental health counseling master's program at the University of Northern Iowa.

**Sedaria LaNora Williams** is a middle-aged, middle-class, cisgender, heterosexual, Christian, African American woman from the South—Memphis, Tennessee. She is a doctoral student at the University of Memphis in counselor education and supervision working on her dissertation. Sedaria earned her bachelor's degree in psychology from Christian Brothers University, master's degree in sports administration from Belhaven University, and a master's degree in clinical mental health counseling from the University of Memphis. Her research areas are application of feminist theory in counseling, athletics and sports therapy, African American women in therapy, and interpersonal therapy for professional and college athletes.

In addition to her academic work, she works in private practice with athletes by adopting feminist principles that challenge stereotypes, specifically about mental health, fostering an environment where all athletes feel respected and supported, and intersectionality that impacts an athlete's experience.

**Joelle Zabotka**, PhD, LCSW, LCADC, is a middle-aged, middle-class, cisgender, heterosexual, Christian, White female. She was raised in Northern New Jersey and now resides on the New Jersey Shore. She is an Associate Professor in the School of Social Work at Monmouth University, New Jersey, teaching at both the undergraduate and graduate levels. Her research interests include clinical work with families and children; people affected by fetal alcohol spectrum disorder; parenting; and clinical applications of feminist theory. She maintains a clinical social work practice focused on children, parents, and families.

www.ingramcontent.com/pod-product-compliance
Lightning Source LLC
Chambersburg PA
CBHW081734270326
41932CB00020B/3269